Springer Series on Ethics, Law, and Aging

Series Editor

Marshall B. Kapp, JD, MPH
Director, Wright State University
Office of Geriatric Medicine
and Gerontology
Wright State University,
Dayton, OH

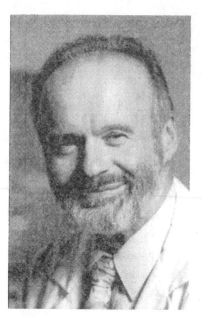

Ladislav Volicer, MD, PhD, is the Clinical Director of the Geriatric Research, Education and Clinical Center (GRECC) located at the E. N. R. M. Veterans Hospital, Bedford, MA, and Medical Director of the Dementia Study Units. He is also the Clinical Core Leader of the Boston University Alzheimer's Disease Center and Professor of Pharmacology and Psychiatry and Assistant Professor of Medicine, Boston University, Boston, MA. Dr. Volicer pioneered the hospice approach to care for persons with late-stage dementia. His research has systematically evaluated the effects of implementation of palliative care options and led to the development of policies to guide hospice care, which have affected U.S. public policy.

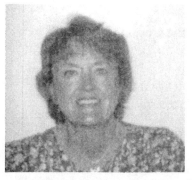

Ann C. Hurley, RN, DNSc, FAAN, is Associate Director for Education and Program Evaluation, Bedford GRECC and Education Core Leader, Boston University Alzheimer's Disease Center. She is Adjunct Associate Professor of Nursing, Northeastern University, Boston, MA, and Visiting Scholar, Boston College School of Nursing. Dr. Hurley has worked with Dr. Volicer in studying the processes and outcomes of providing palliative care to persons with late-stage dementia and to promote evidence-based practice.

Hospice Care for Patients with Advanced Progressive Dementia

Ladislav Volicer, MD, PhD
Ann Hurley, RN, DNSc

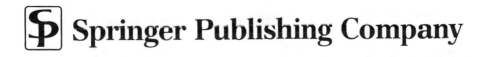

Springer Publishing Company

Springer Publishing Company, Inc.
536 Broadway
New York, NY 10012-3955

Cover design by: Margaret Dunin
Acquisitions Editor: Helvi Gold
Production Editor: Pamela Lankas

00 01 02/5 4 3

Library of Congress Cataloging-in-Publication Data

Hospice care for patients with advanced progressive dementia / [edited
    by] Ladislav Volicer, Ann Hurley.
        p.   cm.
    Includes bibliographical references and index.
    ISBN 0-8261-1162-9
    1. Senile dementia—Patients—Hospice care.   2. Alzheimer's
disease—Patients—Hospice care.   I. Volicer, Ladislav.
II. Hurley, Ann, DSNc.
    [DNLM: 1. Dementia—nursing.   2. Hospice Care—methods.   WM 220
828   1998]
RC522.H67   1998
362.1'9683056—dc21
DNLM/DLC
for Library of Congress   97-32680
                                                            CIP

Printed in the United States of America

Contents

Contributors

Giuseppe Bellelli, MD
Alzheimer's Disease Unit
Istituto S. Cuore-FBF
Geriatrics Research Group
Brescia, Italy

Gary H. Brandeis, MD
E.N. Rogers Memorial Veterans
    Hospital
Bedford, MA 01730
and
Geriatrics Section
Boston University School of
    Medicine,
Boston MA 02118

Paul R. Brenner
Jacob Perlow Hospice
Beth Israel Medical Center
New York, NY, 10003

June Brown, LCSW
Social Work Service
E.N. Rogers Memorial Veterans
Hospital, Bedford, MA 01730

Sandy C. Burgener, PhD, RNC
Indiana University
School of Nursing
Indianapolis, IN 46202

Simone Franzoni, MD
Alzheimer's Disease Unit
Istituto S. Cuore-FBF
Geriatrics Research Group
Brescia, Italy

Giovanni B. Frissoni, MD
Alzheimer's Disease Unit
Istituto S. Cuore-FBF
Geriatrics Research Group
Brescia, Italy

Sara T. Fry, PhD, RN, FAAN
Boston College School of Nursing
Chestnut Hill, MA 02167

Patricia Hanrahan, PhD
Department of Psychiatry
University of Chicago
Chicago, IL 60637

Bruce Jennings, MA
The Hastings Center
Briarcliff Manor, NY 10510

Autumn Klein
Geriatrics Research Education
    Clinical Center
E.N. Rogers Memorial Veterans
    Hospital
Bedford, MA 01730

Christine R. Kovach, PhD, RN
Marquette University College of
  Nursing
Milwaukee, WI 53201-1881

Neil Kowall, MD
Geriatrics Research Education
  Clinical Center
E.N. Rogers Memorial Veterans
  Hospital
Bedford, MA 01730 and Depts. of
  Neurology and Pathology
Boston University School of
  Medicine
Boston, MA 02118

Kim Litzenberg, MA
Department of Psychiatry
University of Chicago
and Illinois State Psychiatric
  Institute
Chicago, IL 60637

Daniel J. Luchins, MD
Department of Psychiatry
University of Chicago
and Illinois State Psychiatric
  Institute
Chicago, IL 60637

Sally A. MacDonald, RN
Nursing Service
E.N. Rogers Memorial Veterans
  Hospital
Bedford, MA 01730

Ellen Mahoney, RN, PhD
Boston College School of Nursing
Chestnut Hill, MA 02167

**Margaret A. Mahoney, PhD, RN,
  CS**
Northeastern University School of
  Nursing
Boston, MA 02115

Judith Morris, RD
Dietary Service
E.N. Rogers Memorial Veterans
  Hospital
Bedford, MA 01730

Stephen G. Post, PhD
Center for Biomedical Ethics
School of Medicine
Case Western Reserve University
Cleveland, OH 44106

**Veronika F. Rempusheski, PhD,
  RN, FAAN**
Center for Nursing Science and
  Scholarly Practice
University of Rochester School of
  Nursing
Rochester, NY 14642

Yvette L. Rheaume, RN
Nursing Service
E.N. Rogers Memorial Veterans
  Hospital
Bedford, MA 01730

Joyce Simard, MSW
Marriott Senior Living Services
Washington, DC 20058

Sally J. Smith, RN, MS, CS
Nursing Service
E.N. Rogers Memorial Veterans
  Hospital
Bedford, MA 01730

Mildred Z. Solomon, EdD
Center for Applied Ethics
Education Development Center
Newton, MA 02158-1060

Victoria Warden, RN
Nursing Service
E.N. Rogers Memorial Veterans
    Hospital
Bedford, MA 01730

Peter J. Whitehouse, MD, PhD
Alzheimer Center
University Hospitals of Cleveland
Cleveland, OH 44120

Introduction

The main goal of the hospice movement, which originated in Great Britain, is to enhance the quality of life of terminally ill persons. Hospices provide a support system for patients and their families, which allows them to live to the fullest in the time remaining before the patient's death. More information about the history of the hospice movement is provided in chapters 6 and 14.

In the beginning, hospices most often served patients with advanced cancer who decided to forgo further aggressive therapies. Later, the success of the hospice movement led to the realization that many persons dying from other chronic diseases would also benefit from hospice services. For instance, many hospices started to include patients with AIDS and the National Hospice organization recently published guidelines for inclusion of noncancer patients in hospice programs. These guideline include patients with heart disease, pulmonary disease, and dementia. This book provides information on the clinical and ethical issues concerning hospice for persons with advanced dementia and gives practical suggestions for implementation of hospice for these individuals.

Caring for patients with a progressive dementia provides many challenges for both family and professional caregivers. In the early stages of the disease, the patient may be able to be cared for at home, although the early stage of dementia may also develop in nursing home residents who are institutionalized for other disabilities. The course of a progressive dementia can be described as the gradual loss of a patient's independence. There are several schemes for the description of the stages of dementia, but we find it most useful to distinguish four such stages: mild, moderate, severe, and terminal (see Figure I.1).

This book focuses on how to care for patients with severe and terminal dementia, because it is at these stages when patients with dementia would most often be included in hospice programs. However, even patients with mild dementia may be treated by a hospice program if they have another terminal condition, for example, cancer. Therefore, hospice workers need to know how to meet the special needs of these patients. Many of the chapters in this book are based on the 10-year experience

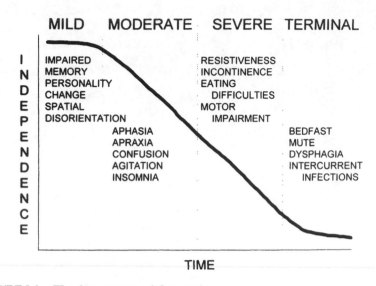

FIGURE I.1   The four stages of dementia.

of the Dementia Special Care Unit at the E. N. Rogers Memorial Veterans Hospital, Bedford, MA, where the first palliative care program in the nation for the management of patients with advanced dementia was developed.

Involvement of patients who are in the terminal stage of progressive dementia in a hospice program benefits both the patients and their family. Patients benefit because a palliative management strategy promotes their comfort and prevents the burden of aggressive medical interventions that do not have long-term benefits. Families benefit from the psychosocial support provided by the hospice program that helps the family caregivers to cope with the relentless deterioration of their loved ones.

The book is divided into three parts. Part I comprises an introductory chapter describing Alzheimer's disease and other progressive dementias, along with chapters devoted to the three main clinical problems encountered during the care for patients with advanced dementia: infections, eating difficulties, and behavioral problems. It concludes with a chapter that discusses the quality of life in patients with late-stage dementia.

Part II addresses ethical aspects and concerns regarding terminal care for patients with dementia. The chapters stress the importance of advance planning and describe the crucial role of the nursing staff in terminal care. This section also describes the impact of Alzheimer's disease on patients' families and society in general.

Part III is devoted to issues dealing with the implementation of hospice care for dementia patients. It describes the acceptance of hospice care, the barriers encountered, and the expected course of terminal dementia. The section ends with reviews of two successful programs that provide hospice care to patients with dementia.

We hope that this book will promote the inclusion of patients with dementia in hospice programs. Hospice care not only would lead to improved quality of life for patients with terminal dementia and their families, but also would save valuable health care resources.

Ladislav Volicer and Ann C. Hurley

PART ONE

Clinical Issues

Alzheimer's Disease and Other Progressive Dementias

Autumn Klein and Neil Kowall

The number of elderly individuals 85 years of age and older in the United States has increased sixfold since 1940 (Rosenwaike & Logue, 1985). The prevalence of dementia in this age group was 23%, with an increase to 58% in those over 95 years of age (Ebly, Parhad, Hogan, & Fung, 1994). This exponential rise in the prevalence of dementia continues until the age of 95 and then plateaus at 48% (Wernicke & Reischies, 1994). Approximately 4 million Americans have Alzheimer's disease (AD), the most common form of dementia, and 19 million Americans say that they have a family member with AD (Cummings & Benson, 1992). Unless a cure is found for AD, there will be 14 million Americans affected by the middle of the next century.

Dementia is characterized by a progressive, multifocal cognitive decline that impairs daily activities. The *Diagnostic and Statistical Manual of Mental Disorder* (DSM-IV: American Psychiatric Association, 1994) classified dementia as an ongoing decline of multiple cognitive deficits with preserved consciousness that can be "due to . . . a general medical condition, the persisting effects of a substance, or multiple etiologies (e.g., the combined effects of cerebrovascular disease and Alzheimer's disease)." These cognitive deficits include memory impairment and one or more of the following: aphasia, apraxia, agnosia, or disturbance in executive function. These changes must be significant enough to impair daily work and social activities. This chapter focuses on the four major causes of progressive dementia: AD, vascular or ischemic dementia

3

(VaD), diffuse Lewy body disease (DLBD), and Pick's disease (PD). There are other rare causes of dementia, such as Creutzfeld–Jakob disease (CJD) and dementia associated with anterior motor neuron degeneration, which will not be discussed here.

A meta-analysis of 47 studies from many countries demonstrated that in subjects 65 years of age and older, the prevalence of dementia doubled every 5.1 years (Jorm, Korten, & Henderson, 1987). When estimating, classifying, or diagnosing different dementias, there is no reliable, reproducible clinical criteria for many dementias, and so patients are not definitively diagnosed until autopsy. Ebly et al. (1994) reported the prevalence of AD among Canadians 85 years of age and older to be 75%, whereas that of VaD was 13%. This left 8.5% of dementias as "unclassified" and 2.7% as "other." In a study of a Swedish population sample of adults 85 years of age and older, one third were found to be demented, but AD and VaD were equally prevalent (Skoog et al., 1993).

Prevalence is also influenced by race and gender. In a study of dementia among institutionalized Blacks and Whites 65 years of age and older in the United States, the prevalence of dementia among Blacks was significantly higher than among Whites, 16.1% versus 3.05% (Heyman et al., 1991). The authors attributed this difference to a higher rate of institutionalization in Blacks, or to a higher rate of cerebrovascular disease in Blacks. Folstein, Bassett, Anthony, Romanoski, and Nestadt (1991) reported that women are more affected by AD than men, but men are more affected by VaD than women. Conversely, Skoog, Nilsson, Palmertz, Andreasson, and Svanborg (1993) reported that men and women are equally affected by AD and VaD. These studies illustrate the complexity and diversity of dementia. Differentiating one dementia from another is difficult because not all of the four major types of dementia have established criteria, making diagnosis difficult. In addition, population samples may influence the prevalence of the different types of dementia. Although many variables affect the prevalence of different types of dementia, each potential dementia patient should be evaluated individually.

DIAGNOSTIC EVALUATION

CLINICAL APPROACH TO THE PATIENT

When examining a person who has the potential to have dementia, problems arise that need special attention. At the time of initial presentation, the patient is often cognitively impaired and cannot provide a reliable personal history. Interviewing a caregiver who has firsthand knowledge is essential in order to obtain an accurate picture of the patient's abilities, deficits, and daily activities. Determining the premorbid physical, intellectual, and cognitive abilities is essential. Sensory deficits not corrected by eyeglasses and hearing aids, for example, may impair a patient's ability to understand and respond to questions asked or pictures presented.

HISTORY

Establishing that the patient has dementia and not delirium is the first crucial point of the evaluation. Delirium is characterized by altered sensorium, confusion, stupor, and fluctuations of consciousness. Clarfeld (1988) determined that 13.2% of patients are misdiagnosed with dementia when they actually have a delirium that can be reversed with early intervention. Characterizing the onset and course of cognitive decline may help to differentiate dementia from delirium. A recent onset increases the probability that delirium or a reversible cause of dementia is present, whereas persistence of symptoms for more than a few weeks or a month will make a diagnosis of dementia more likely. Any delirium or reversible cause of dementia that is not diagnosed and treated promptly may become less reversible with time, however. Reevaluation may clarify the diagnosis to determine if cognitive deficits are stable, fluctuating, or persistent. Fluctuations in cognition are seen in certain progressive dementias, such as DLBD and VaD, and will be discussed later. Drug-induced delirium superimposed on any progressive dementia will also present with fluctuating cognition. Teasing apart these factors depends on taking a careful history of the circumstances surrounding the onset of symptoms. The presence of inflammatory, infectious, or metabolic abnormalities and the use of medications with central nervous system (CNS) side effects favor the presence of delirium. The patient or caregiver should be questioned about environmental or work-related exposures and alcohol consumption.

The patient's past medical history should also be determined. Any history of coronary artery disease, transient ischemic attacks, previous stroke, or hypertension should be considered risk factors for VaD. A history of remote head injury may be associated with AD (Roberts et al., 1994), whereas a history of recent onset of psychoses may suggest DLBD. A family history of dementia increases the patient's risk for having a dementing illness, and a family history of hypertension gives an indication of the risk for VaD.

PHYSICAL EXAMINATION

Although the general physical examination is often normal early in the course of a degenerative dementia, signs of systemic illness are occasionally seen. Altered cognition can be associated with metabolic abnormalities, such as uremia and hypothyroidism, or with inflammatory or demyelinating illnesses, such as systemic lupus erythematosus and multiple sclerosis (Fleming, Adams, & Petersen, 1995). VaD should be considered a potential cause of dementia in patients with coronary artery disease, hypertension, and peripheral vascular disease.

NEUROLOGIC EXAMINATION

Early in the course of a progressive dementia, the neurologic examination may be nonlocalizing and not helpful in establishing a specific diagnosis. Focal neurologic deficits, such as hemiparesis, visual field defects, and loss of deep tendon reflexes may suggest a diagnosis of VaD. Extrapyramidal signs may be seen in many varieties of progressive dementia including AD, Pick's disease, and DLBD. Abnormalities of gait and nystagmus may suggest concomitant alcohol-related cerebellar degeneration. A detailed mental status examination is required of all patients and should include evaluations of orientation, recent and remote memory, language, praxis, visuospatial relations, calculations, and judgment. The Mini Mental Status Examination (MMSE) (Folstein, Folstein, & McHugh, 1975) is commonly performed because it can be done quickly and provides reliable screening results that are used widely. Because age, education, and language may influence the results, the results of the MMSE should not be the sole basis of the diagnosis of dementia.

Additional tests can be done to determine the severity and type of dementia. Given information from the primary caregiver on the patient's decline, the Blessed Dementia Scale (Blessed, Tomlinson, & Roth, 1968) provides a measure to help establish the severity of dementia. The Hachinski Ischemia Scale (Hachinski, Lassen, & Marshall, 1974) can be helpful in distinguishing VaD from other diagnoses, but patients with DLBD may score false positives (McKeith, Fairbairn, Perry, & Thompson, 1994).

BEHAVIORAL CHANGES

Altered cognitive function as a result of depression in the elderly may be misdiagnosed as dementia (Fleming et al., 1995). Typically, patients respond slowly and are disinterested but show no evidence of memory disturbance or behavioral abnormalities. Many neurologists advocate a trial of antidepressants, particularly sertraline, in all cases of early dementia (Fleming et al., 1995). Personality and behavioral changes, disinhibition, indifference, aggression, anger, and lack of motivation are typically seen early in Pick's disease and other frontal dementias, in contrast to the early memory deficits typically found in AD (Cummings & Benson, 1992).

LABORATORY TESTS

Laboratory tests are done primarily to rule out metabolic problems and reversible causes of dementia. Blood tests should include a complete blood count (CBC), blood urea nitrogen (BUN)/creatinine, liver function tests, calcium, thyroid levels, sedimentation rate, electrolytes, serum B_{12} level, and syphilis serology. In addition, metal and drug toxicities may be considered when clinically indicated and a urinalysis done.

Neuroimaging studies using computed tomography (CT) or magnetic resonance imaging (MRI) are highly recommended in a suspected case of dementia. These tests identify structural lesions and potentially reversible causes of dementia, such as brain tumors, subdural hematoma, and normal pressure hydrocephalus. Global atrophy and dilated ventricles, as found in AD, or lobar atrophy, as seen in Pick's disease, can be visualized on CT (Lee, Rao, & Zimmerman, 1992). MRI is best used to visualize small infarcts and other vascular and ischemic changes. If periventricular leukoaraiosis is seen on MRI, a diagnosis of Binswanger's disease should be considered (Erkinjuntti et al., 1984).

A lumbar puncture is only necessary as part of the clinical evaluation to rule out an inflammatory condition confined to the central nervous system, such as meningitis. Other symptoms, such as fever and nuchal rigidity, would suggest meningitis as a potential cause of dementia and warrant this procedure. A new diagnostic test currently available evaluates certain biological markers that have been identified as risk factors associated with AD. In people 60 years of age and older who present with dementia, the test can rule out AD with 95%+ specificity, but it is only 60%+ sensitive. Electroencephalography (EEG) is also not routinely necessary, but in the case of a rapidly progressive dementia with myoclonus, an EEG can help to differentiate CJD from other progressive dementias. In CJD, the EEG would show high-voltage frontal, periodic, sharp waves. In DLBD there may also be high-voltage frontal EEG abnormalities (Crystal, Dickson, Lizardi, Davies, & Wolfson, 1990).

Other tests, such as positron emission tomography (PET), which can be used to measure glucose metabolism and regional blood flow, are used primarily for research purposes and are not widely available. Single positron emission computed tomography (SPECT) is more widely available and may help confirm the diagnosis of AD if the characteristic temporal and parietal hypometabolism is found (Jagust, Reed, Seab, & Budinger, 1990).

ALZHEIMER'S DISEASE

In 1907 Alois Alzheimer described a 51-year-old woman with impaired memory, language, comprehension, and spatial orientation. Motoric functions, such as reflexes and gait coordination, were not impaired, and after a progressive 4-year decline, the woman died. At autopsy, the brain was found to be grossly atrophic with cortical neuronal loss, senile plaques, and neurofibrillary change. These clinical and pathologic features set the precedent for what today bears the name of Alzheimer's disease.

PREVALENCE AND RISK FACTORS

Sample size, nationality, race, sex, and age create many variables that confound studies and make it difficult to estimate the prevalence of AD. Investigators agree, however, that the prevalence of AD increases from 1%–2% in patients under the age of 65 to 40%–50% by the age of 85. Evans et al. (1989) found that 3% of people age 65–74, 18.7% of people age 75–84, and 47.2% of people 85 years of age and older had AD. In a Canadian study, AD was diagnosed in 75% of patients with dementia (Ebly et al., 1994), but in a Swedish study, AD was diagnosed in only 43.5% of dementia patients (Skoog et al., 1993). AD is the diagnosis given to 55.6% of all patients in the Framingham study with dementia age 61–93 (Bachman et al., 1992).

Many possible risk factors for AD have been identified, but there is a lack of consensus in the literature. Age is clearly the major risk factor for AD. Down's syndrome patients who live beyond age 35 or 40 almost always develop AD-type neuropathological changes, but they may not have clinical dementia. Family history is another risk factor. More first-degree relatives of AD patients develop AD than does the general population (Mendez et al., 1992). Less than 10% of all AD cases are inherited as an autosomal dominant trait. Instead, they display early onset and fulminant disease progression. These cases have been linked to single gene mutations on chromosomes 14, 21, and 1, with over two thirds of familial cases caused by mutations on chromosome 14.

Some studies report that female sex is associated with a greater risk for developing AD, but most studies do not support this finding. Bachman et al. (1992) initially reported that the prevalence of AD was 11.7 per 1000 in men compared to 30.1 per 1000 in women age 61–93. However, in a follow up a year later, the prevalence was equal in both sexes (Bachman et al., 1993). The prevalence of AD in Sweden was also shown to be equal between men and women (Skoog et al., 1993).

Educational attainment may also be a risk factor. It has been postulated that education protects against developing AD because education forms additional cortical synapses, and the loss of synapses is the main cause of dementia. Theoretically, less educated people have fewer synapses to lose, so they may show deficits faster or earlier than an educated person. Fratiglioni et al. (1991) showed that less educated Swedes had an increased prevalence of dementia overall, but the prevalence of AD was the same across educational groups. This was attributed to a greater prevalence of alcoholic and "unspecified" dementias in less educated people. More recently, it was shown that in many Eastern and Western countries, education was protective for developing AD (Katzman, 1993).

It has been well established that apolipoprotein E (ApoE) genotype is a major risk factor for developing AD. ApoE has three major allelic forms in the general population designated ApoE2, ApoE3, and ApoE4. It has been shown that the ApoE4 allele is associated with increased risk, whereas the ApoE2 allele appears to be protective (Corder, Saunders, & Risch, 1994). However, only 50% of people with the ApoE4 allele develop AD, so other risk factors must be involved.

Studies suggest that in genetically susceptible patients, head trauma is a risk factor for developing AD. Acute head trauma leads to an immediate increase in the production of amyloid precursor protein (APP), the precursor to beta amyloid (Aß), and Aß is the primary component of senile plaques, a pathologic hallmark found in AD brains (Roberts, Gentleman, Lynch, & Graham, 1991). The potential role of Aß in the pathogenesis of AD is discussed below.

CRITERIA AND CLINICAL DIAGNOSIS

The most widely used criteria are the DSM-IV and those developed by the National Institute of Neurological and Communicative Related Disorders and Stroke and the Alzheimer's Disease and Related Disorders Association (NINCDS-ADRDA) task force established in 1984 (McKhann et al., 1984) (see Table 1.1). The DSM-IV divides AD into early onset (at age 65 years old or below) and late onset (after age 65). Diagnostic criteria for AD include the gradual onset and continuing decline in multiple cognitive deficits that cover both memory impairment and at least one

TABLE 1.1 Diagnostic Criteria for Neurodegenerative Dementias

Criteria	AD	VaD	DLBD	PD
Pattern of cognitive deficits	Early memory loss Progressive decline Aphasia later	Variable Stepwise progression	Variable May have sudden onset Mimics delirium	Memory and visuospatial loss later Early aphasia
Behavior and mood	Indifference Irritability Anxiety Depression	Variable depression	Auditory and visual hallucinations	Early personality changes Kluver–Bücy syndrome Pacing
CT/MRI	Global atrophy	Multiple infarcts of sufficient volume to explain dementia	No change or slight atrophy	Frontotemporal atrophy
EEG	Diffuse slowing Late changes Nonspecific	variable	High-voltage Frontal change	Diffuse slowing Late changes
Pathology	Neurofibrillary tangles Senile plaques	Infarcts	Cortical and brainstem Lewy bodies	Pick bodies Balloned cells Gliosis

of the following: aphasia, apraxia, agnosia, or a disturbance in executive function. These symptoms impair social and occupational functioning but are not due to a delirium, other central nervous system diseases, systemic conditions, or drug-induced conditions. The NINCDS-ADRDA criteria divide AD into probable, possible, and definite AD. Criteria for probable AD include dementia, established by clinical examination and supported by neuropsychological testing, deficits in two or more areas of cognition, progressive worsening of memory and other cognitive functions, no disturbance of consciousness, onset between age 40 and 90, most often after age 65, and absence of other systemic disorders or brain diseases that could account for the progressive deficits in memory and cognition. The clinical diagnosis of possible AD is made on the basis of the dementia syndrome without neurologic, psychiatric, or systemic disorders sufficient to cause dementia. The NINCDS-ADRDA criteria also establish subtypes for research purposes, such as familial occurrence, onset before age 65, presence of trisomy 21, and coexistence of other relevant conditions. The criteria for a definite diagnosis of AD are restricted to the clinical criteria for probable AD and histopathologic evidence from an autopsy or biopsy. The problem with the NINCDS-ADRDA criteria is that, depending on the area of the brain affected and the corresponding presenting symptoms, other dementia syndromes also qualify by these criteria. Pick's disease patients fufill the criteria for probable AD, as could complications of alcoholism and VaD.

Although patients with AD most commonly present with forgetfulness, an inability to learn new material, or naming difficulties, the actual cognitive and functional decline has been progressing for several years before diagnosis. Subjects diagnosed with probable AD have been shown to have significant early memory decline and poor immediate auditory retention span when compared to normal subjects (Linn et al., 1995). When correcting for education, sex, and language, Jacobs et al. (1995) showed that subjects diagnosed with probable AD scored significantly different from control subjects on the Boston Naming Test, Immediate Recall on the Selective Reminding Test, and the Similarities subtest of the Weschler Adult Intelligence Scale–Revised during early testing. These studies support the idea of an actual preclinical phase of AD that may precede the actual diagnosis by up to 13 years.

Usually, patients present to the physician several years after the onset of the disease when a family member recognizes cognitive decline. Due to AD's insidious nature, it is often difficult for people close to the patient to see changes until they become significant enough to impair daily activities. AD is typically divided into three stages, characterized by progressive decline in memory, naming, visuospatial tasks, and activities of daily living (ADLs) (Cummings & Benson, 1992). The first stage of the disease is subtle and can be relatively short, lasting only a year, or it can progress insidiously for several years. Classically, the patient presents with difficulties recalling recent events and learning new material. This is accompanied by cognitive deficits in complex learned behavior. The patient has decreased word-finding abilities characterized by decreased word output, anomia, and repetition. Difficulties in calculation, such as financial management and making change as well as poor insight and judgment, are also present. Visuospatial skills are impaired early on in AD and manifest themselves as disorientation, getting lost, and an inability to copy complex objects.

Personality and behavioral changes are also common in AD (see chapter 4). The first changes seen may be depression and lack of interest in hobbies or activities that were once pleasurable. Physicians often treat the depression, only to have the patient decline again in a few months. This is an indication that an underlying dementia may be present. Patients also become irritable, violent, or apathetic when they were not before. These behavioral changes may not always be present initially but may manifest themselves later. If the patient has delusions or hallucinations early in the course of the illness that are not related to medication use, DLBD should be suspected (McKeith, Fairbairn, Perry, Thompson, & Perry, 1992).

At the mild stage of AD, patients have normal neurologic and physical examinations. Reflexes are intact, and diagnostic tests show a normal EEG, CT, or MRI. If PET or SPECT scans are done at this stage, or even in preclinical stages, a bilateral hypometabolism in temporal and parietal cortices would be evident. Although these patients have impaired social and work activities and show slight deficits in simple ADLs such as dressing and shaving, independent living is generally acceptable. Individual patients may appear to plateau for periods of time or fluctuate on a day-to-day basis, but the clinical course of AD is slowly progressive.

In the moderate stage, patients may lose remote memories in addition to recent ones. Language, calculation, and comprehension are usually impaired, and insight deteriorates rapidly. Patients may get lost in familiar surroundings, and increasing apraxia makes simple tasks difficult. Personality changes may be increasingly difficult to control as patients may become more resistive, aggressive, restless, anxious, or irritable. Although medications can control some of these behaviors, the patient may become too difficult for the caregiver to handle and may require institutionalization. Delusions may become more common at this time, but if the course is rapidly progressive, then DLBD should be suspected. Neurologic examination is still relatively intact, but slowed reflexes are common. EEG shows slowing, and CT or MRI gives indications of ventricular enlargement and diffuse atrophy. Hypometabolism may become more apparent on PET or SPECT. Supervised care may be needed at this stage of the disease, and medications can be administered to obviate sleeping problems, irritability, restlessness, and wandering. Patients become increasingly dependent on others for their ADLs. Eating, dressing, toileting, and all other personal hygiene activities may need to be performed by a caregiver.

The severe stage of AD usually begins with more difficulties in fecal and urinary incontinence, and increasing aggression, anxiety, and irritability. Recent and remote memory is patchy with very little recall. The patient can no longer perform complex learned behaviors, is totally dependent on caregivers, and may require constant supervision. Language is reduced to random, repeated words and syllables, if anything is spoken at all. Abnormal reflexes, seizures, and myoclonic jerks may occur in late stages of AD (Cummings & Benson, 1992). The EEG may be diffusely slowed, and CT or MRI usually shows marked ventricular dilatation and striking cortical atrophy. Patients may lose weight, have rigid limbs and flexed posture, and may be confined to bed for the last few years of the disease. The cause of death is often due to aspiration pneumonia or sepsis due to a urinary tract infection (see chapter 2).

The range of the illness is usually 2 to 20 years, but on average, the illness lasts for 8 years (Cummings & Benson, 1992). If symptoms progress within the course of a few months to a year and show marked EEG changes, other causes, such as CJD should be suspected (Fleming et al., 1995). Myoclonic seizures early in the course of the disease and familial cases may indicate a more rapid downhill progression (Fleming et al., 1995). Atypical presentations of AD can occur, but other progressive illnesses should be weighed more heavily in the differential diagnosis. Early aphasia or behavioral problems alone may indicate Pick's disease (Cummings & Benson, 1992).

PATHOLOGY AND PATHOGENESIS

The brain of an AD patient shows diffuse atrophy of the association areas of the parietal, temporal, and frontal cerebral cortices, greatly enlarged ventricles, and as the disease process progresses, subcortical atrophy. Upon autopsy, the AD brain typically weighs less than 1,000 g.

The neuropathological hallmarks of AD are the neurofibrillary tangle (NFT) and the senile plaque (SP) (Masters & Beyreuther, 1995). NFTs are intraneuronal accumulations of abnormally phosphorylated and oxidized tau protein, a microtubule-associated protein that regulates microtubule stability in axons (McKee, Kosik, & Kowall, 1991). SPs are primarily composed of a central core of amyloid fibrils surrounded by astrocytes and degenerative, or reactive, neuronal processes. This particular form of amyloid, ß amyloid (Aß), is found in SPs and in blood vessels in AD brains, but it is also produced in normal individuals, where it is found in blood and cerebrospinal fluid (CSF). Although a few localized SPs are found in a normal aged brain, they are very abundant and can be found anywhere in the AD brain.

The pathogenesis of AD is an area of intense research. It has been established that certain familial forms of AD are associated with mutations in APP, the precursor molecule from which Aß is cleaved. The excessive synthesis, impaired degradation, or altered processing of APP may then lead to the extracellular deposition seen in AD. Other theories of the pathogenesis of AD are concerned with neurotoxicity through free radical generation of Aß and/or impaired mitochondrial metabolism. Although the true cause of AD is still not known, much research is being done to discover the pathogenesis of this prevalent neurodegenerative disease. It is only with more research that the cause can be elucidated.

VASCULAR OR ISCHEMIC DEMENTIA

The term vascular dementia (VaD) is generally accepted as the preferred designation for dementia caused by vascular insufficiency. Multiple small and/or large brain infarcts are the cause of dementia in about 5% to 10% of patients. Symptoms appear when a certain volume of tissue is infarcted or when a smaller storke is strategically placed. In some cases widespread subcortical leukoencephalopathy or Binswanger's disease is the cause (Babikien & Ropper, 1987). Multi-infarct dementia is an older term used to describe dementia associated with mutiple bilateral supratentorial infarcts (Hachinski et al., 1974). Tomlinson, Blessed, and Ropth (1970) noted that dementia was found only when the volume of brain tissue lost exceeded 100 ml. Clinically, VaD is asssociated with sudden onset of dysfunction in one or more cognitive domains with patchy distribution of deficits and a stepwise deteriorating course. Focal neurologic symptoms such as weakness of an extremity, exaggeration of deep tendon reflexes, an extensor plantar response, or gait abnormalities. Stepwise deterioration or focal findings are not always present. Affective changes and psychotic symptoms may occur, especially depression or delusions. As the disease advances, emotional incontinence and pseudobulbar palsy may be apparent. There is often a history of previous strokes, transient ischemic attacks (TIAs), and risk factors for stroke such as hypertension, coronary artery disease, and atrial fibrillation.

Diagnostic accuracy has improved with the introduction of neuroimaging techniques capable of demonstrating ischemic lesions. The accuracy of the clinical diagnosis of VaD in studies with postmortem follow up varies from 25% to 85%. Further clinicopathologic studies will likely be necessary to confirm the usefulness of ischemic scores such as that of Hachinski et al. (1974) and its modifications as aids in the differential diagnosis between AD and VaD.

PREVALENCE AND RISK FACTORS

Reports on the prevalence of VaD are conflicting and vary according to the population studied. In a meta-analysis done by Jorm, Korten, and Henderson (1987) of 47 different studies on the prevalence of dementia, the prevalence of AD was much greater than that of VaD in the United States, while in Japan and Russia, the prevalence of AD equaled that of VaD. In Canada, 13% of dementias are attributed to VaD, and the proportion of AD to VaD increases after age 65. In Sweden, Skoog et al. (1993) found that the percentage of AD equaled that of VaD after age 65, but VaD patients had a significantly higher 3-year mortality rate. Overall, studies indicate that the prevalence of VaD is lower than that of AD in the United States, but nearly equal or equal in European countries.

VaD occurring with AD, or mixed dementia (MIX), is a category of progressive dementia that is rising in prevalence (Fleming et al., 1995). Folstein et al. (1991) estimated the prevalence of MIX dementia at 0.5% of the population over 65. Clinical presentation and neuroimaging studies are the best way to diagnose VaD and MIX dementia. Dementia accompanied by vascular changes on CT or MRI is not absolutely diagnostic of VaD or MIX dementia since patients may have vascular changes that do not contribute to the dementia. The best way to differentiate MIX dementia from VaD alone is to take a thorough patient history, paying careful attention to the onset and time course of the dementia, in addition to neuroimaging and other clinical features. Even the best efforts at determining the underlying cause of a patient's dementia can be confounded by presentation. The only way that definitive diagnoses can be made is by correlating findings at autopsy with clinical information and neuroimaging results.

Patient history is critical in determining if the patient has VaD over any other progressive dementia. Important points to note are hypertension, hyperlipidemia, TIAs, strokes, diabetes mellitus, and alcohol abuse. Chronic hypertension is by far the most important factor to document and control. Most studies have shown that maleness may also be a risk factor (Folstein et al., 1991; Jorm et al. 1987). If the onset of dementia is before the age of 65, VaD should be strongly considered, unless patient history indicates otherwise.

CRITERIA AND DIAGNOSIS

Since 1975, VaD has been diagnosed using dementia criteria and the Hachinski Ischemic Score (Hachinski et al., 1975). With advances in imaging techniques, however, the Hachinski scale is no longer widely used. Another set of criteria was developed by the California Alzheimer's Disease and Diagnosis Center (Chui, Teng, Henderson, & Moy, 1985), but this is currently not as widely used as the DSM-IV and the criteria developed by the NINCDS with the Association Internationale pour la Recherche et l'Ensignement en Neurosciences (NINCDS-AIREN). The DSM-IV criteria specify that deficits must occur in memory and in one other area of cognitive function enough to impair daily work and social activities. These deficits do not have to be slowly progressive, but must be focal and proven either through examination or laboratory evidence to be etiologically related to the deficit. These are also subdivided into vascular dementia with delirium, depression, delusions, or behavioral disturbances. The newest definitions for VaD, the NINCDS-AIREN criteria, were established in 1993 (Roman et al., 1993). The NINCDS-AIREN criteria, like the NINCDS-ADRDA criteria for AD, are divided into possible, probable, and definite VaD, with definite diagnoses restricted to histopathologic evidence from autopsy. As with DSM-IV criteria, the crux of these criteria is to establish a provable relationship between dementia and cerebrovascular disease as defined by neurologic examination or brain imaging. These criteria generously define vascular dementia as including multi-infarct dementia, strategic single-infarct dementia, small vessel disease with dementia such as Binswanger's disease, hypoperfusion, hemorrhagic dementia, or any combination of the above. The onset of dementia must occur within 3 months after a vascular change that has been substantiated by radiologic imaging, clinical testing, or neuropsychological testing. Unlike older criteria for VaD, these criteria specify that only cognitive impairment due to a stroke, and not physical impairment, be a requirement for the diagnosis of VaD. Patients with aphasia or hemiplegia whose intellectual evaluation was somehow impaired by the stroke were included in older VaD criteria. Drachman (1993) suggested that dementia due to vascular events be differentiated either as primary, and due only to the vascular event, or as stroke with secondary dementia.

The clinical picture of VaD is quite variable, depending on where the lesion occurs, and must be substantiated with imaging and patient history. VaD is typically characterized by stepwise progression and fluctuations in sensorium with patchy intellectual deficits. The pattern of decline is very important to recognize and document. A stepwise or fluctuating progression may also be present in DLBD, but other clinical features discussed below may differentiate the two. Determining VaD as the cause of dementia early in the course of the illness is important since proper pharmacologic treatment of hypertension may save the patient from further functional deterioration.

Hypertension, abnormal electrocardiograms (EKGs), strokes, cardiovascular or renal problems, and thromboembolic disorders may provide clues to the diagnosis. The diagnosis of VaD will be much more likely in a patient with poorly controlled or untreated hypertension or a family history of vascular disease. The location of the vascular lesion is the most important factor in determining clinical presentation and progression. An unusual clinical variant of VaD characterized by progressive subcortical leukoencephalopathy is called Binswanger's disease. The patient has slowly progressive dementia simulating AD with evidence of diffuse white matter abnormalities and periventricular leukoaraiosis on MRI (Erkinjuntti et al., 1984).

DIFFUSE LEWY BODY DISEASE

Lewy bodies are intracellular inclusions that are present in the brainstem of idiopathic Parkinson's disease. In DLBD, Lewy bodies are widely distributed throughout the brain. The occurrence of Lewy bodies in the cortex was first noted by Lipkin in 1959, but the association between cortical Lewy bodies and a dementia syndrome was not made until 1962 by Woodard et al. Because DLBD may first present either with Parkinsonian syndrome or with dementia, it may be misdiagnosed as Parkinson's, VaD, or probable AD. By 1988 DLBD was being more widely considered as a cause of a progressive dementia (Burkhardt et al., 1988). The diagnosis may be missed by pathologists because cortical Lewy bodies can be difficult to recognize in brain sections stained with conventional dyes. Clinical criteria have been formulated and tested, but because of the varied presentation of DLBD and the relatively recent pathological verification of cortical Lewy bodies, these criteria have only recently been acknowledged and applied.

PREVALENCE AND RISK FACTORS

Diffuse Lewy body disease may be the second most common cause of degenerative dementia after AD. DLBD shares several risk factors with

AD and with Parkinson's disease, as might be expected from the clinical presentation. A family history of Parkinson's and a young age of onset of the disease significantly increase a patient's chances of developing DLBD. The ApoE4 allele, discussed earlier as a risk factor for AD, is also a risk factor for DLBD (Helisalmi et al., 1996).

CRITERIA AND CLINICAL DIAGNOSIS

In 1984 Kosaka, Yoshimura, Ikeda, and Budka defined three pathological variants of Lewy body disease. Group A was called DLBD because patients had widespread cortical Lewy bodies. Group C was idiopathic Parkinson's disease because patients had Lewy bodies restricted to the brainstem. Group B patients fell in between these two groups, with some cortical Lewy bodies but fewer Lewy bodies than Group A. In 1990 Kosaka revised his criteria and made only two groups, pure and common DLBD. Pure DLBD patients had Lewy bodies in the cortex but no NFTs or SPs. These patients were much rarer than the common DLBD patients who had AD pathology throughout the brain and Lewy bodies. In 1990 Hansen et al. described a Lewy body variant of AD (LBV-AD) in which only one Lewy body was required in one of several subcortical nuclei and one of several cortical areas in addition to the normal AD pathologic changes. Forstl, Burns, Luthert, Cairns and Levy (1993) further characterized the LBV-AD, noting significantly more frontal atrophy and more neuron loss in the nucleus basalis of Meynert and the substantia nigra.

Clinically, criteria for DLBD has been more difficult to formulate because patients may present with Parkinsonian symptoms, AD-like dementia, or psychiatric disturbances. Mayeux, Stern, and Spanton (1985) classified AD into four subtypes, one of which, the extrapyramidal group, was found to have more severe intellectual and functional decline with psychotic symptoms. Chui et al. (1985) also associated extrapyramidal signs in AD patients with a greater severity of dementia. In an early study of the clinical and pathological features of DLBD, Gibb, Esiri, and Lees (1985) noted cortical and brainstem Lewy bodies and cortical NFTs in demented Parkinson's patients and proposed that this was a spectrum of Parkinson diseases.

There are currently two sets of clinical criteria used for diagnosing DLBD. The Nottingham criteria, composed in 1991 (Byrne, Lennox, Lowe, & Godwin-Austen), identifies patients who present with Parkinson's symptoms. The Newcastle criteria, devised by McKeith et al. (1992), identifies patients who present with dementia or behavioral symptoms. The Newcastle criteria include fluctuating cognitive decline with visual and/ or auditory hallucinations, neuroleptic sensitivity, and transient losses of consciousness. These symptoms progress slowly over a period of time and end with a rapid decline. McKeith et al. (1992) stated that Parkinsonian features, psychotic symptoms, rapid cognitive decline, and reduced survival differentiate DLBD from AD patients. In a follow-up study in 1994, McKeith et al. determined that their criteria were very accurate. However, some pathologically diagnosed DLBD patients were misdiagnosed as having VaD or probable AD. McKeith concluded in his 1994 study that the approach to diagnosing DLBD is a challenge to the physician because the symptoms are multifaceted and require information gathered from several specialists. Neurologic, psychologic, and motoric impairment must be assessed simultaneously and at more frequent intervals than other progressive dementias.

PATHOLOGY AND PATHOGENESIS

In 1912 F. H. Lewy was the first to describe an intracytoplasmic inclusion found in the neurons of the motor nucleus of the vagus and the substantia nigra of Parkinson's patients. With trichrome stain, "classical" Lewy bodies in the brainstem were a round to oval brilliant red, dense core surrounded by a less dense blue halo. This structure pushed the nucleus aside if intracellular, or floated free in the brainstem. Cortical Lewy bodies are smaller, lack a distinct core, stain less intensely blue, and are usually located in the small neurons of layers five and six, although they can be found in any small cortical neurons (Gibb et al., 1985). Lewy bodies are known to be composed of various cellular components. Other pathological changes in DLBD brains are similar to those found in AD brains. SPs and NFTs may or may not be present, but the distribution of Lewy bodies does not follow that of SPs or NFTs. Spongiform change is seen to a lesser degree than in AD and is usually nonspecific.

PICK'S DISEASE

In 1892 Arnold Pick described a 71-year-old man with difficulty recognizing objects, aphasia, and progressive dementia. After the man died a few months later, his brain was noted to have severe frontotemporal atrophy. In 1911 Alzheimer described the histopathology of the brain of a similar patient. He found ovoid intracytoplasmic neuronal inclusions that pushed the nucleus aside and appeared black with silver staining. The name Pick's disease was given to this clinical and pathological presentation. PD has since been characterized as a progressive dementia, usually sporadic but often inherited, that is associated with personality changes and language disturbances and usually begins between ages 40 and 60. Since Pick's description in 1892, several diseases that have a similar clinical presentation have been described. At autopsy, however, each disease presents with unique histopathology and frontotemporal atrophy. Because there is no neuropathological or clinical criteria for PD or related clinical syndromes, this diversity of neuropathology creates much controversy over classifying this group of diseases. Currently, two schools of thought exist that center on Pick bodies, the microscopic hallmark Alzheimer described, and frontotemporal atrophy. Some neuropathologists consider frontotemporal atrophy alone to be the characteristic feature of a larger spectrum of diseases called frontal lobe dementias, or the Pick's spectrum of dementia. PD is considered a subset of frontal lobe dementias and is characterized by Pick bodies, the inclusions described by Alzheimer. Others consider frontotemporal atrophy alone to be Pick's disease. However, it is important to understand that the clinical presentation is similar among all of these diseases and that, until more research is done on the pathogenesis of these diseases, our limited treatments suffice for this spectrum of frontal degenerative dementias.

The PD clinical presentation can be idiopathic or can present secondarily as a result of another disease. The diseases in which dementia is the primary symptom include frontal lobe degeneration of the non-Alzheimer's type (FLD), progressive language dysfunction with frontal lobe atrophy, progresssive subcortical gliosis, and frontal onset of Creutzfeld–Jacob disease. The lobar variant of AD is included in this group because the clinical presentation is similar to PD, but the pathology is like that of AD brains (Cummings & Benson, 1992). There are also diseases that secondarily present with progressive frontal degenerative dementia. These include Huntington's disease, Parkinson's disease, progressive supranuclear palsy, motor neuron disease, or ALS, and sometimes chronic alcoholism. These secondary frontal dementias can be recognized given the clinical information below, but the underlying disease will usually manifest itself before any dementia occurs. While these diseases will not be discussed here because they are quite rare, it is important to remember that they have presentations very similar to PD and should be included in a differential diagnosis.

PREVALENCE AND RISK FACTORS

PD is relatively rare compared to AD and has been estimated at 10 to 15 times less prevalent than AD (Jervis, 1971). The prevalence of dementia classified as non-AD, non-VaD are reported to range from 9.5% (Skoog et al., 1993) to12% (Ebly et al., 1994). Studies by Tissot, Constantinidis, and

Richard (1985) show the prevalence of PD among patients under 65 years of age in a psychiatric hospital to be 1.3%. This figure increases to 3% to 6% in those 65 years of age and older.

It has been known since the time of Arnold Pick that 20% of cases of PD are inherited. Such patients first present between the ages of 40 and 60, a much earlier age than other progressive dementias, except for AD associated with chromosomal abnormalities. The disease is inherited in an autosomal dominant manner. No gene has been linked to PD; thus, screening offsprings of Pick's patients is not yet possible. Recent evidence suggests that ApoE4 is also associated with an increased risk for PD (Schneider, Gearing, Robbins, de l'Aune, & Mirra, 1995).

CRITERIA AND CLINICAL DIAGNOSIS

Although many physicians have documented the progression of PD in individuals and groups of patients, there are no conclusive clinical criteria for PD. Neuropathological criteria are currently being devised. There are two difficulties with creating criteria for PD and the Pick's spectrum of diseases. The number of patients with these symptoms is quite small, and it is difficult to recognize them as having a unique disease entity that is not an atypical form of another neurodegenerative process. PD patients are often misdiagnosed as having probable AD because they fulfill the NINCDS-AIREN criteria. Without an autopsy to verify the diagnosis, as is often the case, it is never known what the patient truly had. Constantinidis, Richard, and Tissot (1974) compiled comprehensive evidence of 32 cases of Pick's lobar atrophy and created three classes of the disease using pathological and clinical criteria. To date, this system seems to be the most accurate for clinical diagnosis and pathological criteria.

The clinical picture of PD is characterized by personality changes and aphasia initially, with later progression of memory and cognitive deficits. Inherited cases, in which symptoms first appear between the ages of 40 and 60, occur much more frequently than inherited cases of AD. Similar to AD, PD most often occurs sporadically and progresses for 8 to 10 years (Cummings & Benson, 1992).

Subtle changes in personality indicate the onset of the disease. Often patients will act out of character and will show altered behavior. The patient may be apathetic or euphoric. Favorite activities and hobbies may no longer interest the patient. They may become disinhibited, making socially inappropriate comments or blunt emotional remarks, and may act on them, embarrassing and shocking family members or caregivers. The Pick's patient may not become incontinent until late in the disease, but they may urinate or defecate anywhere due to their impaired social behavior. Patients may also become sexually or physically aggressive and manifest exhibitionist tendencies. The mouth becomes a fixation point for many PD patients. Initially the PD patient may eat excessively, becoming gluttonous and gaining a tremendous amount of weight. These features mimic the Kluver–Bücy syndrome, in which amygdaloid lesions cause hypersexuality, hyperorality, and decreased fear. This may reflect the temporal lobe involvement in PD. These characteristics present insidiously and may occur more frequently as the disease progresses (Cummings & Benson, 1992).

Exploration to the point of obsession and compulsion to find objects or people is a unique sign of PD. Patients may take 5- or 6-mile walks every day, pointedly searching for someone or something. This manifests itself as roaming or pacing behavior. The patient will walk around rooms in the house or circle the hallways of the nursing home (Mendez et al., 1993). Emotional lability, especially depression, and affective changes are commonly seen in PD patients. These may be difficult to differentiate from simple senile depression or other psychotic episodes. Progression of these clinical symptoms is the differentiating feature of PD. Speech is markedly affected early in PD. Word finding is usually the most obvious symptom, resulting in decreased speech output, reiteration, decreased word fluency, and circumlocution. The patient may later become palilalic or echolalic, constantly repeating one or two words, while in the final stages of the disease, the patient is incomprehensible or mute (Cummings & Benson, 1992).

Memory and visuospatial tasks, often the first deficits recognized in AD, are usually preserved in the early stages of PD. Deterioration of these faculties may begin in the middle stage of the disease, but often it is not until the later stages of the disease that the patient loses recent and immediate memory. This varies greatly from patient to patient, but preservation of memory and visuospatial tasks are highly suggestive of a frontal dementia. Although it has been found (Knopman et al., 1989) that PD patients score similarly to AD patients on the MMSE and that PD patients are indistinguishable from AD patients early in the disease process, there are certain clinical features that may help to differentiate PD from AD. Mendez, Selwood, Mastri, and Frey (1993) showed PD patients to have a presenile onset (before age 65), an initial personality change, hyperoral behavior, disinhibition, and roaming behavior significantly more than AD.

Constantinidis et al. (1974) divided 32 PD patients into four groups—A, B, C1, and C2—based on correlations between their clinical and pathological findings. A variety of clinical signs, both pyramidal and extrapyramidal, were used to differentiate the groups. Pyramidal signs include spastic paralysis, hyperreactive reflexes, and a present Babinski sign, whereas extrapyramidal signs include flaccid paralysis and hypotonic reflexes. All except group C1 showed the "PES syndrome" (palilalia, echolalia, and stereotypic activity) and gluttony. Group A lacked pyramidal and extrapyramidal signs, but group B showed pyramidal and extrapyramidal signs. Group C was divided into C1 and C2 because of pathological criteria that are described later. Group C1 had clinical features similar to group A, whereas group C2 clinically resembled group B. These are the most comprehensive criteria currently available for classifying PD patients.

PATHOLOGY AND PATHOGENESIS

Grossly, the brain of a PD patient weighs less than 1,000 grams, has asymmetric lobar atrophy, most often right hemisphere greater than left, and ventricular dilatation (Adams & Duchen, 1992). Although any single gyrus can be affected, the anterior frontal and temporal lobes are most commonly affected, with the parietal lobes rarely involved. These degenerative changes, often called knife-edged atrophy, can be seen on a CT scan and include both gray and white matter. Studies have shown that PD patients have decreased blood flow in areas of the brain where gyral atrophy has been identified on CT (Friedland et al., 1993).

The pathological definition of Pick's disease is frontal or temporal lobar atrophy. Microscopically, Pick bodies and Pick cells (ballooned neurons) often accompany the atrophy. Pick bodies are ovoid to round intracytoplasmic, argentophilic structures that are equal in size to the nucleus. They are primarily found in layers 2, 3, and 6 of the medial temporal lobes and in the hippocampus in layers 2, 3, and 6 (Gibb et al., 1985). Pick bodies are rarely found in subcortical structures and, unlike SPs and Lewy bodies, they are never found in normal aged brains. Since Pick bodies are not surrounded by a membrane, they are not considered to be an inclusion or have a viral etiology. Many of the components of Pick bodies are found in the brains of patients with Alzheimer's disease, raising questions about a common etiology of these neurodegenerative disorders.

Ballooned neurons, or Pick cells, are argentophilic, inflated neurons that appear to be dying or going through a transition to a Pick body. They are found in layers 3 and 5 of the frontal cortex, the basal ganglia, and the substantia nigra. Evidence of heavy astrocytic gliosis in cortical and subcortical white matter and the random array of neurofilaments and neurotubules indicate that ballooned neurons may be a reaction to axonal damage and, in some cases, a loss of myelin (Constantidis et al., 1974).

The four pathological groups of Constantidis et al. (1974) were defined according to the presence or absence of "neuronal swellings" (ballooned cells), Pick bodies, and localization of atrophy. Group A had both neuronal swellings and Pick bodies. Atrophy began primarily in the temporal pole with gliosis and proportional white matter demyelination. Pick bodies were found primarily but not exclusively in the hippocampus. Group B had neuronal swellings, including the proximal part of the axon, but no Pick bodies. Atrophy was found in the frontal lobe, often extending to the precentral gyrus. Gliosis in these cases was unaccompanied by white matter demyelination. Group C was defined by the presence of atrophy and gliosis but the absence of *both* neuronal swellings *and* Pick bodies. Within this group, two populations were seen. Group C1 had temporal atrophy and closely resembled group A in the areas of the brain affected. Group C2 had frontal atrophy and closely resembled group B in the distribution of pathology, but the white matter was severely demyelinated.

CONCLUSIONS

The clinical features of the diseases associated with progressive dementia that have been discussed in this chapter depend more on the pattern of regional cortical involvement than on the specific nature of the underlying pathology. AD usually affects temporal structures early in its course, leading to a memory disorder, which is the most common initial complaint. In those unusual cases with a frontal predominance of pathology, behavioral changes occur similar to those seen in PD. Rarely AD or PD affects cortical language areas in isolation, and, again, symptoms depend on the region damaged, not the underlying process. Similarly, clinical management depends more on specific symptomatology than on the etiology. Behavioral disturbances in a patient with AD or PD are treated identically. However, DLBD is associated with neuroleptic sensitivity, which limits the therapeutic options available to treat the hallucinations that often occur in these patients. Unfortunately, the management of patients with these devastating illnesses is not likely to significantly improve until rational therapies are devised based on a better understanding of disease pathogenesis. At present, patients with a terminal phase of any of these diseases would equally qualify and benefit from palliative treatment and hospice involvement.

REFERENCES

Adams, J. H., & Duchen, L. W. (1992). *Greenfield's neuropathology.* (5th ed.). New York: Oxford University Press

American Psychiatric Association. (1994). *Diagnostic and statistical manual of mental disorders* (4th ed). Washington, DC: American Psychiatric Press.

Babikian, V., & Ropper, A. H. (1987). Binswanger's disease: A review. *Stroke, 18,* 2–12.

Bachman, D. L., Wolf, P. A., Linn, R. T., Knoefel, J. E., Cobb, J. L., Belanger, A. J., D'Agnostino, R. B., & White, L. R. (1992). Prevalence of dementia and probable senile dementia of the Alzheimer type in the Framingham study. *Neurology, 42,* 115–119.

Bachman, D. L., Wolf, P. A., Linn, R. T., Knoefel, J. E., Cobb, J. L., Belanger, A. J., White, L. R., & D'Agnostino, R. B. (1993) Incidence of dementia and probable AD in a general population: The Framingham study. *Neurology, 43,* 515–519.

Blessed, G., Tomlinson, B. E., & Roth, M. (1968). The association between quantitative measures of dementia, and of senile change in the cerebral grey matter of elderly subjects. *British Journal of Psychiatry, 114,* 797–811.

Burkhardt, C. R., Filley, C. M., Kleinschmidt-DeMasters, B. K., de la Monte, S., Norenberg, M. D., & Schenk, S. A. (1988). Diffuse Lewy body disease and progressive dementia. *Neurology, 38,* 1520–1528.

Chui, H. C., Teng, E. L., Henderson, V. W., & Moy, A. C. (1985). Clinical subtypes of dementia of the Alzheimer's type. *Neurology, 35,* 1544–1550.

Clarfield, A. M. (1988). The reversible dementias: Do they reverse? *Annals of Internal Medicine, 109,* 476–486.

Constantinidis, J., Richard, J., & Tissot, R. (1974). Pick's Disease: Histological and clinical correlations. *European Neurology, 11,* 208–217.

Corder, E. H., Saunders, A. M., & Risch, N. J. (1994). Protective effect of apolipoprotein E type 2 allele for late onset Alzheimer's disease. *Nature Genetics, 7,* 180–184.

Crystal, H. A., Dickson, D. W., Lizardi, J. E., Davies, P., & Wolfson, L. I. (1990). Antemortem diagnosis of diffuse Lewy body disease. *Neurology, 40,* 1523–1528.

Cummings, J. L., & Benson, D. F. (1992). *Dementia: A clinical approach* (2nd ed.). Boston: Butterworth-Heinemann.

Drachman, D. A. (1993). New criteria for the diagnosis of vascular dementia: Do we know enough yet? *Neurology, 43,* 243–245.

Ebly, E. M., Parhad, I. M., Hogan, D. B., & Fung, T. S. (1994). Prevalence and types of dementia in the very old: Results from the Canadian Study of Health and Aging. *Neurology, 44,* 1593–1600.

Erkinjuntti, T., Sipponen, J. T., Iivanainen, M., Ketonen, L., Sulkava, R., & Sepponen, R. E. (1984). Cerebral NMR & CT imaging in dementia. *Journal of Computer Assisted Tomography, 8,* 614–618.

Evans, D. A., Funkenstein, H. H., Albert, M. S., Scherr, P. A., Cook, N. R., Chown, M. J., Hebert, L. E., Hennekens, C. H., & Taylor, J. O. (1989). Prevalence of

Alzheimer's Disease in a community population of older persons: Higher than previously reported. *Journal of the American Medical Association, 262,* 2551–2556.

Fleming, K. C., Adams, A. C., & Petersen, R. C. (1995). Dementia: Diagnosis and evaluation. *Mayo Clinic Proceedings, 70,* 1093–1107.

Folstein, K. C., Folstein, S. E., & McHugh, P. R. (1975). Mini-Mental State: A practical method for grading the cognitive state of patients for the clinician. *Journal of Psychiatric Research, 12,* 323–329.

Folstein, M. F., Bassett, S. S., Anthony, J. C., Romanoski, A. J., & Nestadt, G. R. (1991). Dementia: Case Ascertainment in a Community Survey. *Journal of Gerontology; 46,* M132–138.

Forstl, H., Burns, A., Luthert, P., Cairns, N., & Levy, R. (1993). The Lewy body variant of Alzheimer's disease. Clinical and pathological findings. *British Journal of Psychiatry, 162,* 385–392.

Fratiglioni, L., Grut, M., Forsell, Y., Viitanen, M., Grafstrom, M., Holmen, K., Ericsson, K., Backman, L., Ahlbom, A., & Winblad, B. (1991). Prevalence of AD and other dementias in an elderly urban population: Relationship with age, sex, and education. *Neurology, 41,* 1886–1892.

Friedland, R. P., Koss, E., Lerner, A., Hedera, P., Ellis, W., Dronkers, N., Ober, B. A., & Jagust, W. J., (1993). Functional imaging, the frontal lobes, and dementia. *Dementia, 4,* 192–203.

Gibb, W. R. G. , Esiri, M. M., & Lees, A. J . (1985). Clinical and pathological features of diffuse Lewy body disease (Lewy body dementia). *Brain, 110,* 1131–1153.

Hachinski, V. C., Iliff, L. D., Zilhka, E., DuBoulay, G. H., McAllister, V. L., Marshall, J., Russell, R. W., & Symon, L. (1975). Cerebral blood flow in dementia. *Archives of Neurology, 32,* 632–637.

Hachinski, V. C., Lassen, N. A., & Marshall, J. (1974). Multi-infarct dementia, a cause of mental deterioration in the elderly. *Lancet, 2,* 207–210.

Hansen, L., Salmon, D., Galasko, D., Masliah, E., Katzman, R., DeTeresa, R., Thal, L., Pay, M. M., Hofstetter, R., Klauber, M., Rice, V., Butters, N., & Alford, M. (1990). The Lewy body variant of Alzheimer's disease: A clinical and pathologic entity. *Neurology, 40,* 1–8.

Helisalmi, S., Linnaranta, K., Lehtovirta, M., Mannermaa, A., Heinonen, O., Ryynanen, M., Reikkinen, Sr., P., & Soininen, H. (1996). Apolipoprotein E polymorphism in patients with different neurodegenerative disorders. *Neuroscience Letters, 205,* 61–64.

Heyman, A., Fillenbaum, G., Prosnitz, B., Raiford, K., Burchett, B., & Clark, C. (1991). Estimated prevalence of dementia among elderly black and white community residents. *Archives of Neurology, 48,* 594–598.

Jacobs, D. M., Sano, M., Dooneief, G., Marder, K., Bell, K. L., & Stern, Y. (1995). Neuropsychological detection and characterization of preclinical Alzheimer's disease. *Neurology, 45,* 957–962.

Jagust, W. J., Reed, B. R., Seab, J. P., & Budinger, T. F. (1990). Alzheimer's disease: Age at onset and single-photon emission computed tomographic patterns of regional cerebral blood flow. *Archives of Neurology, 47,* 628–633.

Jervis, G. A. (1971). Pick's disease. In J. Minckler (Ed.), *Pathology of the nervous system.* (Vol. 2, pp. 1395–1404). New York: McGraw-Hill.

Jorm, A. F., Korten, A. E., & Henderson, A. S. (1987). The prevalence of dementia: A quantitative integration of the literature. *Acta Psychiatria Scandinavia, 76,* 465–479.

Katzman, R. (1993). Education and the prevalence of dementia and Alzheimer's disease. *Neurology, 43,* 13–20.

Knopman, D. S., Christensen, K. J., Schut, L. J., Harbaugh, R. E., Reeder, T., Ngo, T., & Frey, W. (1989). The spectrum of imaging and neuropsychological findings in Pick's disease. *Neurology, 39,* 362–368.

Kosaka, K. (1990). Diffuse Lewy body disease in Japan. *Journal of Neurology, 237,* 197–204.

Kosaka, K., Yoshimura, M., Ikeda, K., & Budka, H. (1984). Diffuse type of Lewy body disease: Progressive dementia with abundant cortical Lewy bodies and senile changes of varying degree. A new disease? *Clinical Neuropathology, 3,* 185–192.

Lee, S. H., Rao, K. C. V. G., & Zimmerman, R. A. (1992). *Cranial MRI and CT.* New York: McGraw-Hill.

Linn, R. T., Wolf, P. A., Bachman, D. L., Knoefel, J. E., Cobb, J. L., Belanger, A. J., Kaplan, E. F., & D'Agnostino, R. B. (1995). The "preclinical phase" of probable AD: A 13-year prospective study of the Framingham cohort. *Archives of Neurology, 52,* 485–490.

Lipkin, L. E. (1959). Cytoplasmic inclusions in ganglion cells associated with parkinsonian states. *American Journal of Pathology, 35,* 1117–1133.

Masters, C. L., & Beyreuther, K. (1995). Molecular neuropathology of Alzheimer's disease. [Review]. *Arzneimittel Forschung, 45,* 410–412.

Mayeux, R., Stern, Y., & Spanton, S. (1985). Heterogeneity in dementia of the Alzheimer's type: Evidence of subgroups. *Neurology, 35,* 453–461.

McKee, A. C., Kosik, K. S., & Kowall, N. W. (1991) Neuritic pathology and dementia in Alzheimer's disease. *Annals of Neurology, 30,* 156–165.

McKeith, I., Fairbairn, A., Perry, R., Thompson, P., & Perry, E. (1992). Neuroleptic sensitivity in patients with senile dementia of the Lewy body type. *British Medical Journal, 305,* 673–678.

McKhann, G., Drachmann, D., Folstein, M., Katzman, R., Price, D., & Stadlan, E. M. (1984). Clinical diagnosis of Alzheimer's disease: Report of the NINCDS-ARDA Work Group under the auspices of Department of Health and Human Services Task Force on Alzheimer's Disease. *Neurology, 34,* 939–944.

Mendez, M. F., Selwood, A., Mastri, A. R., & Frey, W. H. (1993). Pick's disease versus Alzheimer's disease: A comparison of clinical characteristics. *Neurology, 43,* 289–292.

Mendez, M. F., Underwood, K. L., Zander, B. A., Mastri, A. R., Sung, J. H., & Frey, W. H. (1992). Risk factors in AD: A clinicopathological study. *Neurology, 42,* 770–775.

Reiman, E. M., Caselli, R. J., Yun, L. S., Chen, K., Bandy, D., Minoshima, S., Thibodeau, S. N., & Osbourne, D. (1996). Preclinical evidence of Alzheimer's disease in persons homozygous for the e4 allele for apolipoprotein E. *New England Journal of Medicine, 334,* 752–758.

Roberts, G. W., Gentleman, S. M., Lynch, A., Murray, L., Landon, M., & Graham, D.I. (1991). ßA4 amyloid protein deposition in brain after severe head injury: Implications for the pathogenesis of Alzheimer's disease. *Journal of Neurology, Neurosurgery, & Psychiatry, 57,* 419–425.

Roman, G. C., Tatemichi, T. K., Erkinjuntti, T., Cummings, J. L., Masdeu, J. C., Garcia, J. H., Arnaducci, L., Orgogozo, J. M., Brun, A., Hofman, A. et al. (1993). Vascular dementia: Diagnostic criteria for research studies. Report of the NINCDS-AIREN International Workshop. *Neurology, 43,* 250–260.

Rosenwaike, I., & Logue, B. (1985). *The extreme aged in America: A portrait of an expanding population.* Westport, CT: Greenwood Press.

Schneider, J. A., Gearing, M., Robbins, R. S., de l'Aune, W., & Mirra, S. S. (1995). Apolipoprotein E genotype in diverse neurodegenerative diseases. *Annals of Neurology, 38,* 131–135.

Skoog, I., Nilsson, L., Palmertz, B., Andreasson, L.A., & Svanborg, A. (1993). A population-based study of dementia in 85-year olds. *New England Journal of Medicine, 328,* 153–158.

Tissot, R., Constantinidis, J., & Richard, J. (1985). Pick's disease. In J. A. M. Frederiks (Ed.), *Handbook of clinical neurology* (vol. 2., pp. 223–246). Amsterdam: Elsevier.

Tomlinson, B. E., Blessed G., & Ropth, M. (1970). Observations on the brains of demented old people. *Journal of Neurological Sciences, 35,* 1025–1029.

Wernicke, T. F., & Reischies, F. M. (1994). Prevalence of dementia in old age: Clinical diagnoses in subjects aged 95 years and older. *Neurology, 44,* 250–253.

Wisniewski, H. M., & Wegiel, J. (1995). The neuropathology of Alzheimer's disease [Review]. *Neuroimaging Clinics of North America, 5,* 45–57.

Woodard, J. S. (1962). Concentric hyaline inclusion body formation in mental disease analysis of twenty-seven cases. *Journal of Neuropathology and Experimental Neurology, 20,* 442–449.

Infections in Advanced Dementia

Ladislav Volicer, Gary H. Brandeis, and Ann C. Hurley

Infections are a common complication of advanced dementia and are the most frequent cause of death of patients in the terminal stage of the disease. Bronchopneumonia was the cause of death in 54% to 59% of Alzheimer patients and in 69% of patients with multi-infarct dementia (Molsa, Marttila, & Rinne, 1986; Sulkava, Haltia, Paetav, Wikstrom, & Palo, 1983). An analysis of 174 death certificates of individuals enrolled in an Alzheimer's Disease Research Center cohort showed that pneumonia was the primary cause of death in 24% and a contributing factor in 44% of deaths, whereas urinary tract infection was a contributing factor in 6% and sepsis in 5% of deaths (Olichney, Hofstetter, Galasko, Thal, & Katzman, 1995). These numbers probably underestimate true rates of infections because cardiorespiratory arrest and respiratory arrest/failure, which were the primary cause of death in 25% of individuals, might also have been secondary to an infectious episode. The frequency with which pneumonia contributes to death increases with the severity of dementia (Kukull et al., 1994), and several kinds of infections (septicemia, acute upper respiratory infections, pneumococcal pneumonia, bronchopneumonia, kidney infections, and cystitis) are listed more often on death certificates of people who died with the diagnosis of dementia than on certificates of case controls (Chandra, Bharucha, & Schoenberg, 1986).

Relatively little is known about the prevalence of infections in patients with advanced dementia who are cared for at home (Collins & Ogle,

1994). However, a large amount of information is available about infections in nursing homes [for a review, see Olive and Berk, (1992)], but few studies specifically explore infections in patients suffering from advanced dementia. It was reported that 28% to 33% of nursing home residents hospitalized for pneumonia carried the diagnosis of dementia (Gabow et al., 1985; Marrie, Durant, & Kwan, 1986) and an even larger number (53%) showed confusion during the hospitalization (Marrie et al., 1986).

In two studies that monitored the occurrence of infections in 175 patients with advanced dementia cared for at a Dementia Special Care Unit, the proportions of patients developing at least one febrile episode were 25% and 31% per year, respectively (Fabiszewski, Volicer, & Volicer, 1990; Volicer, Hurley, Fabiszewski, Montgomery, & Volicer, 1993). Many of these patients had multiple fever episodes with an average of 2.5 fevers per year. The most common symptoms during the fever episodes were respiratory (46%), urinary (31%), systemic (15%), and a combination of respiratory and urinary symptoms (8%) (Fabiszewski, et al., 1990). Despite a complete diagnostic evaluation, the exact cause of the fever episode was not identified in 30% of patients. During the 34 months when infections were monitored 41 patients died, 21 had respiratory symptoms, and two additional patients had been asymptomatic but had a diagnosis of pneumonia on autopsy (Fabiszewski et al., 1990). Thus penumonia accounted for 56% of deaths in this patient population.

CONTRIBUTING FACTORS

Several factors contribute to the high incidence of infections and their severity in patients with advanced dementia: changes in immune function, difficulty in diagnosing an infectious process, incontinence, decreased mobility, and a propensity for aspiration of food, liquids, and respiratory secretions.

CHANGES IN IMMUNE FUNCTION

Immune responses to foreign antigens decline with age. This is due mainly to the loss of thymic and T-lymphocyte function (for a review, see Ben-Yehuda & Weksler (1992)). This loss increases sensitivity to infections in elderly individuals, including patients with dementia. The incidence of pneumonia and influenza requiring hospitalization increases from 35 per 100,000 persons 15 to 40 years old, to 93 per 100,000 persons 45 to 64 years old, to 310 per 100,000 persons 65 and older (Barker, 1986).

In addition to this age-related increase in sensitivity to infections, demented patients have further immunological deficiencies. Cell-mediated immunity, measured by skin responses to seven different antigens, was absent in 60% of nursing home residents requiring assistance with their daily activities, 42% of self-sufficient nursing home residents, and only 18% of senior citizens living at home (Marrie, Johnson, & Durant, 1988). Another study showed that anergy increased overall mortality, and the incidence of pneumonia was almost three times higher in anergic individuals than in residents responding to at least one of four antigens (Wayne, Rhyne, Garry, & Goodwin, 1990).

Cytokine secretion by mononuclear cells is also influenced by Alzheimer's disease, but the effect varies during the progression of dementia. Patients with a mild stage of dementia have decreased secretion of interleukin-3 and of tumor necrosis factor, whereas patients with moderate to severe dementia have an increased secretion of interleukin-2 and gamma interferon when compared to age-matched controls (see Figure 2.1; Huberman et al., 1994). The increase of gamma interferon secretion is probably due to increased interleukin-2 secretion, because interleukin is an interferon inducer, and the increase of interleukin-2 secretion is due to an increase in the CD4$^+$ cell population. The decreased tumor necrosis factor secretion in patients with mild dementia may play a role in pathogenesis of Alzheimer's disease because tumor necrosis factors protect neurons agains amyloid toxicity (Barger et al., 1995).

Dementia also affects the endocrine function of the thymus. It was reported that reactivation of plasma thymulin in vitro by addition of zinc was less effective in dementia patients than in age-matched controls (Licastro et al., 1990). The T8$^+$ cell–mediated suppression of allogenic B-cell responses, which declines during aging, was reported to be further impaired in Alzheimer patients compared to age-matched controls (Skias, Bania, Reder, Luchins, & Antel, 1985). In contrast, concavalin A-induced suppressor activity directed toward an autologous mitogen-induced predominantly T-cell response, which is increased during aging, is further increased in Alzheimer patients (Miller, Neighbors, Katzman, Aronson, & Lipkowitz, 1981). This finding may reflect a heightened sensitivity of responder cells to suppressor influences rather than activity of the suppressor cells.

DIFFICULTY IN DIAGNOSING AN INFECTIOUS PROCESS

The severity of infections may be increased by a delay or lack of treatment in the early stages of the infectious process. Two factors contribute to the difficulty in identifying a possible infectious process: an altered

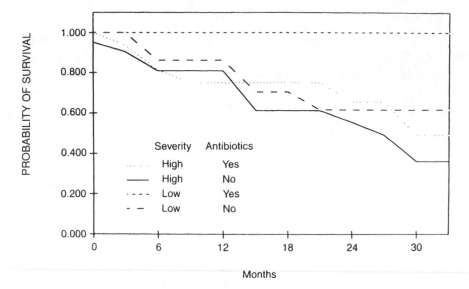

FIGURE 2.1 Survival analysis of four groups of patients with Alzheimer's disease divided according to the severity of the disease indicated by the Social Contact subscale of the MACC Behavioral Adjustiment Scale and according to the use of antibiotics in treatment of fever episodes.

From "Effect of antibiotic treatment on outcome of fevers in institutionalized Alzheimer Patients," by K. J. Fabiszewski, B. Volicer, and L. Volicer, 1990, *Journal of the American Medical Association, 263,* pp. 3168–3172. Copyright 1990, American Medical Association. Reproduced with permission.

clinical presentation and an inability of patients to report symptoms. The altered clinical presentation includes decreased perception of pain and absence of a fever response to an infection (Norman & Toledo, 1992). In some cases, the only evidence of an infectious process is a behavioral change, increased confusion, or diminished eating ability. A study investigating clinical features in 50 consecutive institution- acquired bacterial pneumonias in an elderly population reported that fever occurred only in 80%, cough in 75%, and sputum production in 40% of cases (Bentley, 1984).

Severe aphasia prevents the reporting of symptoms by the patient, but even patients with mild dementia are less likely to complain. It was reported that individuals with mild dementia are less likely to report cough, rash, gastrointestinal symptoms, and joint pain than cognitively intact controls (McCormick et al., 1994). Therefore, frequent clinical assessments of demented patients are necessary to detect signs and symptoms of emerging infectious processes.

INCONTINENCE

Incontinence is an inevitable consequence of cognitive impairment in patients with severe dementia. Initially, patients may not be able to find a bathroom, may not recognize the urge to void, or the urge to void occurs so suddenly that they are unable to prevent leakage (Resnick, Subbarao, & Laurino, 1989). This can be managed by prompted voiding (Ouslander et al., 1995) or toileting patients every 2 hours or after meals. Prompted voiding is more effective in preventing urinary incontinence than routine toileting in patients who can still benefit from it, but it is difficult to maintain this program in a longterm care setting (Schnelle, McNees, Crooks, & Ouslander, 1995). However, even toileting eventually becomes ineffective because the patients do not recognize placement on a toilet as a stimulus for evacuation. With the progression of dementia, a patient may also become afraid to sit on a toilet or become unable to sit down safely.

Factors that predispose the demented, infirm patient to urinary incontinence also predispose to urinary tract infection. As a person ages, changes in the bladder—both normal and pathological—coupled with changes in the immune system can lead to bacteriuria. If the person is not able to fully empty the bladder because of outlet obstruction, detrusor hyperactivity with impaired contractility, or underactive detrusor, increased postvoid residual follows, which predisposes to bacteriuria. The presence of bacteria in the urine can lead to overt infection. This is of major concern since it is estimated that half of demented, institutionalized elderly are bacteriuric (Nicolle, 1994).

Other changes, such as decreased estrogen in women, can impact on the urethra's ability to close, which helps prevent bacteria from entering the bladder. In men, changes in prostatic fluid may make it easier for bacteria to migrate up the urethra (Nicolle, 1994). In patients who have both urinary and fecal incontinence, pathogens are present in close proximity to the urethra, the port of entry. Once inside the urethra, these pathogens colonize the bladder. If the normal defensive mechanisms are impaired, this colonization leads to bacteriuria and infection. The presence of bacteriuria in elderly men was reported to be associated with both urinary and bowel incontinence. Eighty-two percent of men with urinary incontinence and 92% of men with bowel incontinence had intermittent or continuous bacteriuria (Nicolle et al., 1987).

Ouslander, Greengold, and Chen (1987a) studied the frequency of urinary tract infections (UTIs) among male nursing home patients. In two combined groups of continent residents (*n* = 71), 8% developed symptomatic UTIs during 468 months of follow-up, resulting in 0.02 UTI per patient-month at risk. In the incontinent patient group, not using external catheter (*n* = 13), one patient developed 3 UTIs, resulting in 0.05 UTI per patient-month at risk. The incidence of UTIs was even greater in patients managed by the use of external catheters; 0.07 UTI per patient-month in patients who wore external catheters only during the night and 0.08 UTI per patient-month with continuous use. The proportion of patients who developed at least one symptomatic UTI increased from 8% of the continent residents to 16% of patients who wore an external catheter at night only and to 40% of patients who wore an external catheter continuously. However, these data cannot exclude the possibility that this increase was due to a higher incidence of stool incontinence, which was 0% in patients not using external catheters, 21% in patients using external catheters only during the night, and 70% in patients using external catheters continuously. Others have noted that stool incontinence increased the incidence of bacteriuria, although the presence of bacteriuria was not associated with increased mortality (Nicolle et al., 1987).

DECREASED MOBILITY

Decreased ability to ambulate occurs in most patients with severe dementia. Patients may not be able to ambulate safely because of perceptual problems, which make them unaware of obstacles in their path. They also may develop an abnormal gait, either broad based or extremely narrow based (scissoring). Patients often become unable to turn around and may lean to one side. Many of the gait problems could be caused or aggravated by psychoactive medications. This is especially true for neuroleptics (e.g., haloperidol), but dystonia may develop even with other medications (e.g., trazodone).

It was reported that the chance for the development of UTIs is 3.4 times higher and for development of lower respiratory infections is 6.6 times higher than the chance for development of infections in an ambulatory individual (Magaziner et al., 1991). Each day of bed confinement increased the risk of development of pneumonia by 10%. Continuous lateral rotational therapy, which provided more turning than a typical turning protocol of every 2 hours, decreased the incidence of pneumonia, urinary tract infection, and sepsis (Sahn, 1991). Decreased mobility is also a risk factor for the development of deep vein thrombosis and pressure ulcers.

Pressure ulcers can be a significant source of morbidity for patients with advanced dementia. As patients become less mobile and more bed- or chair-bound, the risk for pressure ulcer formation increases. Once a break in the skin occurs, a patient becomes vulnerable to invasion by bacteria. This may result in local colonization of the ulcer, local infection, or systemic infection. Local colonization of an ulcer with bacteria will impede healing. Local infection such as cellulitis, osteomyelitis, or even infection of neighboring sites such as joint spaces can occur. Systemically, tetanus and sepsis with a high mortality rate can result (Evans, Andrews, Chutka, Fleming, & Garness, 1995). The causative organism is often difficult to obtain, unless a quantitative biopsy culture is performed, because swab cultures can be misleading (Bergstrom et al., 1994). Thus treatment with multiple antibiotics is usually prescribed to cover mixed infections, which may include aerobic and anaerobic organisms. Moreover, infected pressure ulcers heal very poorly despite enormous effort.

ASPIRATION

As dementia progresses, a patient may develop swallowing difficulties leading to choking on food and liquids (see chapter 3). These swallowing difficulties may result in aspiration of food or liquids and the development of aspiration pneumonia.

Aspiration pneumonia may also result from aspiration of upper respiratory secretions and/or stomach contents. Aspiration of pharyngeal secretions occur during sleep in 45% of normal subjects and in 70% of subjects with depressed consciousness (Huxley, Viroslav, Gray, & Pierce, 1978). A pneumonia results when aspirated bacteria are not effectively cleared because of impaired clearance mechanisms or because of large amounts of aspirated secretions. Stomach content may be aspirated during vomiting and can induce chemical pneumonitis, which is characterized by a sudden onset of respiratory distress, absence of sputum production, and diffuse rales (Marrie, 1992). Pharmacological inhibition of gastric acid secretion leads to colonization of the stomach by gram-negative bacilli, which could further increase the danger of stomach content aspiration (Driks et al., 1987).

Difficulty with oropharyngeal secretions was identified as the most important risk factor for development of pneumonia in both acute care and long-term care settings (Harkness, Bentley, & Roghmann, 1990). Another important factor for predicting pneumonia in the long-term care setting was the presence of an unusual event, which included increased confusion and agitation. These events could indicate the presence of delirium but are also common symptoms of dementia. The presence of nasogastric or gastric tube feeding increased the incidence of pneumonia threefold in an acute care setting, and 120-fold in the long-term care setting (Harkness et al., 1990).

PREVENTION

Some of the risk factors mentioned previously can be influenced by management strategies. Meticulous nursing care, which keeps the skin clean and dry despite incontinence, may minimize the risk of infection connected with incontinence. Kinesiotherapy or physical therapy programs, which maintain patients' ambulation as long as possible, decrease patients' immobility and delay bedfast status. Aspiration of food and liquids may be minimized by the adjustment of diet texture and by using thickened liquids.

Several stategies, which are used to limit infections in the general population, are also useful in dementia patients. The incidence of upper respiratory infections, which was higher on a Dementia Special Care Unit than on a traditional unit, was decreased by reducing the size of activity groups and by staff education about prevention strategies: encouraging staff to stay home when sick, frequent staff and resident hand washing, and frequent cleaning of commonly touched items such as doorknobs and armrests (Perls & Herget, 1995).

Avoidance of internal urinary catheters is the most important prevention strategy for UTIs (Ouslander, Greengold, & Chen, 1987b). Antimicrobial prophylaxis is effective in decreasing the recurrence of UTIs but is potentially toxic and leads to the development of antibiotic-resistant bacteria (Lipsky, 1989). Therefore, prophylaxis is recommended only in patients with frequent UTIs (3 or more per year) or in patients with special risks. Administration of estrogen for atrophic vaginitis decreases the frequency of symptomatic cystitis in elderly women prone to this recurrent disease (Parsons & Schmidt, 1982).

Residual urine in the bladder after voiding, caused by bladder outlet obstruction, an underactive detrusor or detrusor hyperactivity with impaired contractility, promotes bacteriuria. Reducing the reservoir associated with increased bladder volume will lessen the potential for colonization/infection of the bladder. The approach to treatment should be tailored to patient needs and staff capabilities. In general, treatment should follow a stepped approach. The feasibility of behavioral, pharmaceutical, and surgical options should be assessed for each person. The first treatment step should be behavioral in nature. The Crede maneuver, which involves massaging the abdomen to push fluid out, should be tried. However, this may not be possible in a severely demented population. Another method is clean intermittent straight catheterization, which will decrease the amount of urine in the bladder when performed on a regular basis. Use of an indwelling catheter reduces bladder volume but leaves an open conduit for bacteria to enter the bladder. The bladder is usually colonized within 30 days with bacteria in patients with an indwelling catheter.

The second treatment option is medications. Medications that enhance bladder contraction, such as urecholine, can be tried, but their efficacy is questionable (Urinary Incontinence in Adults Guideline Update Panel, 1996). Discontinuation of medications that inhibit bladder contraction (e.g., drugs with anticholinergic effects) can lead to decreased bladder volume, because the bladder's ability to empty will improve. Administration of doxazosin or finasteride may improve bladder emptying in patients with an outlet obstruction. The third treatment option is surgery. For example, prostatectomy may resolve an obstruction resulting in decreased residual volume. A combination of the three treatment modalities may be needed to maximally treat a patient.

VACCINATION

Influenza and pneumococcal vaccines are routinely recommended for elderly frail individuals (Centers for Disease Control, 1989; Centers for Disease Control and Prevention, 1995).

Influenza usually occurs during the winter season. Infection in patients with advanced dementia can have a very high mortality rate. In fact, influenza routinely ranks among the top 10 yearly causes of death in the United States (White & Fenner, 1994). The Centers for Disease Control and Prevention recommend influenza vaccination for populations at risk, which includes the severely demented, especially if institutionalized (Centers for Disease Control and Prevention, 1995). Even with high vaccination rates, however, outbreaks of disease occur. Furthermore, for the institutionalized elderly, the data on prevention of clinical disease are unclear. As stated earlier, the immune system changes with age and dementia impair the ability to develop antibodies (Gross, Hermogenes, Saeks, Lau, & Levandowski, 1995); these changes may affect vaccine efficacy for the infirm elderly.

Patriarca, Weber, Parker, Hall, and Kendal, (1985) reviewed an influenza outbreak in Michigan nursing homes in 1982–1983 and found that unvaccinated residents were more likely to become ill, be hospitalized, or die.

Similarly, Gross et al. (1988) found that influenza vaccination decreased the mortality rate by 59% in a New York nursing home. In another study, Cartter, Rensullo, Helgerson, Marin, and Jekel (1990), in a study of Connecticut nursing homes, found that vaccination did not prevent clinical illness from influenza. Similar findings were reported by Saah et al. (1986) in a study of a New York nursing home. However, the researchers did find that vaccination decreased deaths from pneumonia. The effectiveness of influenza vaccination may be lower in patients with advanced dementia. In a study of 105 patients living in a Dementia Special Care Unit, Brandeis et al. found that vaccination did not prevent the outbreak of clinical influenza nor did vaccination have an effect on mortality that resulted from influenza (unpublished results). Thus, although the current national policy recommends influenza vaccination for this population, its effectiveness may be limited.

The incidence of pneumococcal pneumonia increases with age and is higher in nursing home residents than in community-residing older persons (Bentley, 1996). This type of pneumonia is often associated with bacteremia, and antibiotic treatment is not always effective (Austrian & Gold, 1964). There is a disagreement about the effectiveness of vaccination against pneumococcal infections (Hirschmann & Lipsky, 1994). Randomized prospective studies have failed to show an evidence for decreased frequency of pneumonias or decreased mortality. Some retrospective studies have reported a protective effect, but the effectiveness decreases with age. The protective efficacy when vaccinated within 3 years ranged from 93% in patients under the age of 55 to 46% in patients age 85 and older (Shapiro et al., 1991). Antibody levels also decay faster in older individuals (Riley & Douglas, 1981), thus further decreasing the effectiveness of immunization.

Repeated immunization is not recommended, because adverse reactions correlate with increased antibody levels and additional doses of pneumococcal vaccine provide a poor booster response (Borgano et al., 1978). Vaccine-associated reactions, which occur in about 10% to 15% of elderly vaccinees, include discomfort, erythema, and induration. Less common reactions are fever, headache, myalgias, and chills (Bentley et al., 1981). Vaccination is recommended for all individuals over the age of 65, but only once in a lifetime unless the individual is at a high risk (e.g., as a result of nephrotic syndrome, renal failure, organ transplantation, or immunodefficiency) (Centers for Disease Control, 1989). Since protection may persist at most 6 years and effectiveness decreases with age, pneumococcal vaccination is not able to eliminate pneumococcal pneumonia in elderly demented individuals.

TREATMENT

Because several risk factors for the development of infections discussed earlier are inevitable consequences of dementia progression, an infection can be considered a clinical feature of advanced dementia, and not just an unrelated intercurrent disease. The persistence of risk factors results in the development of many infections, relapse after succesful treatment, and infections that gradually become more and more difficult to treat. Thus the treatment of infections might inflict an increasing degree of burden on the patient without any long-term beneficial effect regarding the course of dementia. The stress of an infection on the already compromised brain may accelerate the progression of dementia. It was recently found that this progression is not slowed down by an aggressive treatment (Hurley, Volicer, & Volicer, 1996). It is, therefore, important to weigh the risks and benefits of different management strategies.

ANTIBIOTICS

An empirical oral administration of antibiotics is commonly used in the treatment of demented individuals presenting with signs and symptoms of an infection (Marrie, 1992). However, it should be recognized that such a treatment may lead to serious side effects, such as allergic reactions, rash, diarrhea, and blood dyscrasias, including agranulocytosis (International Agranulocytosis and Aplastic Anemia Study Group, 1989). At the same time, many fever episodes, which in noncommunicative dementia patients have to be considered as a sign of infection, resolve spontaneously without antibiotic treatment. Even when a complete diagnostic work-up was performed, the source of a fever was not identified in 30% of patients (Fabiszewski et al., 1990). This makes automatic antibiotic administration for all fever episodes questionable.

The effectiveness of antibiotic therapy depends on the severity of the dementia. It was reported that patients with feeding dependence and the need for a mechanically altered diet had significantly higher rates of treatment failure than patients with unimpaired eating abilities when treated for pneumonia in a long-term care setting (Degelau, Gray, Straub, & Luxenberg, 1995). Although the cognitive status of these individuals was not known, feeding dependence and a need for altered diets are inevitable consequences of dementia progression (see chapter 3). When patients on a Dementia Special Care Unit were divided according to dementia severity, patients with high severity of dementia receiving aggressive treatment, which included intravenous antibiotics and respiratory support, did not have a significantly longer survival than the patients who received comfort measures only (see Figure 2.1) (Fabiszewski et al., 1990). This lack of difference in survival of very advanced patients was true when several clinical indicators (speech ability including communication and social contact measures, muscle rigidity and decreased mobility, and feeding dependence) were used to classify patients into high and low severity groups.

Fabiszewski et al. (1990) found that aggressive treatment of fever episodes was successful in preventing death from the infection in all patients with low severity of dementia, whereas patients with low severity who were not treated with antibiotics had a mortality rate similar to patients with high severity of dementia. This "treatment success," however, has to be weighed against the burden imposed by aggressive treatment. Many patients were exposed to the stress of transfer to an unfamiliar acute care setting and to invasive diagnostic procedures, which often included suctioning of the sputum. Twenty percent of fever episodes, which were treated with antibiotics, required repeated intramuscular injections, which are quite painful. Intravenous antibiotic therapy, which was used in 16% of fever episodes, required mechanical or chemical restraints to prevent the patients from removing intravenous tubing. In addition, administration of aminoglycosides and cephalosporins required additional laboratory analyses involving blood drawing and predisposed the patients to renal failure and ototoxicity.

COMFORT MEASURES

The increased burden imposed on the patient by the aggressive treatment of an infection could be justified if it promotes patients' comfort or shortens the duration of the infection. However, in this case study, the duration of fever was similar in patients treated with antibiotics and patients treated with comfort measures only (Fabiszewski et al., 1990). In addition, patients' discomfort, measured by an observational scale (Hurley, Volicer, Hanrahan, Houde, & Volicer, 1992), was similar in patients treated with antibiotics and in patients treated by comfort measures only (see Figure 2.2) (Hurley, Volicer, Mahoney, & Volicer, 1993). In this later study, patients were categorized according to the treatment strategy used to manage the fever episode. During a basal condition, in the absence of a fever, the discomfort levels were similar in both palliative and aggressive care groups on the Dementia Special Care Unit (DSCU), and higher in patients hospitalized on a traditional long-term

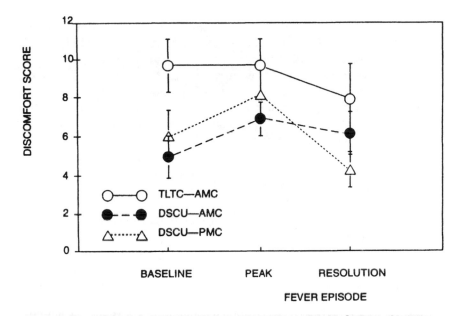

FIGURE 2.2   Discomfort during a fever episode. Peak observations were made 3 to 5 days and resolution observations 8 to 11 days after the onset of a fever episode. TLTC-AMC = traditional long-term care with antibiotics, DSCU-AMC = Dementia Special Care Unit with antibiotics, DSCU-PMC = Dementia Special Care Unit without antibiotics.

From "Palliative Fever Management in Nursing Science," by A. C. Hurley, B. Volicer, and L. Volicer, 1993, *Advances in Nursing Science, 16*, 21–32. Copyright 1993, Aspen Publishers, Inc. Reproduced with permission.

care unit. Discomfort levels increased during the first 3 to 5 days of a fever episode in patients on the DSCU and returned to the basal level during the resolution period (9 to 11 days after the onset of fever). This increase was similar in patients treated with antibiotics and patients treated with comfort measures. There was no evidence that antibiotic treatment would lead to faster resolution of discomfort caused by the fever episode. Thus these data indicate that antibiotic treatment neither extends the survival of patients with severe dementia nor decreases discomfort induced by a fever episode.

Comfort measures useful during a fever episode include antipyretics (mostly acetaminophen), which were used more often on the DSCU than in the traditional setting (Hurley et al., 1993), and analgesics (oral morphine sulphate), which were used more often in patients receiving palliative treatment than in patients treated with antibiotics (Fabiszewski et al., 1990). Morphine has the additional benefit of reducing tachypnea. Low-flow oxygen therapy is also effective in decreasing dyspnea in patients dying with pneumonia. An additional advantage of the palliative treatment is the avoidance of overhydration caused by intravenous therapy, which leads to increased respiratory secretions requiring frequent suctioning. If increased secretions are present, atropine administration is effective in improving patient's comfort. (For a further description of the terminal stage of Alzheimer's disease, see chapter 13.)

CONCLUSIONS

Because there is no agreed-upon standard to guide the treatment of infections in late-stage dementia, clinicians face clinical, ethical, and health policy dilemmas concerning the use of aggressive medical interventions that may or may not extend a patient's life. Attempts to prevent or treat infections are a paradigm for the balance between the burdens and benefits in patients with late-stage dementia. To forgo aggressive interventions that do not ultimately result in improvement of the underlying dementia may be considered ethically justifiable as well as more compassionate than striving to extend survival at all costs. The empirical evidence reported earlier in this chapter revealed that providing palliative care for infections prevents patients from undergoing invasive diagnostic work-ups and treatments, does not accelerate the progression of advanced Alzheimer's disease, is associated with lower observed discomfort, and is not associated with higher rates of mortality for more advanced patients.

Clinicians should consider recommending that the treatment of infections in patients with advanced dementia consist of palliative management. A palliative approach to care for patients with advanced dementia not only benefits patients by decreasing their discomfort but also saves valuable medical care resources (Volicer et al., 1994). It can be further argued from a principled ethical perspective that aggressive care should not even be offered because it is not indicated on the basis of survival time or retarding the progression of dementia and places an extra burden on both the patient and society. "Ordinary" treatments such as vaccines and antibiotics may violate the fundamental principle of "do no harm" at the end of life. Whitehouse, Post, and Sachs (1996) stated that "we must recognize that it is not only immoral to provide ineffective and distressing care, but also a waste of social resources."

REFERENCES

Austrian, R., & Gold, J. (1964). Pneumococcal bacteremia with especial reference to bacteremic pneumococcal pneumonia. *Annals of Internal Medicine, 60,* 759.

Barger, S. W., Hörster, D., Furukawa, K., Goodman, Y., Krieglstein, J., & Mattson, M. P. (1995). Tumor necrosis factors Á and Ã protect neurons against amyloid Ã-peptide toxicity: Evidence for involvement of a kappa-binding factor and attenuation of peroxide and Ca^{2+} accumulation. *Proceedings of the National Academy of Sciences USA, 92,* 9328–9332.

Barker, W. H. (1986). Excess pneumonia and influenza associated hospitalization during influenza epidemics in the United States. *American Journal of Public Health, 76,* 761.

Bentley, D. W. (1984). Bacterial pneumonia in the elderly: Clinical features, diagnosis, etiology, and treatment. *Gerontology, 30,* 297–307.

Bentley, D. W. (1996). Vaccinations. *Clinics in Geriatric Medicine, 8,* 745–760.

Bentley, D. W., Ha, K., Mamot, K., Moon, D., Moore, L., Poletto, P., & Springett, A. (1981). Pneumococcal vaccine in the institutionalized elderly: Design of a nonrandomized trial and preliminary results. *Review of Infectious Diseases, 3* (Suppl.), 571–581.

Ben-Yehuda, A., & Weksler, M. E. (1992). Host resistance and the immune system. *Clinics in Geriatric Medicine, 8,* 701–711.

Bergstrom, N., Allman, R. M., Alvarez, D. M., Bennett, M. A., Carlson, C. E., Frantz, R. A., Garber, S. L., Jackson, B. S., Kaminski, M. V., Jr., Kemp, M. G., Kronskop, T. A., Lewis, V. L., Maklebust, J., Margolis, D. J., Marvel, E. M., Regent, S. I., Rodelaver, G. T., Salcidor, R., Xakellis, G. L., & Yarkory, G. M. (1994). *Treatment of pressure ulcers* (Clinical Practice Guideline No. 15, AHCPR Publication No. 95–0652) Washington, DC: U.S. Department of Health and Human Services.

Borgano, J. M., McLean, A. A., Vella, P. P., Woodhour, A. F., Carepa, I., Davidson, W. L., & Hilleman, M. R. (1978). Vaccination and revaccination with polyvalent pneumococcal polysaccharide vaccines in adults and infants. *Proceedings of the Society for Experimental Biology and Medicine, 157,* 148–154.

Cartter, M. L., Rensullo, P. O., Helgerson, S. D., Marin, S. M., & Jekel, J. F. (1990). Influenza outbreaks in nursing homes: How effective is influenza vaccine in the institutionalized elderly? *Infection Control and Hospital Epidemiology, 11,* 473–478.

Centers for Disease Control. (1989). Pneumococcal polysaccharide vaccine. *Morbidity and Mortality Weekly Report, 38,* 64.

Centers for Disease Control and Prevention. (1995). Prevention and control of influenza: Recommendation of the advisory committee on immunization practices (ACIP). *Morbidity and Mortality Weekly Report, 44,* 1–22.

Chandra, V., Bharucha, N. E., & Schoenberg, B. S. (1986). Conditions associated with Alzheimer's disease at death: Case-control study. *Neurology, 36,* 209–211.

Collins, C., & Ogle, K. (1994). Patterns of predeath service use by dementia patients with a family caregiver. *Journal of the American Geriatrics Society, 42,* 719–722.

Degelau, J., Guay, D., Straub, K., & Luxenberg, M. G. (1995). Effectiveness of oral antibiotic treatment in nursing home–acquired pneumonia. *Journal of the American Geriatrics Society, 43,* 245–251.

Driks, M. R., Craven, D. E., Celli, B. R., Manning, M., Burke, R. A., Garvin, G. M., Kunches, L. M., Farber, H. W., Wedel, S. A., & McCabe, W. R. (1987). Nosocomial pneumonia in intubated patients given sucralfate as compared with antacids or histamine type 2 blockers: The role of gastric colonization. *New England Journal of Medicine, 317,* 1376–1382.

Evans, J. M., Andrews, K. L., Chutka, D. S., Fleming, K. C., & Garness, S. L. (1995). Pressure ulcers: Prevention and management. *Mayo Clinic Proceedings, 70,* 789–799.

Fabiszewski, K. J., Volicer, B., & Volicer, L. (1990). Effect of antibiotic treatment on outcome of fevers in institutionalized Alzheimer patients. *Journal of the American Medical Association, 263,* 3168–3172.

Gabow, P. A., Hutt, D. M., Baker, S., Craig, S. R., Gordon, J. B., & Lezotte, D. C. (1985). Comparison of hospitalization between nursing home and community residents. *Journal of the American Geriatrics Society, 33,* 524–529.

Gross, P. A., Hermogenes, A. W., Sacks, H. S., Lau, J., & Levandowski, R. A. (1995). The efficacy of influenza vaccine in elderly persons: A meta-analysis and review of the literature. *Annals of Internal Medicine, 123,* 518–527.

Gross, P. A., Quinnan, G. V., Rodstein, M., LaMontagne, J. R., Kaslow, R. A., Saah, A. J., Wallenstein, S., Neufeld, R., Denning, C., & Gaerlan, P. (1988). Association of influenza immunization with reduction in mortality in an elderly population. *Archives of Internal Medicine, 148,* 562–565.

Harkness, G. A., Bentley, D. W., & Roghmann, K. J. (1990). Risk factors for nosocomial pneumonia in the elderly. *American Journal of Medicine, 89,* 457–463.

Hirschmann, J. V., & Lipsky, B. A. (1994). The pneumococcal vaccine after 15 years of use. *Archives of Internal Medicine, 154,* 373–377.

Huberman, M., Shalit, F., Roth-Deri, I., Gutman, B., Brodie, C., Kott, E., & Sredni, B. (1994). Correlation of cytokine secretion by mononuclear cells of Alzheimer patients and their disease stage. *Journal of Neuroimmunology, 52,* 147–152.

Hurley, A. C., Volicer, B. J., Hanrahan, P., Houde, S., & Volicer, L. (1992). Assessment of discomfort in advanced Alzheimer patients. *Research in Nursing and Health, 15,* 369–377.

Hurley, A. C., Volicer, B., Mahoney, M. A., & Volicer, L. (1993). Palliative fever management in Alzheimer patients: Quality plus fiscal responsibility. *Advances in Nursing Science, 16,* 21–32.

Hurley, A. C., Volicer, B. J., & Volicer, L. (1996). Effect of fever-management strategy on the progression of dementia of the Alzheimer type. *Alzheimer Disease and Associated Disorders, 10,* 5–10.

Huxley, E. J., Viroslav, J., Gray, W. R., & Pierce, A. K. (1978). Pharyngeal aspiration in normal adults and patients with depressed consciousness. *American Journal of Medicine, 64,* 564–568.

International Agranulocytosis and Aplastic Anemia Study Group. (1989). Anti-infective drug use in relation to the risk of agranulocytosis and aplastic anemia. *Archives of Internal Medicine, 149,* 1036–1040.

Kukull, W. A., Brenner, D. E., Speck, C. E., Nochlin, D., Bowen, J., McCormick, W., Teri, L., Pfanschmidt, M. L., & Larson, E. B. (1994). Causes of death associated with Alzheimer disease: Variation by level of cognitive impairment before death. *Journal of the American Geriatrics Society, 4*(II), 723–726.

Licastro, F., Savorani, G., Sarti, G., Salsi, A., Cavazzuti, F., Zanichelli, L., Tucci, G., Mocchegiani, E., & Fabris, N. (1990). Zinc and thymic hormone-dependent immunity in normal aging and in patients with senile dementia of the Alzheimer type. *Journal of Neuroimmunology, 27,* 201–208.

Lipsky, B. A. (1989). Urinary tract infections in men: Epidemiology, pathophysiology, diagnosis, and treatment. *Annals of Internal Medicine, 110,* 138–150.

Magaziner, J., Tenney, J. H., DeForge, B., Hebel, R., Munice, H. L., & Warren, J. W. (1991). Prevalence and characteristics of nursing home–acquired infections in the aged. *Journal of the American Geriatrics Society, 39,* 1071–1078.

Marrie, T. J. (1992). Pneumonia. *Clinics in Geriatric Medicine, 8,* 721–734.

Marrie, T. J., Durant, H., & Kwan, C. (1986). Nursing home–acquired pneumonia: A case-control study. *Journal of the American Geriatrics Society, 34,* 697–702.

Marrie, T. J., Johnson, S., & Durant, H. (1988). Cell-mediated immunity of healthy adult Nova Scotians in various age groups compared with nursing home and hospitalized senior citizens. *Journal of Allergy and Clinical Immunology, 81,* 836–844.

McCormick, W. C., Kukull, W. A., Van Belle, G., Bowen, J. D., Teri, L., & Larson, E. B. (1994). Symptom patterns and comorbidity in the early stages of Alzheimer's disease. *Journal of the American Geriatrics Society, 42,* 517–521.

Miller, A. E., Neighbour, P. A., Katzman, R., Aronson, M., & Lipkowitz, R. (1981). Immunological studies in senile dementia of the Alzheimer type: Evidence for enhanced suppressor cell activity. *Annals of Neurology, 10,* 506–510.

Molsa, P. K., Marttila, R. J., & Rinne, U. K. (1986). Survival and cause of death in Alzheimer's disease and multi-infarct dementia. *Acta Neurologia Scandinavica, 74,* 103–107.

Nicolle, L. E. (1994). Urinary tract infection. In P. D. O'Donnell (Ed.), *Geriatric urology* (pp. 399–412). Boston: Little, Brown.

Nicolle, L. E., Henderson, E., Bjornson, J., McIntyre, M., Harding, G. K. M., & MacDonell, J. (1987). The association of bacteriuria with resident characteristics and survival in elderly institutionalized men. *Annals of Internal Medicine, 106,* 682–686.

Norman, D. C., & Toledo, S. D. (1992). Infections in elderly persons: An altered clinical presentation. *Clinics in Geriatric Medicine, 8,* 713–719.

Olichney, J. M., Hofstetter, C. R., Galasko, D., Thal, L. J., & Katzman, R. (1995). Death certificate reporting of dementia and mortality in an Alzheimer's disease research center cohort. *Journal of the American Geriatrics Society, 43,* 890–893.

Olive, K. E., & Berk, S. L. (1992). Infections in the nursing home. *Clinics in Geriatric Medicine, 8,* 821–834.

Ouslander, J. G., Greengold, B., & Chen, S. (1987a). External catheter use and urinary tract infections among incontinent male nursing home patients. *Journal of the American Geriatrics Society, 35,* 1063–1070.

Ouslander, J. G., Greengold, B., & Chen, S. (1987b). Complications of chronic indwelling urinary catheters among male nursing home patients: A prospective study. *Journal of Urology, 138,* 1191–1195.

Ouslander, J. G., Schnelle, J. F., Uman, G., Fingold, S., Nigam, J. G., Tuico, E., & Bates-Jensen, B. (1995). Predictors of successful prompted voiding among incontinent nursing home residents. *Journal of the American Medical Association, 273,* 1366–1370.

Parsons, C. L., & Schmidt, J. D. (1982). Control of current lower urinary tract infection in the postmenopausal women. *Journal of Urology, 128,* 1224.

Patriarca, P. A., Weber, J. A., Parker, R. A., Hall, W. N., & Kendal, A. P. (1985). Efficacy of influenza vaccine in nursing homes. *Journal of the American Medical Association, 253,* 1136–1139.

Perls, T. T., & Herget, M. (1995). Higher respiratory infection rates on an Alzheimer's special care unit and successful intervention. *Journal of the American Geriatrics Society, 43,* 1341–1344.

Resnick, N. M., Subbarao, V. Y., & Laurino, E. (1989). The pathophysiology of urinary incontinence among institutionalized elderly persons. *New England Journal of Medicine, 320,* 1–7.

Riley, I. D., & Douglas, R. M. (1981). An epidemiologic approach to pneumococcal disease. *Review of Infectious Diseases, 3,* 233.

Saah, A. J., Neufeld, R., Rodstein, M., LaMontagne, J. R., Blackwelder, W. C., Gross, P., Quinnan, G., & Kaslow, R. A. (1986). Influenza vaccine and pneumonia mortality in a nursing home population. *Archives of Internal Medicine, 146,* 2353–2357.

Sahn, S. A. (1991). Continuous lateral rotational therapy and nosocomial pneumonia. *Chest, 99,* 1263–1267.

Schnelle, J. F., McNees, P., Crooks, V., & Ouslander, J. G. (1995). The use of a computer-based model to implement an incontinence management program. *Gerontologist, 35,* 656–665.

Shapiro, E. D., Berg, A. T., Austrian, R., Schroeder, D., Parcells, V., Margolis, A., Adair, R. K., & Clemens, J. D. (1991). The protective efficacy of polyvalent pneumococcal polysaccharide vaccine. *New England Journal of Medicine, 325,* 1453–1460.

Skias, D., Bania, M., Reder, A. T., Luchins, D., & Antel, J. P. (1985). Senile dementia of Alzheimer's type (SDAT): Reduced T8+-cell-mediated suppressor activity. *Neurology, 35,* 1635–1638.

Sulkava, R., Haltia, M., Paetau, A., Wikstrom, J., & Palo, J. (1983). Accuracy of clinical diagnosis in primary degenerative dementia: correlation with neuropathological findings. *Journal of Neurology and Neurosurgical Psychiatry, 46,* 9–13.

Urinary Incontinence in Adults Guideline Update Panel. (1996). *Urinary incontinence in adults: Acute and chronic management* (AHCPR Publication No. 96-0682). Rockville, MD: U.S. Department of Health and Human Services.

Volicer, B. J., Hurley, A., Fabiszewski, K. J., Montgomery, P., & Volicer, L. (1993). Predicting short-term survival for patients with advanced Alzheimer's disease. *Journal of the American Geriatrics Society, 41,* 535–540.

Volicer, L., Collard, A., Hurley, A., Bishop, C., Kern, D., & Karon, S. (1994). Impact of special care unit for patients with advanced Alzheimer's disease on patients' discomfort and costs. *Journal of the American Geriatrics Society, 42,* 597–603.

Wayne, S. J., Rhyne, R. L., Garry, P. J., & Goodwin, J. S. (1990). Cell-mediated immunity as a predictor of morbidity and mortality in subjects over 60. *Journal of Gerontology: Medical Sciences, 45,* M45–M48.

White, D. O., & Fenner, F. J. (1994). Orthomyxoviridae. In *Medical Virology* (4th ed., pp. 489–499). New York: Academic Press.

Whitehouse, P. J., Post, S. G., & Sachs, G. A. (1996). Dementia care at the end of life: Empirical research and international collaboration. *Alzheimer Disease and Associated Disorders, 10,* 3–4.

Overcoming Eating Difficulties in the Severely Demented

Giovanni B. Frissoni, Simone Franzoni,
Giuseppe Bellelli, Judith Morris,
and Victoria Warden

Throughout the course of all dementing disorders, patients are at risk for developing nutritional problems (Trabucchi, 1992). In the early stage of Alzheimer's disease, memory impairment, poor judgment, and apraxia predispose patients to eating difficulties. In the late stages of the disease, behavioral and neuromuscular conditions may cause eating difficulties.

Despite the eating difficulties caused by dementia, dementia in the elderly is not necessarily associated with malnutrition and decreased life expectancy. In fact, a study carried out in an institution where staff provided intensive feeding assistance found that demented patients (mean age of 85 years) had similar nutritional status and mortality rates as did the nondemented patients of the same age and somatic health, except for smaller triceps skinfold thickness in the demented (Franzoni, Frisoni, Boffelli, Rozzini, & Trabucchi, 1996). The cumulative annual death rate in the demented (0.23 death/year) was similar to the nondemented (0.22 death/year). Unadjusted survival by Kaplan-Meyer analysis was similar in the two groups, and this similarity was retained when adjusted for age, gender, cognition, triceps skinfold thickness, and number of drugs in a Cox regression model. These data suggest that malnutrition is not an unavoidable correlate of dementia. The clinically relevant conclusion is that dementia in very old age does not necessarily decrease survival, and that when appropriate dietary intake with feeding assistance is provided to the demented, malnutrition need not develop (Franzoni et al., 1996; Morley, 1996).

Previously, Volicer et al. (1989) had found that the mortality rate of patients with moderate and severe Alzheimer's disease was similar in patients who experienced eating difficulties and in patients who could be fed without problems. They reported that weight loss by itself did not increase mortality, which was similar in patients with body weights below and above 80% of ideal body weight. The study by Volicer et al. was also conducted at an institution where staff provided intensive feeding assistance and used nutrient-dense diets (Warden, 1989).

Patients with advanced Alzheimer's disease must have their special needs met to avoid malnutrition. In this chapter, we will explain the pathogenesis of the most common feeding and nutritional problems encountered in the care of the severely demented and suggest treatment strategies to manage these problems.

UNIQUE PROBLEMS PRESENTED BY DEMENTIA

COGNITIVE IMPAIRMENT

Cognitive impairments that result from the progression of Alzheimer's disease are manifested by multiple symptoms that in combination make patients dependent on others for their basic needs. Specific threats to maintaining eating independence are agnosia, apraxia, and aphasia. However, patients may develop more functional dependence than can be explained by the disease. Therefore, caregivers need to assess patients' abilities and develop individualized treatment plans, recognizing the need to provide help for patients who are experiencing problems that interfere with their ability to eat independently.

Preventing Excess Dependence

Apraxia prevents demented patients from recognizing and properly using utensils, so that patients are at risk of losing their independence in eating. A few simple strategies can be used to maintain independence at mealtime. Proper utensils and finger foods can maintain self-feeding for as long as possible for individual patients. A deep dish (plate with a raised rim) and the use of spoons help to keep the food more manageable. It is best to use one large spoon because it is the least likely to cause injury during feeding, can be easily manipulated by patients, and provides more ease of feeding when caregivers offer some assistance. At certain stages of the disease, straws can be helpful for drinking liquids. Small cups (6–8 oz size) are easier to use than a cup with a handle, and paper cups that can mold to form a spout are helpful when caregivers are assisting. Finger foods, such as soft sandwiches cut in quarters, french fries, and meat nuggets, should be used when the manipulation of eating utensils becomes increasingly difficult due to apraxia. Nonfood items such as paper napkins should be removed from the table to eliminate the risk of patients ingesting them. Assistance to promote self-feeding should be provided, such as opening milk cartons. One course should be presented at a time, and the quantity of food placed in front of each patient should be limited. Some patients may be distracted during mealtime and need constant cueing (e.g., "bite," "drink"). Other patients may need coaxing and reassurance throughout the mealtime.

Impact of Setting

Some studies have found that an unpleasant meal environment was an important negative factor in nutrition in the institutional setting (Steen, 1992). In one study, the dining room of a nursing home was changed from a very sterile environment to one typical of the 1940s when these patients had their most active period (Elmsthäl, Blabolil, Fex, Küller, & Steen, 1987). Dietary intake of carbohydrates and proteins increased by 25%, and physical activity, conversation, facial expression, and social interest also improved. Although not all subjects in the Elmsthäl et al. study were demented, it can be hypothesized that the overlearned recollections thus aroused might be generalizable to stimulate eating behaviors in demented individuals.

In some settings an insufficient number of staff might be responsible for some of the malnutrition observed in the demented and for some cases of food refusal. Morley (1995) underscored the fact that a lack of time spent feeding institutionalized demented patients may increase the potential risk of anorexia and malnutrition. In one study 18 minutes per day were spent feeding demented patients in a nursing home compared to 99 minutes per day when these patients were kept at home (Hu, Huang, & Cartwright, 1986). A recent observation suggested that institutionalized demented patients can have food intake similar to that of their nondemented peers in a specific setting that allows for an appropriate patient/caregiver ratio (Franzoni et al., 1996; Morley, 1996).

Eaton, Mitchell-Bonair, and Friedmann (1986) investigated touch as a therapeutic tool and a method for improving nutritional intake of elderly demented patients. Tactile sensation is often retained in the late stages of dementia, when other senses are impaired.

BEHAVIORAL DISTURBANCES

Behavioral disturbances, alone or in combination with neuromuscular impairment of the swallowing muscles and somatic diseases, are frequently associated with the development of severe eating difficulties in the demented.

Wandering

Wandering is a prevalent disturbance in the demented, occurring in as much as 25% of nursing home residents (Teri et al., 1992). Wandering is frequently associated with increased psychomotor activity. The two symptoms have a double effect on nutritional status, on the one hand by increasing energy expenditures and on the other by interfering with feeding. Patients who wander cannot sit for longer than a few minutes, continuously try to stand and stop eating, and require significant effort by the caregiver and nursing home staff to make them continue eating. Sometimes patients who wander around the tables at the beginning of the meal eat from the trays of others patients and then refuse to eat their own food. Patients who pace constantly are exhausted at mealtime and thus may have a poor appetite. Because of the calories expended pacing for several miles a day, high-calorie foods and nutritional supplements should be provided (Rheaume, Riley, & Volicer, 1987). Providing rest periods during the day helps to conserve calories, and arranging these patients in lounge chairs with tray tables enables them to sit for the duration of their meal.

Agitation

Agitation is an unpleasant state of excitement often precipitated by external stimuli. Meals can be associated with increased agitation because three senses are stimulated simultaneously: visual, acoustic (staff activity, setting tables, moving chairs, distributing trays), and olfactory (food smells). Therefore, noises from dishes and glasses and staff voices should be kept to the lowest possible level. Environmental stimuli that may increase confusion, such as fast movements, too many plates on the table, too many foods on a tray, and overcrowding of the room, should be reduced.

Manifestations of agitation during mealtimes vary. Patients who have hallucinations or delusions may fear that caregivers or neighbors will take food from their dishes, misunderstand the actions of others, and quarrel with them. Agitation can increase when the customary table seat of one patient in the dining room is occupied by another one. Patients known to become agitated at mealtimes should be provided a clear separation of their table space. As a rule, seats should be permanently reserved for each patient. Some patients can become agitated if there is an excessive delay between courses; others may become agitated when staff members try to help them. Self-feeding may be more efficient if nutrient-dense finger foods are available.

Environmental interventions should be examined for possibly reducing agitation during meals. For instance, since increased agitation in the late afternoon or evening, so-called sundown syndrome, might be due to reduced illumination (Little, Satlin, Sunderland, & Volicer, 1994), it may be appropriate to provide all dining rooms with daylight-level artificial illumination for all meals.

Patients with dementia might have sight alterations and difficulties in perceiving the contrast of colors and shades. A relaxing but contrasting color of the tablecloths, dishes, and glasses may help patients to recognize eating tools.

Relaxing music has been found to buffer the general noise level typical of nursing home dining rooms and to exert a calming effect, thus reducing agitated behavior in these patients (Goddaer & Abraham, 1994). Appropriate music may be helpful to remind patients about the timing of meals.

Food Refusal

Food refusal is a highly prevalent disturbance in institutionalized patients. A study of eating difficulties observed among 73 male patients receiving long-term care for dementia found that 36 subjects refused food, while 23 had at least one occurrence of choking during mealtime (Volicer et al., 1989). Of those who refused feeding, 89% turned their head away when fed, 78% kept their mouth shut, 72% pushed the spoon or hand away, and 39% spat food. Patients may also cover their mouth or let food run out of their mouth.

Patients need to be carefully assessed to identify possible causes for food refusal. Some causes may be ameliorable to treatment. When patients refuse to eat, depression or a decision to "give up" and die should be considered in the pathogenesis of the eating disturbance. Volicer, Rheaume, and Cyr (1994) found that treatment with sertraline improved affect in 8 out of 10 severely demented patients who were identified by the staff as being clinically depressed, and diminished food refusal in 5 of 6 patients who also refused food. Serotonin may play a role in the sense of hunger (Miller, Darby, Swartz, Yener, & Mena, 1994), and the first three authors of this chapter have observed that hunger stimulants such as cyproheptadine sometimes increase appetite in the demented individuals. Food refusal can follow dysphagic episodes due to excessive quickness in feeding patients, somatic diseases, pain, and taste alterations (see the discussion that follows).

In addition to alleviating problems and removing the negative conditions that may have caused food refusal, staff members can take some positive steps to increase food intake. First, it is important to identify which foods patients like. In the later stages of the disease, patients tend to develop a "sweet tooth." If ice cream is a favorite, the staff should offer it at each meal. Alternating a spoonful of the preferred food (ice cream, puddings, or pureed fruit) with a spoonful of the main meal may increase overall intake. A large spoonful of the main meal with a little ice cream on the tip of the spoon may also encourage eating. If either clenching teeth or refusal to open the mouth is a problem, the pureed food may be thinned into a liquid soup that the patient can drink. Lip pursing is another hindrance to feeding. Putting small amounts of food on the lips can encourage opening of the mouth to facilitate giving a spoonful of food. The caregiver can also anticipate opening of the mouth after the patient swallows and give another spoonful. Lifting the lip gently may also cue mouth opening.

The fourth and fifth authors of this chapter were members of an interdisciplinary team that wrote the script and developed a videotape to illustrate these procedures. This training tape, *Natural Feeding for Patients with Alzheimer's Disease,* is available in all VA Medical Center libraries as well as by interlibrary loan or purchase from the National Technical Information Service.

POUCHING AND DYSPHAGIA

It is a common clinical observation that some patients linger on chewing food for an excessively long time (pouching) or take food in their mouth but swallow only on command (Volicer et al., 1989). The pathogenesis of this behavior is unknown, but it seems to occur in the stage that precedes dysphagia, which is due to neuromuscular problems of the pharyngeal musculature. Therefore, pouching might be interpreted as an early sign of dysphagia. This is supported by the observation that small amounts of soft-textured foods, which can be more easily propelled by the pharyngeal muscles, can reduce pouching (Groher & McKaig, 1995).

Regardless of whether or not pouching occurred, dysphagia commonly develops in the late stages of dementia. The term *dysphagia* literally indicates subjective difficulty during swallowing. Dysphagia in the person with dementia who cannot report such difficulty is assessed by staff members who observe elaborate, labored, and difficult swallowing that may be accompanied by choking. Epidemiological studies of dysphagia in the demented are scanty. In a cross-sectional study of 73 male patients who were receiving long-term care for dementia, 23 had choking episodes (Volicer et al. 1989); all choked on liquids and nearly all (96%) on solids.

Although dysphagia is considered a risk factor for the development of aspiration pneumonia, Volicer et al. (1989) found that the mortality rate was similar in patients who choked on food and liquids and in those who were able to be fed without choking. Dysphagia is believed to exist in patients with Alzheimer's disease as a result of degenerative changes in the corticobulbar tracts and cranial nerve nuclei (Volicer et al., 1989).

Acute Dysphagia

Dysphagia can appear suddenly, in a matter of hours or days. In this case, the suspicion should always be raised that somatic causes (e.g., pneumonia and urinary tract infections), even if not readily apparent, may be responsible. Reversibility of acute dysphagia must always be considered possible. In these cases, temporary placement of a nasogastric tube and enteral feeding might be considered, but after the acute event is over, a return to oral feeding should always be tried (Volicer, Rheaume, Riley, Karner, & Glennon, 1990).

Chronic Dysphagia

Although somatic causes should always be considered, when dysphagia develops progressively over weeks or months, the cause is usually the relentless progression of the brain disease. The development and progression of chronic dysphagia often follows a similar course across patients, suggesting that the brain lesions leading to the neuromuscular impairment occur in relatively fixed sites and with relatively fixed timing. Dysphagia for liquids appears first. In the early stages of dysphagia for liquids, small amounts of liquids can still be swallowed in elaborate and repetitive sips. In this stage, drinking with a straw in small sips with the head slightly flexed is still possible, although movements of the glottis can be markedly reduced. Small amounts of liquids may also be able to pass into the esophagus by the effect of gravity, and without inducing a complete swallowing reflex. To avoid choking on thin liquids, substitutions of semisolid foods such as yogurt, pudding, applesauce, and ice cream that have a high water content but do not induce choking should be used. Thin liquids may be thickened by mixing them with semisolid foods or by using a commercially available thickening product.

In the late stage of the disease, patients may pouch solid food but may be able to swallow smaller amounts of foods with softer textures (pureed or mashed). In this phase, dysphagia for solid foods (meat, pasta, or bread) typically develops. Patients may also develop dysphagia for pureed and mashed foods. Some patients may even hold the pureed food in their mouths, neither chewing nor swallowing, possibly not recognizing the substance as food. Thinning the food with milk or a nutritional supplement often encourages eating and swallowing.

Our clinical observation indicates that in the late stages of dysphagia some patients may have greater difficulty swallowing pureed than mashed foods, suggesting that a more consistent texture of the bolus might help in its passage through the pharynx. Groher and McKaig (1995) reported that many patients who were receiving pureed food could be advanced to a mechanical soft diet, and that even some patients who previously were tube fed could receive a mechanical soft diet. Matthews (1988) suggested that foods that form a bolus in the mouth and do not break apart might be appropriate for some patients. Thick, even gelatinous foods might be sometimes advisable.

Foods with appropriate consistency and smell–taste properties that can induce salivation should be preferred. The sitting position in the chair or bed allows for the assistance of gravity and good alignment of the alimentary canal to facilitate swallowing. When feeding those at risk for choking, the head of the bed should be elevated at least 45°. The patient's head should be slightly forward, supported if needed by pillows. Patients should be fed slowly and the swallowing of each mouthful or sip of liquid should be assessed before offering another. Some patients can hold a great deal of food in their mouths or in the backs of their throats, causing choking. Others may need to swallow several times before all food is gone from their mouths. Cueing is most often necessary to remind patients to chew and/or swallow. Touching or gently stroking the throat may help initiate swallowing. To improve the patient's focus for eating, the caregiver should try to maintain eye contact, preferably by standing or sitting in front of the patient. A patient's facial expressions should be observed for signs of distress. Feeding should be discontinued if distress is present and resumed when the patient appears comfortable. Food and fluids that are too hot or too cold may precipitate choking in some patients. If dry mouth is a problem, the mouth should be moistened with some fluids or mouth care given before feeding. In all cases, however, the choice of the appropriate texture of food should be tailored to the individual patient and continuously evaluated and modified over the disease course as necessary.

SOMATIC DISEASES

In addition to episodic dysphagia caused by acute somatic diseases and head trauma, a number of diseases affecting the mouth and gastrointestinal tract can also cause food refusal and swallowing difficulty. Candidiasis of the mouth can cause pain on chewing, swallowing difficulty, and food refusal. Dentition is another problem. Often, patients with eating problems had lost or broken teeth. Morales, Gonzales, and Santolaria (1989) found that demented patients with a loss of more than 50% of their teeth have less muscular and fatty areas of the arm as well as a greater degree of temporal muscle atrophy . Although a diet that provides adequate energy and nutrients can be furnished with pureed or mechanically altered food, it may be that the ability to chew food increases patients' willingness to eat. Although this hypothesis is untested, it might be advisable to allow patients with denture devices to use them, at least as long as they are able to keep their dentures safely in their mouths.

Decayed dental roots, ulcers, or gum diseases may cause food refusal. The repetitive movements of the jaws that are sometimes present in the demented can lead to ulcers of the lips and in the anterior part of the jaws if decayed teeth or roots are present. Removal of diseased or broken teeth can promote healing of the ulcer and decrease food refusal. Pain may also be causing food refusal. Pressure sores can generate pain when the patient is in a sitting position, causing the patient to be less prone to consume food while sitting. Appropriately shaped cushions to alleviate pressure can be useful in this case. Acute fecal impaction and urinary retention can also precipitate food refusal.

Alterations in Taste and Smell

It is a relatively frequent observation that many severely demented patients refuse some foods but not others. The changes of gustatory function in dementia are not clear (Huff et al., 1987; Schiffman, Clark, & Warwick, 1990). In contrast, it is generally accepted that central and peripheral components of the olfactory function are impaired in different stages of the disease. The recognition of smell stimuli (for which integrity of central nervous olfactory structures is needed) is impaired early in the disease course when smell detection threshold (for which integrity of peripheral nervous olfactory structures is needed) is normal. Smell detection is impaired only in the later stages, indicating an increased threshold (Koss, Weiffenbach, Haxby, & Frieland, 1988).

These observations fit the clinical observation that severely demented patients who refuse many foods will sometimes accept particular foods. The relevance of food palatability was demonstrated by Eaton et al. (1986), who found that specific menu items were consumed more completely by demented than by nondemented elders. This suggests that palatability of foods can positively affect nutritional intake.

Iatrogenesis

Many drugs may cause eating difficulties in the demented elderly (Cusack, 1995). Drugs that are most commonly involved are those that affect cognitive/behavioral functioning (anticholinergics and sedatives), salivation (anticholinergics), and motor speed (sedatives and neuroleptics). Restlessness, depression, confusion, constipation, and extrapyramidal side effects can cause problems in bringing food to the mouth, chewing, or swallowing. In addition, other drugs such as diuretics, beta-blockers, digoxin, and antihyperlipidemics can cause anorexia (Morley, 1995). Drugs that have a noxious action on the gastric mucosa (i.e., aspirin and no-steroidal anti-inflammatory agents) may also cause anorexia.

Demented patients often receive neuroleptics, which can increase eating difficulties by their anticholinergic effects and by the relaxation of muscles involved in the swallowing process. A prolonged use of high doses of these drugs may lead to a severe condition of malnutrition. Rohrbaugh and Siegal (1989) described a case of reversible weight loss associated with neuroleptic use in a patient with advanced dementia of the Alzheimer type. Neuroleptic-induced tardive dyskinesia (tongue thrusting) can interfere with feeding. In these patients, placing the spoon carefully and using adaptive spoons and long spout cups can be helpful.

NUTRITIONAL SUPPORT

Consensus is emerging that nutritional support, including enteral feeding, is a form of medical treatment. This is an important shift from the previous view that nutritional support is a mandatory humane act (Peck,

Cohen, & Mulvihill, 1990; Zanetti et al., 1996). Therefore, guidelines for nutritional support should consider both medical and ethical issues. It should be recognized that food and liquid refusal is common in patients dying of a terminal illness. McCann, Hall, and Groth-Juncker (1994) have reported lack of hunger or thirst in cognitively intact patients receiving narcotics.

Caloric needs of the person with Alzheimer's disease change as symptoms and manifestations of the disease change. Pacing, previous weight loss, and infection can all increase caloric needs. Pacing may increase caloric requirements by as much as 1,600 calories per day above maintenance levels (Rheaume et al., 1987). At the other end of the spectrum, the bedfast patient seems to require fewer calories over the years to maintain weight, and careful monitoring is necessary to prevent inappropriate weight gain. A decrease in muscle mass may also contribute to a decline in caloric needs. The clinical experience of the last two authors of this chapter indicates that the dementia patient may have lower ideal body weight (IBW) requirements than most rule-of-thumb guidelines suggest. Of significant importance for bedfast patients is the need to preserve sufficient subcutaneous tissue to afford protection against skin breakdown and pressure sores as well as maintain adequate nutritional intake to preserve protein stores and provide nutrients. In addition, it has been shown that institutionalized patients with lower food intake have poorer long-term prognosis even after all the known predictors of mortality have been accounted for (Frisoni et al., 1995). Some composite indices, combining both biochemical and anthropometric measures, have been proposed to detect malnutrition (Bianchetti, Rozzini, Carabellese, Zanetti, & Trabucchi, 1990; Buzby, Mullen, Matthews, Hobbs, & Rosato, 1980; Frisoni et al., 1994).

The type of diet can affect constipation, and the prevalence of constipation increases with age. Cognitive impairment interferes with the ability to recognize, acknowledge, and communicate the urge to defecate. Variable intake of nutrition and hydration and decreased physical mobility, associated with the later stages of dementia, increase the risk for constipation. Prevention of constipation is the best course, but when it does occur, attempts should be made to recognize and alleviate its underlying cause to prevent impaction. Treatments may include providing more fluids, ensuring adequate dietary fiber, and administering stool softeners. The initial intervention should include natural methods of bowel stimulation using food. Prune juice and bran cereal each provide additional fiber and may suffice. However, the ability to increase dietary fiber is limited with dementia patients due to chewing difficulties as well as the potential for choking. The use of a commercially available product such as prune pudding may be appropriate for patients who have a wide range of texture tolerance. One such product contains fruit puree (plum and apple), dextrose and pectin. The caloric value of 1 tbsp is 35 calories, so that a 1/2 cup serving equals 280 calories. This product is a good consistency for most patients, even those who may no longer tolerate pureed foods, and if taken daily, the product contributes to bowel regularity.

DIET MODIFICATIONS

Food volume distribution is a consideration when planning meals. Alzheimer patients are often more alert and cooperative in the morning and tend to decline as the day progresses. Patients tolerate a higher level of texture as well as an increased volume of food during the first two meals of the day. Individualization of the diet to accommodate these variations is another important factor contributing to optimal nutritional intake. Attention to volume adjustment of the meal is also important. Calorically dense foods with minimal volume decrease feeding time required to consume adequate nutrients. For example, a breakfast of a regular-texture diet consisting of fried eggs, sausage, and toast may be appropriate for the same person who may only be able to tolerate a pureed diet consistency by the evening meal. High-density foods are easily incorporated into the pureed diet. For example, the addition of thickeners such as margarine, cheese, instant mashed potatoes, and nonfat dry milk will enhance the caloric value as well as improve the consistency without increasing the volume significantly. Once again, this type of individualization enhances the ability to maintain natural feeding techniques for a prolonged period. Adjusting the texture of the diet is central to maintaining adequate nutritional intake throughout all the stages of Alzheimer's disease.

Mastication apraxia (chewing impairment) is one of most common of the eating difficulties and occurs fairly early in the progression of the disease. Poor-fitting dentures or lack of dentition may be a contributor but rarely is the only cause of the decline in the chewing process. At this point, chopped or ground foods are usually necessary, and a combination of ground meats augmented by finger foods may be appropriate.

Other behaviors that necessitate texture adjustment are pocketing and pouching of food. In these behaviors the patient holds food in his or her mouth for a long period without swallowing or continues to chew incessantly without swallowing. At this point the texture of the diet needs to be downgraded. A regular diet texture may need to be reduced to a mechanical, or a mechanical may need to be reduced to a pureed. It is not always necessary to automatically downgrade the texture to pureed or liquids; a slow progression is always preferred. The length of time that the patient can be maintained on any texture level varies depending on the individual. Texture adjustments incorporate nutrient density and volume of food as well as ease of consumption to minimize the need for oral manipulation of the food.

An Adult puree diet or Special Adult puree diet (SAP) (see Table 3.1) meets the needs of a chair-to-bed patient. It is a high-density, low-volume diet of 1,700 calories. The largest amount of food should be offered during the day and lesser amounts in the evening when the patients are more tired and weaker. These diets are well tolerated by patients, have been successful in maintaining patient weight, take less staff time for feeding, and are cost effective (Warden, 1989).

When patients are at danger of choking on food or liquids, a diet adjustment is necessary. The elimination of certain foods that have been associated with episodes of choking is one method of intervention. The Bedford (MA) VA Medical Center has developed an Alzheimer Mechanical Diet (see Table 3.2) that eliminates food items that require more than minimal oral manipulation or could easily be stuffed into the mouth and

TABLE 3.1   Adult Pureed Special Diet

Purpose: This diet is designed for difficult-to-feed patients with end-stage Alzheimer's disease.

Diet principles: The low-volume, nutrient-dense diet is designed to facilitate feeding. Meals are planned to accommodate a decreased attention span, especially at the evening meal. The diet can be individualized according to a patient's tolerance.

Approximate composition:

Kilocalories:	1,850
Protein:	70 g
Carbohydrate:	260 g
Fat:	65 g
Sodium:	93.3 mEq (2,148 mg)
Potassium:	80.7 mEq (3,155 mg)

Suggested meal pattern:

Breakfast	Noon	Evening
8 oz Ensure Plus	8 oz pureed meat	Ensure Plus
2x hot cereal	Pureed potato/starch	Pudding
2x margarine	Gravy or sauce	Pureed fruit
2x sugar	Pureed vegetable	
Juice	Pureed dessert	
Milk	Milk	

TABLE 3.2   Alzheimer Mechanical Diet

Purpose: This diet is designed for Alzheimer patients with chewing difficulties.

Diet principles: The diet follows the regular menu with alterations in consistency. Certain food items that have been shown to be a choking risk for Alzheimer patients are restricted. This diet can be individualized according to each patient's tolerance.

Approximate composition:

Kilocalories:	2,400
Protein:	100 g
Carbohydrate:	315 g
Fat:	80 g
Sodium	214 mEq (5,540 mg)
Potassium	101 mEq (3,935 mg)

Suggested meal pattern:

Breakfast	Noon	Evening
4 oz juice	4 oz juice/salad	4 oz juice/salad
6 oz hot cereal	2 oz ground meat/sub	3 oz ground meat/sub
1 scrambled egg	Potato/sub	Potato/sub
2 slices buttered toast	Vegetable	Vegetable
2 sugar packets	Dessert/fruit	Dessert/fruit
8 oz milk	8 oz milk	8 oz milk

Restricted Items:

Beverages: No alcohol, no coffee or tea unless specifically requested.

Bread: No plain bagged bread, muffins, biscuits, rolls, danish, donuts, crackers, hard crusts, dates, nuts, popcorn, French toast, pancakes. (May have toast for breakfast. For entrees served on toast, substitute with bread.)

Cereals: Same as regular mechanical diet.

Desserts: No donuts, cookies, or brownies. No desserts with nuts, dates, or raisins.

Fats: No peanut butter, bacon, nuts, or olives.

Fruits and fruit juices: Same as regular mechanical diet, except no grapes.

Cheese: None.

Eggs: None.

Fish: No fried fish or fish with bones.

Meat entrees: Same as regular mechanical diet, except no meatballs.

Poultry: Same as regular mechanical diet, except no chicken with bones.

Milk products: None.

Potatoes: No crispy fried potatoes, potato chips, whole boiled potatoes, corn chips, spaghetti.

Soups: None.

Sweets: No individual candy, candy with nuts (sugar packet at breakfast only).

Vegetables and vegetable juices: Same as regular mechanical diet, except no whole kernel corn.

Miscellaneous: Same as regular mechanical diet, except no condiments or olives.

precipitate choking. Individualization is very important, however, as texture tolerance may vary considerably from meal to meal and person to person.

NUTRITIONAL SUPPLEMENTS

The role of nutritional supplements for Alzheimer patients is extremely important. The term *supplement* refers to enhancements of the basic diet. They can be available in a variety of mediums, but the common characteristics are that supplements add calories and nutrients in an easily accessible manner. A sandwich supplement can offer an alternative when the main entree is poorly accepted or can provide extra calories in addition to the main entree. A moist sandwich such as peanut butter and jelly or other popular sandwich selections of tuna, egg, and chicken salad, as long as any celery added is finely chopped, are preferred by patients. Puddings and milk shakes are also appropriate and provide the sweetness that patients often prefer.

Commercial supplements are well tolerated and offer a variety of enhancements to the diet. For example, Ensure®, Ensure Plus®, and 2 Cal® are products that are utilized for almost every patient at the Dementia Special Care Unit at the Bedford (MA) VA Medical Center at one time or another. These supplements provide a sweet, slightly thickened, nutrient-dense palatable beverage. They provide extra calories, replace a poorly accepted meal, and are well tolerated when eating difficulties are evident. During periods of decline or even illness the use of commercial supplements is crucial for weight maintenance. Often liquids are better tolerated than solids at various periods throughout the disease progression. The choice of product depends on the degree of weight loss or food refusal. Each product varies in level of caloric and nutrient density, typically ranging from 1 calorie to 2 calories per cc. As the appetite wanes, more concentrated products are appropriate. Appetite and food refusal are never a constant. Thus a patient's weight must be monitored at least monthly to be able to track the appropriateness of the supplement being provided.

As the patient's swallowing impairment progresses, the texture of the diet will need periodic adjustment. Often food items need to be thickened or even thinned depending on the individual. The commercial supplements can be used to accomplish this by mixing them with pureed potatoes, vegetables, meat, or milk. Fruit-flavored yogurt is excellent as a thickener. It can be mixed with a variety foods, including the commercial supplements. Many later-stage Alzheimer patients are maintained on a mixture of Ensure Plus, yogurt, juice, and ice cream administered in a paper cup. Other products used for thickeners are applesauce, cornstarch, gelatin, and commercial products such as Thicket-it and Sysco Classic thickening agent. Often components of the pureed diet are thickened by the addition of instant mashed potatoes, cheese, or cornstarch to produce a firmer consistency. Offering juices mixed with applesauce or commercial thickeners may be necessary to provide additional fluids. Cranberry juice is popular and has the additional benefit of providing acid ash, which helps to prevent urinary tract infections. Commercially thickened juices are available in syrup and honey consistencies. The powdered thickeners can be added to items to individualize the consistency.

TUBE FEEDING

Tube feedings are similar to other medical treatments in that a benefit/burden analysis should be made. The ethical principles that guide the decision-making process are beneficence and the need for respect for patient autonomy (see chapters 6 and 7). Demented patients can perceive discomfort and can potentially be burdened by tube feedings. Patients can feel the tube and may try to pull it out, necessitating keeping their hands physically restrained (Meyers & Grodin, 1991). The use of restraints may increase the risk of pressure sores and pneumonia. If the decision is made to place a gastrostomy tube, endoscopic or surgical placement is required with their attendant risks. These risks include operative hemorrhage, peritoneal leakage of tube feedings and gastric contents with resultant peritonitis, wound infection, and leakage of gastric contents around the stoma (Meyers & Grodin, 1991). However, temporary tube feeding may be beneficial in patients developing dysphagia during an acute illness.

Even the percutaneous enteral gastrostomy (PEG) has a number of potentially adverse effects. Ciocon, Silverstone, Graver, & Foley (1988) reported the occurrence of local wound infections, peritonitis, painful insertion sites, wound dehiscence, hemorrhage, prolonged ileus, pyloric obstruction, and gastric prolapse. The patient incurs the danger of anesthesia, as well as the risk of diarrhea and associated dehydration. Moreover, hospitalization for either gastrostomy or jejunostomy is a stressful experience for demented aged patients and increases the need for skilled nursing services (Peck et al., 1990).

Furthermore, there is debate in the literature as to whether tube feeding can maintain skin integrity by enhanced protein intake (Campbell-Taylor & Fisher, 1987; Lo & Dornbrand, 1984). Peck et al. (1990) compared

71 tube-fed patients with 56 demented patients fed naturally and found that 21% of the patients with feeding tubes developed decubiti versus 14% of patients who were fed by natural means. Also questioned is the capability of gastrostomy and jejunostomy to avoid aspiration. The Campbell-Taylor and Fisher (1987) and Peck et al. (1990) groups both found that aspiration pneumonia occurred more frequently in the tube-fed group, and that the frequency of pneumonia was no different with respect to tube (nasogastric or gastrostomy).

Peck et al. (1990) claimed that patients who spend all or most of their time in a recumbent position have a higher probability of aspiration pneumonia if tube-fed than if carefully spoon-fed. However, the data that support that claim included dissimilar lengths of institutionalization in the two groups in which the length of stay of tube-fed patients was twice that of patients who were spoon-fed, which raises the possibility that dementia severity might be an important confounding factor. Temporary tube feeding may be considered when dysphagia develops acutely. Volicer et al. (1990) demonstrated that it was possible to resume natural feeding in 5 of 6 patients with DAT (dementia of the Alzheimer type) who had chronic feeding tubes. Similarly, Leff, Cheuvront, and Russell (1994) reported that it was possible to wean 7 out of 15 patients from tube feeding after admission to a nursing home. These patients clearly had an improvement in quality of life by being able to taste food again and having increased caregiver interaction during feeding. Longitudinal studies of demented nursing home residents are needed to clarify the complications related to the feeding and the effect of tube feeding on the length of survival in patients with progressive dementia.

CONCLUSIONS

The investigation of eating problems in late-stage dementia has been pursued actively at many centers, by both clinicians and academicians. Drawing on this expertise, it is possible to provide adequate nutrition and calories throughout the progressive stages of Alzheimer's disease until the terminal phase.

Both staff members and families need to be prepared for the time when patients will be unable to drink even water by mouth. Families and caregivers should receive appropriate information and counseling regarding nutritional strategies. Ethical and medical issues are involved in this choice, as well as personal beliefs and cultural backgrounds. The role of the health worker is to implement all these factors to guide patients and families through the ultimate steps of the disease.

REFERENCES

Bianchetti, A., Rozzini, R., Carabellese, C., Zanetti, O., & Trabucchi, M. (1990). Nutritional intake, socioeconomic conditions, and heatlth status in a large elderly population. *Journal of the American Geriatrics Society, 38,* 521–526.

Buzby, G. P., Mullen, J. L., Matthews, D. C., Hobbs, C. L., & Rosato, E. F. (1980). Prognostic nutritional index in gastrointestinal surgery. *American Journal of Surgery, 139,* 160–167.

Campbell-Taylor, I., & Fisher, R. H. (1987). The clinical case against tube feeding in the palliative care of the elderly. *Journal of the American Geriatrics Society, 35,* 1100–1104.

Ciocon, J. O., Silverstone, F. A., Graver, L. M., & Foley, C. J. (1988). Tube feedings in elderly patients. Indications, benefits, and complications. *Archives of Internal Medicine, 148,* 429–433.

Cusack, B. J. (1995). Clinical pharmacology. In W. B. Abrams, M. H. Beers, & R. Berkow (Eds.),*The Merck manual of geriatric* (2nd ed.). Whitehouse Station, NJ: Merck & Co.

Eaton, M., Mitchell-Bonair, I. L., & Friedmann, E. (1986). The effect of touch on nutritional intake of chronic organic brain syndrome patients. *Journal of Gerontology, 41,* 611–616.

Elmsthäl, S., Blabolil, V., Fex, G., Kuller, R., & Steen, B. (1987). Hospital nutrition in geriatric long-term care medicine: I. Effects of a changed meal environment. *Comprehensive Gerontology, 1,* 29–33.

Franzoni, S., Frisoni, G. B., Boffelli, S., Rozzini, R., & Trabucchi, M. (1996). Good nutritional oral intake is associated with equal survival in demented and non demented very old patients. *Journal of the American Geriatrics Society, 44,* 1403–1404.

Frisoni, G. B., Franzoni, S., Rozzini, R., Ferrucci, L., Boffelli, S., & Trabucchi, M. (1994). A nutritional index predicting mortality in the nursing home. *Journal of the American Geriatric Society, 42,* 1167–1172.

Frisoni, G. B., Franzoni, S., Rozzini, R., Ferrucci, L., Boffelli, S., & Trabucchi, M. (1995). Food intake and mortality in the frail elderly. *Journal of Gerontology, 4,* M203–210.

Goddaer, J., & Abraham, I. L. (1994). Effects on relaxing music on agitation during meals among nursing home residents with severe cognitive impairment. *Archives of Psychiatric Nursing, 3,* 150–158.

Groher, M. E., & McKaig, T. N. (1995). Dysphagia and dietary levels in skilled nursing facilities. *Journal of the American Geriatrics Society, 43,* 528–532.

Hu, T. H., Huang, L., & Cartwright, W. S. (1986). Evaluation of the cost of caring for the senile demented elderly: A pilot study. *Gerontologist, 26,* 158–163.

Huff, F. J., Boller, F., Lucchelli, F., Querriera, R., Beyer, J., & Belle, S. (1987). The neurologic examination in patients with probable Alzheimer's disease. *Archives of Neurology, 44,* 929–932.

Koss, E., Weiffenbach, J. M., Haxby, J. V., & Frieland, R. P. (1988). Olfactory detection and identification performance are dissociated in early Alzheimer's disease. *Neurology, 38,* 1228–1232.

Leff, B., Cheuvront, N., & Russell, W. (1994). Discontinuing feeding tubes in a community nursing home. *Gerontologist, 34,* 130–133.

Little, J. T., Satlin, A., Sunderland, T., & Volicer, L. (1994). Sundown syndrome in severely demented patients with probable Alzheimer's disease. *Journal of Geriatric Psychiatry Neurology, 8,* 103–106.

Lo, B., & Dornbrand, L. (1984). Guiding the hand that feeds: Caring for the demented elderly. *New England Journal of Medicine, 311,* 402–408.

Matthews, L. E. (1988). Techniques for feeding the person with dysphagia. *Journal of Nutrition for the Elderly, 8,* 59–63.

McCann, R. M., Hall, W. J. & Groth-Juncker, A. (1994). Comfort care for terminally ill patients: The appropriate use of nutrition and hydration. *Journal of the American Medical Association, 272,* 1263–1266.

Meyers, R. M., & Grodin, M. A. (1991). Decision making regarding the initiation of tube feedings in the severely demented elderly: A review. *Journal of the American Geriatrics Society, 39,* 526–531.

Miller, B., Darby, A. L., Swartz, J. R., Yener, G. G., & Mena, I. (1994). Dietary changes, compulsions and sexual behavior in frontotemporal degeneration. *Dementia, 6,* 195–199.

Morales, R. P., Gonzales, R. E., & Santolaria, F. F. (1989). The relationship between psychophysical involution in the elderly subjects and his nutritional status. *Nutritional Hospital, 5,* 276–282.

Morley, J. E. (1995). The role of nutrition in the prevention of age-associated diseases. In J. E. Morley, Z. Glick, & L. Z. Rubenstein (Eds.), *Geriatric nutrition* (pp. 67–73). New York: Raven Press.

Morley, J. E. (1996). Dementia is not necessarily a cause of undernutrition. *Journal of the American Geriatrics Society, 44,* 1403–1404.

Peck, A., Cohen, C. E., & Mulvihill, M. N. (1990). Long-term enteral feeding of aged demented nursing home patients. *Journal of the American Geriatrics Society, 38,* 1195–1198.

Rheaume, Y., Riley, M., & Volicer, L. (1987). Meeting nutritional needs of Alzheimer's patients who pace constantly. *Journal of Nutrition for the Elderly, 7,* 43–52.

Rohrbaugh, R. M., & Siegal, A. P. (1989). Reversible anorexia and rapid weight loss associated with neuroleptic administration in Alzheimer's disease. *Journal of Geriatric Psychiatry Neurology, 1,* 45–47.

Schiffman, S. S., Clark, C. M., & Warwick, Z. S. (1990). Gustatory and olfactory dysfunction in dementia: not specific to Alzheimer's disease. *Neurobiology of Aging, 11,* 597–600.

Steen, B. (1992). Practical aspect of nutrition of the elderly in institutions. *Nutrition of the Elderly, 29,* 211–217.

Teri, L., Rabins, P., Whitehouse, P., Berg, L., Reisberg, B., Sunderland, T., Eichelman, B., & Phelps, C. (1992). Management of behavior disturbance in Alzheimer disease: current knowledge and future directions. *Alzheimer Disease and Associated Disorders, 2,* 77–88.

Trabucchi, M. (1992). *Invecchiamento della specie e vecchiaia della persona.* Milano: Franco Angeli.

Volicer, L., Rheaume, Y., Riley, M. E., Karner, J., & Glennon, M. (1990). Discontinuation of tube feeding in patients with dementia of the Alzheimer type. *American Journal of Alzheimer's Care and Related Disorders and Research, 4,* 22–25.
Volicer, L., Rheaume, Y., & Cyr, D. (1994). Treatment of depression in advanced Alzheimer's disease using sertraline. *Journal of Geriatric Psychiatry and Neurology, 7,* 227–229.
Volicer, L., Seltzer, B., Rheaume, Y., Karner, J., Glennon, M., Riley, M.E., & Crino, P.B. (1989). Eating difficulties in patients with probable dementia of the Alzheimer type. *Journal of Geriatric Psychiatry and Neurology, 2,* 169–176.
Warden, V. J. (1989). Waste not, want not. *Geriatric Nursing , 10,* 21–211.
Zanetti, O., Bianchetti, A., Zanetti, E., Magni, E., Frisoni, G. B., & Trabucchi, M. (in press). Geriatric nurses' attitudes towards the use of nasogastric feeding tubes in demented patients. *International Journal of Geriatric Psychiatry.*

Behavioral Symptoms of Dementia

Ladislav Volicer, Ann C. Hurley, and Ellen Mahoney

T he involvement of patients with advanced progressive dementia in a hospice program brings program staff in contact with a different patient population than the most commonly served patients in hospice programs—patients with terminal cancer. There are two main differences. First, patients with dementia cannot decide about involvement in a hospice program themselves, and this involvement has to be initiated by their proxies (see chapter 9). The second difference is the communication deficit and behavioral problems that dementia patients exhibit. Hospice staff have to know that the management of behavioral problems in dementia patients is as important as the management of pain in cancer patients. Patients' care plans need to reflect that such problems have been carefully assessed and that there is an interdisciplinary approach to management of these symptoms.

The primary symptoms of dementia are memory problems and other cognitive impairments that interfere with daily living activities (Corey-Bloom et al., 1995). These include both comprehension problems and functional deficits due to apraxia. In addition, most demented patients exhibit one or more secondary behavioral symptoms that could be either disruptive or nondisruptive. A nondisruptive behavioral problem is apathy, which is exhibited by many patients.

There is no unified terminology for the description of disruptive behavioral problems. Different investigators use several labels for these symptoms, including agitation, aggressiveness, and combativeness. Disruptive behavior is very common in nursing home residents. For instance, Cohen-Mansfield (1988) reported that two "agitated behaviors," which included physical and verbal aggression, occurred at least once a week in 87% of demented nursing home residents, while Ryden, Bossenmaier, and McLachlan (1991) found "aggressive behavior" to be present in 86%. In large probability samples drawn from all nursing home residents (not only those with dementia), estimates of the prevalence of disruptive behaviors range from 26% to 64% (Jackson et al., 1989; Zimmer, Watson, & Treat, 1984).

Management of the disruptive behaviors is important not only because they could endanger the safety of the patient, other residents, and staff, but also because these behaviors are often reflections of the patient's discomfort. Furthermore, the recent trend toward understanding the perspective of the person with dementia suggests that the behavioral symptoms may be more disabling than the historically emphasized cognitive decline. In a recent review of interventions for treating behavioral problems, Beck and Shue (1994) emphasized the importance of a conceptual framework, which encompasses biologic as well as psychosocial explanations, for understanding and managing disruptive behaviors.

The management of secondary behavioral symptoms of dementia requires a careful evaluation of the patient. It cannot be assumed that the behavior is a symptom of dementia just because the patient is demented. The behavior may be a consequence of discomfort caused by a physical illness, which the patient cannot report because of a speech impairment. Conditions such as pain, infections, cardiovascular insufficiency, constipation, dyspnea, and liver or kidney failure may lead to behavioral symptoms that can be readily alleviated by correcting the underlying problem. Interestingly, in qualitative interviews with nursing staff on our Dementia Special Care Units, we found that expert nurses consider change in behavioral symptoms (increase or decrease) to presage overt physical illness (Mahoney et al., unpublished data). Some symptoms are the first overt indication of an infection (Hurley, Volicer, Mahoney, & Volicer, 1993).

However, no reversible medical problem can be found in most cases. These patients have to be evaluated carefully to determine which aspects of the dementing process are triggering the behavioral symptoms. This evaluation is very important because the secondary symptoms can be managed more effectively by treating the underlying process rather than by trying to block the behavioral consequences themselves.

Several levels of the processes can be distinguished (see Figure 4.1). At the core of the symptoms is, of course, the dementing process itself.

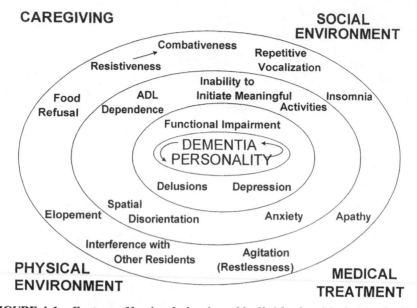

FIGURE 4.1   Factors affecting behavior of individuals with dementia: Personality, primary, secondary, and peripheral consequences of dementia, and interaction between the individual and environmental influences.

This process directly causes not only functional impairment, but may also cause delusions/hallucinations and depression. These primary consequences in turn lead to spatial disorientation, anxiety, dependence in activities of daily living (ADL), and the inability to initiate meaningful activities. Behavioral symptoms, such as agitation or "aggressive behavior," are peripheral expressions of these more basic processes.

All processes at a more basic level influence the next levels in a comprehensive way. Thus delusions may result in spatial disorientation, anxiety, and ADL dependence, while depression may lead to anxiety, and the inability to initiate meaningful activities. Similarly, spatial disorientation may lead to elopement attempts, combativeness, interference with other patients, and agitation. The inability to initiate meaningful activities may lead to apathy, repetitive vocalization, agitation, and insomnia. Therefore, not only are there multiple possible etiologies for specific behavioral symptoms, but the scope of therapeutic effectiveness is broader when interventions are directed closer to the core. The relationships of the underlying processes to behavioral symptoms may differ from patient to patient, and could even differ in the same patient at different times. The effective management of behavioral symptoms thus requires careful and comprehensive evaluation of all possible contributing factors.

Viewed in this way, behaviors are understood as symptoms of an underlying process, or a meaningful response to an environment that may be perceived as threatening, uncomfortable, confusing, or beyond control (Burgener, Jirovec, Murrell, & Barton, 1992; Gwyther, 1994; Sloane et al., 1995). The basic tenant of ethology, that all behavior has meaning (Eibl-Eibesfeldt, 1989), guides the practitioner to search for etiology as a target for preventive and therapeutic care. This conceptual framework emphasizes biologic factors, but the role of the environment must also be considered. Behavior is the outcome of the interaction between personal and environmental systems, which include the physical environment, the social environment, caregiving strategies, and management of intercurrent diseases.

The physical environment includes such factors as the level of lighting, temperature, noise, and decor. Low-level lighting increases confusion and may participate in "sundowning," heightened level of agitation that some patients exhibit in late afternoon. The extremes of temperature and a high noise level are likely to increase agitation, whereas a homelike atmosphere has a calming effect. The social environment includes other residents and visitors, as well as staff members and volunteers involved in patients' activities. Providing care for patients on a locked unit with homogeneous patient population minimizes such problems as elopement and interference with other residents.

Caregiving strategies should include a gentle approach and sensitivity to nonverbal communication (Volicer, Hurley, & Mahoney, 1995). These behavioral interventions are facilitated by shifting the emphasis from high-technology care striving for survival at all costs to care oriented toward assuring a patient's comfort. Aggressive medical interventions, such as cardiopulmonary resuscitation, intravenous therapy, and tube feeding, may not be appropriate in a late-stage dementia (Volicer, 1993). All of these interventions may produce a high degree of discomfort, which leads to agitation and other problem behaviors.

Empirical evidence of the contextual nature of behavior is beginning to accumulate, in support of earlier theoretical insights about the role of the physical and social environment in shaping behavior in people with dementia (Hall & Buckwalter, 1987; Lawton & Nahemow, 1973). Behavior has been found to vary as a function of setting, activity, complexity of demands, and the nature of caregiver-patient interactive behaviors (Beck, 1988; Burgener et al., 1992; Burgio et al., 1994; Cohen-Mansfield & Werner,

1995). Therefore, the first approach to the management of behavioral symptoms of dementia should be a well-designed behavioral intervention.

DEMENTIA

The dementia is at the core of all behavioral problems. A progressive dementia causes the loss of nerve cells and other irreversible brain changes. This leads to the development of cognitive impairments, which include memory deficit, poor judgment, and other impairments that will be described below. There is a complex interaction between dementia and the patient's premorbid personality. Although generally there is a significant correlation between premorbid and morbid personality traits (Kleban, Brody, & Lawton, 1971), a personality change may be the first symptom of dementia. The patient's personality may change for better or worse. Although on average patients become less extroverted and less conscientious and more neurotic (Chatterjee, Strauss, Smyth, & White-house, 1992), some families report that their relative, who was always a very distant and cold person, became much more warm and loving in the early stages of the disease. Conversely, a patient who was always a perfect gentleman may become verbally abusive and even strike out at his wife.

In contrast, other patients not only retain their premorbid personality, but the personality characteristics are magnified by the development of dementia. Thus individuals with a more hostile premorbid personality are more likely to develop paranoid delusions, whereas individuals who were neurotic are more likely to become depressed (Chatterjee et al., 1992). Some of the most difficult patients are those whose job involved controlling other people, such as police officers. They sometimes become very resistant to any input from caregivers and are quick to defend themselves from a perceived physical danger by subduing a caregiver. It was reported that women with an "aggressive" premorbid personality benefit most from an individual evaluation and intensive treatment (Kleban, et al., 1971).

Currently, there are few pharmacological options for the treatment of progressive dementias. Tacrine (Cognex) is approved for treatment of dementia of the Alzheimer type and may be beneficial in diffuse Lewy body disease (DLBD). Tacrine acts by inhibiting the breakdown of acetylcholine, one of the chemicals in the brain that the nerve cells use to communicate with each other. Acetylcholine is important for memory processes, which are disrupted even in healthy individuals who are given drugs that block acetylcholine effect (Beatty, Butters, & Janowsky, 1986).

A postmortem examination of the brains of Alzheimer patients showed that the number of nerve cells that use acetylcholine was markedly reduced (Mountjoy, 1986). This led to an acetylcholine deficit, which may have been responsible for the memory problems. Inhibition of acetylcholine breakdown by tacrine will enhance the functioning of the remaining cells and may improve memory and other cognitive functions.

However, this effect is present only in earlier stages of dementia when there are still some remaining cells. Additionally, many patients do not tolerate effective doses of tacrine because they develop liver toxicity (Watkins, Zimmerman, Knapp, Gracon, & Lewis, 1994). Even in patients who tolerate the therapy, tacrine merely delays the progression of dementia, on the average by 6 months (Knapp et al., 1994). Low-dose aspirin therapy may be effective in delaying the progression of a multi-infarct dementia (Grotta, 1987) by decreasing blood clotting, but aspirin therapy is not completely effective.

Despite these limitations in the treatment of the dementing process, there are therapeutic strategies that can be applied to treat some consequences of dementia in the encircling levels. The goals of therapeutic intervention include maintaining the dignity of patient and caregiver, preventing excess disability, and maximizing function, comfort, and quality of life (Hall, et al., 1995; Hurley, Hanrahan, Houde, & Volicer, 1992). The creation of a therapeutic environment underlies all of the interventions and is based on knowing the person's preferences, abilities, and usual patterns of response; modifying the environment to maximize safety and autonomy; and planning to avoid known triggers of behavioral symptoms. These include fatigue, multiple competing stimuli, physical stressors such as hunger or need to eliminate, changes in routine, and excess demands.

DELUSIONS AND HALLUCINATIONS

Delusions are very common in all stages of dementia. Paranoid delusions are sometimes the first symptom of progressive dementia observed in a long-term care setting, because other impairments may not be detected in a sheltered nursing home environment. In some patients, delusions can be managed by distracting the patient and involving him or her in an activity. It is important to respond to a patient's feelings rather than argue or correct. Paranoid delusions, such as believing that things are lost or that food is poisoned, usually respond well to a low dose of neuroleptics. Neuroleptics have been widely used to treat psychiatric symptoms of dementia, although controlled clinical trials are limited. The framework proposed here may identify relevant outcomes for future study, including behaviors that may improve, as well as those that may decline as a result of side effects such as sedation, anticholinergic symptoms, or muscle rigidity.

All neuroleptics are equally effective in this patient population, although at different dosages. However, neuroleptics differ significantly in their side effects. Drugs such as haloperidol (Haldol) and fluphenazine (Prolixin) have a high incidence of extrapyramidal side effects, resulting in blunt affect, muscle rigidity, and dystonia. In contrast, thioridazine (Mellaril) and mesoridazine (Serentil) may cause postural hypotension, cardiac arrhythmias, and sedation. In between are thiothixene (Navane) and perphenazine (Trilafon), which may have both types of side effects, but to a lesser extent. The choice of neuroleptics should be guided by the current risk factors for side effects that the patient has. A patient with preexisting muscle rigidity should not receive haloperidol, and a patient with significant cardiovascular comorbidity should not be treated with thioridazine. A new neuroleptic, risperidone (Risperdal), has fewer side effects than the older neuroleptic. However, it has a very long duration of action, which may lead to a buildup of its level in the body and overmedication.

A patient may sometimes refuse medications, which makes treatment more difficult. Auditory hallucinations, which consist of hearing voices of other patients or staff criticizing the patient, are also common. Hallucinations are more common in patients with DLBD. These patients are more sensitive to the side effects of older neuroleptics and may respond better to risperidone.

As the dementia progresses, a patient becomes more confused and often develops delusions regarding his or her circumstances. The resident may believe that he or she is working in the nursing home, is at school, or is in his or her parents' house. The patient may also develop delusions regarding another patient or staff, whom he or she believes is a relative who should obey the patient. Such delusions may lead to spatial disorientation and anxiety; elopement, interference with other patients, and agitation may ensue. Demented patients suffering from delusions may also misinterpret staff members' caregiving activities and resist such efforts. The presence of hallucinations and delusions was found to explain about one fourth of the variance in aggressive behavior of Alzheimer patients (Aarsland, Cummings, Yenner, & Miller, 1996).

DEPRESSION

Making the diagnosis of depression in a demented individual is very difficult. Several symptoms of major depressive disorder are commonly seen during some of the stages of a progressive dementia, and the assessment is complicated by speech and comprehension difficulties. Therefore, the estimates of depression in demented patients vary from 15% to 57% (Lazarus, Newton, Cohler, Lesser, & Schwein, 1987). Sometimes depression is the first symptom of dementia, and most patients who develop their first episode of depression in old age eventually develop dementia (Emery & Oxman, 1992). The diagnosis of depression in a demented patient can be made by carefully monitoring the patient's expression, obtaining information about episodes of tearfulness and crying from the staff, and evaluating eating and sleeping patterns. Angry affect, which is common even in younger depressed patients (Apter et al., 1990), may be the main symptom of depression. "Anger attacks," which were inhibited by antidepressant treatment, were described in middle-aged individuals (Fava et al., 1993) and may also occur in some demented patients. The symptoms of depression may differ according to gender, with males exhibiting more apathy and vegetative signs, and females showing more reclusiveness and emotional lability (Ott, Tate, Gordon, & Heindel, 1996).

Depression leads to anxiety and contributes to the inability to initiate meaningful activities. Through these processes or directly, the condition may play a role in food refusal, resistiveness, apathy, insomnia, and agitation. Thus a large proportion of behavioral symptoms may be caused or worsened by an underlying depression. Behavioral approaches to the treatment of depression include using positive feedback and maintaining interaction with the environment. Antidepressant treatment has improved the mood of patients, even those with advanced dementia, and increased food intake in patients who previously refused food (Volicer, Rheaume, & Cyr, 1994).

Although older tricyclic antidepressants (such as desipramine) are effective in this patient population, they frequently have anticholinergic and cardiovascular side effects. The newer specific serotonin reuptake inhibitors (SSRIs) have fewer side effects (e.g., sertraline [Zoloft] and paroxetine [Paxil]) and allow for the safe treatment of depression even in very old patients who have other concurrent diseases. Some antidepressants (e.g., trazodone [Desyrel] and doxepin [Sinequan]) have sedation as one of their side effects. This effect could be utilized in the treatment of insomnia in demented patients who also are depressed. Trazodone was also found to decrease irritability, anxiety, restlessness, and affective disturbance when administered 3 times a day (Lebert, Pasquier, & Petit, 1994).

Depression in dementia patients is persistent, especially in those with vascular dementia (Ballard, Patel, Solis, Lowe, & Wilcock, 1996). Therefore, the antidepressant treatment should be long term, for a year or longer. The effectiveness of SSRIs may decrease with prolonged administration, but they regain their effectiveness if the dose is increased and there is no need for switching to a different antidepressant.

FUNCTIONAL IMPAIRMENT

Functional impairment of a demented patient is related to both cognitive and physical impairments. Cognitive impairment includes the inability to use tools (apraxia) or to recognize objects (agnosia) as well as speech impairment (aphasia). Physical impairment, such as a paralysis due to stroke, aggravates the consequences of dementia. Therefore, it is important to maintain an adequate physical condition even in a patient with dementia. This includes rehabilitation after injury, such as hip fracture, or stroke. Rehabilitation is of course limited by the inability of the patient to follow directions and remember instructions. Rehabilitation also may become counterproductive if it leads to discomfort and fatigue. Some strategies that have been found helpful in treating other populations may still be applied. For example, people with apraxia may be able to imitate, even when unable to initiate an activity. Once started, they may be able to continue unaided.

An important function that is lost in late-stage dementia is the ability to walk, followed by the loss of the ability to stand. Residents either develop an unsteady gait or lose the ability to recognize and react safely to objects in their path. Some residents also develop leg contractures, which impair their mobility. To prevent contractures, patients should be encouraged to walk as much as possible and spend limited periods of time sitting in a chair. Kinesiotherapy promotes the ability to walk and prevents deconditioning and the development of contractures. It is also helpful to have railings along the walls and provide unobstructed path for walking. Functional impairments lead to dependence in activities of daily living and an inability to initiate meaningful activities. This can result in apathy, repetitive vocalization, and resistiveness to care.

ANXIETY

Anxiety is a symptom of depression, but it can also be induced by delusions and hallucinations. Functional impairment may also lead to increased anxiety if caregiving activities, such as using a Hoyer lift, frighten the patient. Anxiety, in turn, can lead to agitation and restlessness, repetitive vocalization, insomnia, and resistive behavior. Anxiety is minimized by a gentle, calm approach by caregivers, by maintaining eye contact, and by explaining to the patient what is being done. The resident must not only be safe but also feel safe.

The phenomenon of anxiety/fear has been described in a manner compatible with the conceptual framework proposed here. For example, Sloane et al. (1995) described "fearful fantasies and beliefs" associated with bathing. Ryden and Feldt (1992) identified fear as an antecedent to aggressive behaviors, and nursing staff attribute behaviors such as grabbing to a resident's fear of falling. In each of these examples, interventions that target the resident's possible feelings should be evaluated. Clinical evidence supports use of environmental cues and relaxation techniques such as music (Snyder, Egan, & Burns, 1995a; Tabloski, McKinnon-Howe, & Remington, 1995).

Trying to correct a patient's delusions seldom succeeds in decreasing anxiety and may precipitate a catastrophic reaction. Gentle distraction and involvement in some activity are usually more effective in reducing anxiety. If not effective, short-acting benzodiazepines (e.g., lorazepam [Ativan]) may be used to calm the patient. Another antianxiety medication is buspirone (Buspar), which, however, has a delayed onset of effect.

SPATIAL DISORIENTATION

Delusions and spatial memory deficits combine to prevent a patient from remembering the location of his or her room, the bathroom, and other facilities. Spatial disorientation may also lead to entry into the rooms of other patients and nursing station/office areas. Signs and visual aids (e.g., a picture of a toilet on the bathroom door or shadow boxes containing personal objects outside residents' rooms) may be helpful in early-stage dementia but lose their effectiveness as the disease progresses. Half-doors are quite effective in preventing patients' access to certain areas while allowing staff to maintain visual control. However, half-doors cannot be the only doors, because full-length doors are required for fire protection.

INABILITY TO INITIATE MEANINGFUL ACTIVITIES

Functional impairment and depression may lead to a decreased ability to initiate meaningful activities. A patient may lose interest in reading and watching TV, and an aphasia may make communication with other patients difficult. Therefore, there is a need for more organized programs that stimulate activity and that take into consideration both a patient's remaining abilities and impairments. However, depression often results in a patient being reluctant to leave his or her room. The lack of meaningful activity may result in apathy, repetitive vocalization, and agitation/restlessness. Teri and Logsdon (1991) identified a wide range of activities meaningful to people with dementia.

The prevention of behavioral symptoms in dementia patients requires special activity programming. The activities should take advantage of a patient's remaining strengths and abilities and be designed to provide positive feedback. Activities should be organized 7 days a week and should be integrated into each patient's daily routine. Patients need to have their days structured and filled with meaningful activities to give their lives purpose. Activity programming should include all staff members because one person could not engage the patients throughout the day and evening hours (Bowlby, 1993).

DEPENDENCE IN ACTIVITIES OF DAILY LIVING

Functional impairments and apraxia make a patient unable to dress, bathe, groom himself or herself and to use a bathroom. The onset of incontinence may be delayed by employing signs pointing to the location of a bathroom and by regular toileting. However, continence is almost invariably lost once a patient loses the ability to ambulate. Eventually, the patient also loses the ability to feed himself or herself and has to be fed by the staff. This dependence may lead to food refusal and resistiveness to care.

Dependence may be decreased by making the ADL activities easier for the patient to do. Loose-fitting clothes that are easy to put on (such as sweat suits) facilitate dressing. Presenting food items one at a time decreases patient confusion and helps maintain independent eating (see chapter 3). It is preferable to maintain a patient's ability as long as possible by cueing and helping the resident instead of doing the activity for him or her. Caregivers are challenged to find the therapeutic path between excess disability and excess demands, as both of these have been associated with negative outcomes for people with dementia (Beck, Heacock, Mercer, Walton, & Shook, 1991; Sloane et al., 1995).

RESISTIVENESS–COMBATIVENESS CONTINUUM

Because a resident is unable to perform ADLs, the ADLs are "imposed" by the staff. Staff members decide when a patient goes to bed and gets up, when he or she needs to be cleaned, and when the resident needs food or liquids. Although demented, a patient may not agree with staff timing and/or goals. Therefore, he or she may refuse help and impede care. If staff members insist on providing care, the patient may refuse to cooperate or may actively resist. This resistiveness could escalate to a combative behavior, which may be a way of defending the self against unwanted physical contact. This combativeness, which is often called an aggressive behavior, occurs predominantly during hands-on care involving touching the patient (Ryden & Feldt, 1992).

This refusal is often only temporary, and the patient may cooperate if staff members repeat their approach after a short period of time, allowing the patient to forget that he or she did not actually want to cooperate. Another effective strategy is distraction of the patient away from the caregiving process. This may be accomplished by having two staff members working as a team. One of the staff members provides distraction by talking or joking with the patient, while the other staff member provides the care (e.g., cleaning).

Delusions and hallucinations may also contribute to resistiveness. Neuroleptics are quite effective in preventing resistive behavior, although this is not confirmed by clinical studies (Helms, 1985). This apparent lack of therapeutic effectiveness is most likely due to poor measurement tools used in these studies, which did not specifically target resistive behavior.

AGITATION–APATHY CONTINUUM

Agitation is an increase of a physical and verbal activity, which does not have an obvious goal. It may express itself as restlessness, repetitive vocalization, and insomnia. Apathy is the opposite extreme of an undesirable patient's state. It may be defined as an absence of any evidence of engagement with the environment expressed by immobility, lack of verbal engagement, inattention to the environment, lack of meaningful eye contact, and sad or "lost" facial expression. Agitation was observed in 60% of Alzheimer patients, whereas apathy was observed in 72% (Mega, Cummings, Fiorello, & Gornbein, 1996). This demonstrates that often periods of agitation alternate with periods of apathy, when the patient does not maintain any contact with the environment. Both of these behavioral symptoms may have a similar cause: lack of meaningful activities. Agitation may also be caused by delusions or hallucinations. A resident may believe that he or she has to do something or be somewhere, and become agitated when this is not possible.

The treatment of an underlying cause of agitation is always more effective than any attempts to decrease agitation by sedating the patient. Attempts to reduce agitation by sedatives have the additional problem of side effects from sedatives that persist much longer than the behavior the drugs were used to treat. In some cases, an increased activity may actually be beneficial. This is true especially for pacing, which allows the patient to exercise, improves sleep, and prevents constipation. Repetitive vocalization is the most difficult behavioral symptom to treat. Repeated requests for help may be very disruptive for both the other patients and the staff. Staff intervention is often not effective in stopping the vocalization, which may be caused by a release of vocal motor activity from the higher brain function, similar to purposeless pacing.

Agitation that is not affected by other treatments sometimes responds to the administration of such anticonvulsants/mood stabilizers as valproic acid (Depakote) and carbamazepine (Tegretol). Used to decrease agitation, these drugs may be effective in blood concentrations lower than those required to prevent seizures. Valproic acid is also effective in decreasing myoclonic movements, which sometimes interfere with feeding and other care.

ELOPEMENT AND INTERFERENCE WITH OTHER PATIENTS

These symptoms may be caused by spatial disorientation, but could also be due to delusions and hallucinations. Alarm systems that indicate an unauthorized exit are disturbing to other patients and require the staff to prevent the patient from exiting. This usually leads to agitation on the part of the patient and interferes with regular care activities. The best way of securing an outside door is a key pad system. Alternatively, disguising exits by painting them the same color as the wall or by covering up the door handle may be sufficient (Dickinson, McLain-Kark, & Marshall-Baker, 1995), but this method should be combined with alarms for added safety. However, disguising the doors may not be possible if these are fire exits. Another strategy is to have the doors locked either at all times or when a patient who presents an elopement risk approaches them. This is more easily accomplished if all patients on a unit are demented. The homogeneous grouping of dementia patients has other advantages, such as eliminating problems with intrusion into other patients' rooms, which is upsetting to cognitively intact patients.

Many behavioral symptoms are more easily managed on a Special Care Dementia Unit. Such a unit can design programs specific for cognitively impaired patients and provide special training for the staff. It is easier for staff members to approach patients in a similar way instead of switching to a different approach when dealing with cognitively intact residents. Use of restraints can be minimized if the environment is modified to make it safe for patients who wander, are likely to touch everything, and may put inedible things in their mouths.

In developing a typology of nursing interventions, Eisenhauer (1994) observed that interventions usually are not diagnosis-specific. Therefore, a nursing diagnosis alone does not direct the choice of intervention, and different interventions can be chosen for the same diagnosis. This analysis applies to research in behavior management as well. For example, music as an intervention has been used for the treatment of symptoms such as anxiety, agitation, and food refusal, while "validation therapy" has been recommended for cognitive impairment, aggressiveness, and depression. Meanwhile, the development of behavior-specific treatments has been recommended as a research priority in order to advance the scientific basis of care for persons with dementia (Teri et al., 1992). The model of problem behaviors shown in Figure 4.1, may help to untangle this web by providing a framework for studying relationships among behaviors, by distinguishing between preventive and symptom-management strategies, and by identifying relevant outcomes for the evaluation of treatment efficacy.

Behavioral interventions designed to improve the quality of care and quality of life of persons with dementia and their caregivers are catalogued in several recent articles. Hall et al. (1995) developed an in-home standardized care plan based on the Progressively Lowered Stress Threshold model to direct caregiver education. Although specifically designed for community-based use, the care plan is both theoretically and empirically driven, and the problems addressed, including loss of stress tolerance, decreased ability to perceive multiple stimuli, communication loss, and fearfulness, are applicable in long-term care settings as well. Rantz and McShane (1995) used focus groups of experienced nursing home staff to describe some effective interventions for residents with chronic confusion. Four categories of interventions, with specific examples of each, were identified in this exploratory study: interpreting reality, maintaining normalcy, meeting basic needs, and managing behavior disturbances. Although not behavior-specific, strategies such as identifying the trigger or using redirection are applicable to many behavioral symptoms. The researchers recommend using psychotropic drugs in low doses *if* functional abilities are maintained or improved while behavior disturbances are reduced. Practical suggestions for coping with a spectrum of behavioral problems in people with dementia are summarized by Carlson, Fleming, Smith, and Evans (1995).

Specific ADLs that are common contexts for behavioral symptoms have been the focus for several studies. Sloane et al. (1995) reported the results of a multidisciplinary consensus conference on techniques to reduce disruptive behaviors during bathing. They addressed environmental characteristics for bathing areas, helpful communication techniques for persons with dementia, approaches for preparing and bathing nursing home residents, and suggestions for managing specific problems that arise. Beck and associates (Beck, 1988; Beck et al., 1993; Vogelpohl, Beck, Heacock, & Mercer, 1996) focused on preventing excess disability and promoting independent dressing in people with cognitive impairment. Seven levels of assistance with dressing were described: stimulus control, initial verbal prompt, repeated verbal prompt, gestures or modeling, occasional physical guidance, complete physical guidance, and complete assistance. Feeding has been studied by Phillips and Van Ort (1993), who have identified both contextual and behavioral interventions to promote functional feeding (Van Ort & Phillips, 1995).

Some interventions for specific behavioral symptoms have been researched, but with nonsignificant results. Analysis of these studies is useful, however, to identify methodological as well as theoretical issues. For example, hand massage and therapeutic touch were compared to presence only in a crossover design in 17 residents with a history of agitation (Snyder, Egan, & Burns, 1995b). Significant differences were reported in the level of relaxation from pre- to postintervention, but there was no decrease in observed agitation, as had been hypothesized. While acknowledging the potential bias of research data collected by the interventionist, key methodological issues in developing empirical support for behavioral interventions are identified. In another study with nonsignificant results, a sensory integration program administered to 40 institutional residents with dementia did not decrease disruptive behaviors or increase functional abilities as hypothesized (Robichaud, Hebert, & Desrosiers, 1994). These researchers questioned whether modifying the frequency of sessions, the number of subjects, and the measurement instruments would lead to similar results and cautioned that further study is necessary before labeling the sensory integration program ineffective. Attention to nonsignificant results contributes to further understanding (Shea, 1996) and should be encouraged as a stimulus to further questions. For example, the finding that a 5-minute hand massage was more effective in producing relaxation in the morning than in the afternoon raises the question of higher levels of stress/fatigue decreasing the effectiveness of an intervention (Snyder et al., 1995b).

More study is needed about the required characteristics of interventions, such as frequency, intensity, complexity, context, sequencing, and implementation strategies (Brooten & Naylor, 1995; Tripp-Reimer, Wood-worth, McCloskey, & Bulechek, 1996), and the best match of patients, behaviors, caregivers, and interventions for maximal efficacy (Teri et al., 1992). Recent attention to specific behaviors, patterns of behavior, behavioral syndromes, and sequences of behavior (Burgio et al., 1994; Kolanowski, 1995; Mahoney, Hurley, & Volicer, unpublished data), as well as research methodologies that account for individual variability in behavior, hold promise for continued development of the knowledge base to guide practice.

Years ago, Irene Burnside (1979), a noted gerontological nurse, observed that calm, functional resident behaviors were related to stable staff and routines, generous use of affection, skilled nonverbal behavior, and qualified nursing staff. While more systematic research is needed that links specific behaviors, interventions, and outcomes in individuals with dementia, empirical evidence supports "knowing the patient" and educating staff members. Consistency in the caregiving relationship can be meaningful for both the caregiver and the patient. Getting to know the patient well and trying to understand the meaning of behavior takes time, commitment, and creativity. Developing and evaluating interventions also ideally take place over time. Frequent changes in caregiving personnel can interfere with the human connection, which is integral to the caregiving relationship and precludes the ability to know the patient well enough to provide skillful and compassionate care. For the patient with dementia, consistency in the caregiving relationship is helpful. Requirements to change and to take in and work with new input can be very challenging for the person with cognitive and functional impairments. The patient benefits from the consistent and human connection.

REFERENCES

Aarsland, D., Cummings, J. L., Yenner, G., & Miller, B. (1996). Relationship of aggressive behavior to other neuropsychiatric symptoms in patients with Alzheimer's disease. *American Journal of Psychiatry, 153,* 243–247.

Apter, A., Van Praag, H. M., Plutchik, R., Sevy, S., Korn, M., & Brown, S.-L. (1990). Interrelationships among anxiety, aggression, impulsivity, and mood: A serotonergically linked cluster. *Psychiatry Research, 32,* 191–199.

Ballard, C. G., Patel, A., Solis, M., Lowe, K., & Wilcock, G. (1996). A one-year follow-up study of depression in dementia sufferers. *British Journal of Psychiatry, 168,* 287–291.

Beatty, W., Butters, N., & Janowsky, D. (1986). Patterns of memory failure after scopolamine treatment: Implications for cholinergic hypotheses of dementia. *Behavioral and Neural Biology, 45,* 196–211.

Beck, C. (1988). Measurement of dressing performance in persons with dementia. *American Journal of Alzheimer's Care, 3*(3), 21–25.

Beck, C., Heacock, P., Mercer, S., Walton, C., & Shook, J. (1991). Dressing for success: Promoting independence among cognitively impaired elderly. *Journal of Psychosocial Nursing, 29,* 30–35.

Beck, C. K., & Shue, V. M. (1994). Interventions for treating disruptive behavior in demented elderly people. *Nursing Clinics of North America, 29,* 143–155.

Bowlby, C. (1993). *Therapeutic activities with persons disabled by Alzheimer's disease and related disorders.* Gaithersburg, MD: Aspen Publishers.

Brooten, D., & Naylor, M. D. (1995). Nurses' effect on changing patient outcomes. *Image: Journal of Nursing Scholarship, 27,* 95–99.

Burgener, S. C., Jirovec, M., Murrell, L., & Barton, D. (1992). Caregiver and environmental variables related to difficult behaviors in institutionalized, demented elderly persons. *Journal of Gerontology: Psychological Sciences, 47,* P242–P249.

Burgio, L. D., Scilley, K., Hardin, M., Janosky, J., Bonino, P., Slater, S. C., & Engberg, R. (1994). Studying disruptive vocalization and contextual factors in the nursing home using computer-assisted real-time observation. *Journal of Gerontology, 49,* P230–P239.

Burnside, I. M. (1979). Alzheimer's disease: An overview. *Journal of Gerontological Nursing, 5*(4), 14–20.

Carlson, D. L., Fleming, K. C., Smith, G. E., & Evans, J. M. (1995). Management of dementia-related behavioral disturbances: A nonpharmacologic approach. *Mayo Clinic Proceedings, 70,* 1108–1115.

Chatterjee, A., Strauss, M. E., Smyth, K. A., & Whitehouse, P. J. (1992). Personality changes in Alzheimer's disease. *Archives of Neurology, 49,* 486–491.

Cohen-Mansfield, J. (1988). Agitated behavior and cognitive functioning in nursing home residents: Preliminary results. *Clinical Gerontologist, 7*(3/4), 11–22.

Cohen-Mansfield, J., & Werner, P. (1995). Environmental influences on agitation: an integrative summary of an observational study. *American Journal of Alzheimer's Care, 10*(1), 32–39.

Corey-Bloom, J., Thal, L. J., Galasko, D., Folstein, M., Drachman, D., Raskind, M., & Lanska, D. J. (1995). Diagnosis and evaluation of dementia. *Neurology, 45,* 211–218.

Dickinson, J. I., McLain-Kark, J., & Marshall-Baker, A. (1995). The effects of visual barriers on exiting behavior in a dementia care unit. *Gerontologist, 35,* 127–130.

Eibl-Eibesfeldt, I. (1989). *Human ethology.* New York: Aldine de Gruyter.

Eisenhauer, L. A. (1994). A typology of nursing therapeutics. *Image: Journal of Nursing Scholarship, 26,* 261–264.

Emery, V. O., & Oxman, T. E. (1992). Update on the dementia spectrum of depression. *American Journal of Psychiatry, 149,* 305–317.

Fava, M., Rosenbaum, J. F., Pava, J. A., McCarthy, M. K., Steingard, R. J., & Bouffides, E. (1993). Anger attacks in unipolar depression: 1. Clinical correlates and response to fluoxetine treatment. *American Journal of Psychiatry, 150,* 1158–1163.

Grotta, J. C. (1987). Current medical and surgical therapy for cerebrovascular disease. *New England Journal of Medicine, 317,* 1505–1516.

Gwyther, L. (1994). Managing challenging behaviors at home. *Alzheimer Disease and Associated Disorders, 8*(3), 110–112.

Hall, G. R., & Buckwalter, K. C. (1987). Progressively lowered stress threshold: A conceptual model for care of adults with Alzheimer's disease. *Archives of Psychiatric Nursing, 1,* 399–406.

Hall, G. R., Buckwalter, K. C., Stolley, J. M., Gerdner, L. A., Garrand, L., Ridgeway, S., & Crump, S. (1995). Standardized care plan: Managing Alzheimer's patients at home. *Journal of Gerontological Nursing, 21*(1), 37–47.

Helms, P. M. (1985). Efficacy of antipsychotics in the treatment of the behavioral complications of dementia: Review of the literature. *Journal of the American Geriatrics Society, 33,* 206–209.

Hurley, A. C., Volicer, B. J., Hanrahan, P. A., Houde, S., & Volicer, L. (1992). Assessment of discomfort in advanced Alzheimer patients. *Research in Nursing and Health, 15,* 369–377.

Hurley, A. C., Volicer, B., Mahoney, M. A., & Volicer, L. (1993). Palliative fever management in Alzheimer patients: Quality plus fiscal responsibility. *Advances in Nursing Science, 16,* 21–32.

Jackson, M. E., Drugovich, M. L., Fretwell, M. D., Spector, W. D., Sternberg, J., & Rosenstein, R. B. (1989). Prevalence and correlates of disruptive behavior in the nursing home. *Journal of Aging and Health, 1*(3), 349–369.

Kleban, M. H., Brody, E. M. & Lawton, M. P. (1971). Personality traits in the mentally impaired aged and their relationship to improvements in current functioning. *Gerontologist, 11,* 134–140.

Knapp, M. J., Knopman, D. S., Solomon, P. R., Pendlebury, W. W., Davis, C. S., & Gracon, S. I. (1994). A 30-week randomized controlled trial of high-dose-tacrine in patients with Alzheimer's disease. *Journal of the American Medical Association, 271,* 985–991.

Kolanowski, A. M. (1995). Disturbing behaviors in demented elders: A concept synthesis. *Archives of Psychiatric Nursing, 9*(4), 188–194.

Lawton, M. P., & Nahemow, L. E. (1973). Ecology and the aging process. In C. Eisdorfer & M. P. Lawton (Eds.), *Psychology of adult development and aging.* Washington, DC: American Psychological Association.

Lazarus, L. W., Newton, N., Cohler, B., Lesser, J., & Schwein, C. (1987). Frequency and presentation of depressive symptoms in patients with primary degenerative dementia. *American Journal of Psychiatry, 144,* 41–45.

Lebert, F., Pasquier, F., & Petit, H. (1994). Behavioral effects of trazodonein Alzheimer's disease. *Journal of Clinical Psychiatry, 55,* 536–538.

Mega, M. S., Cummings, J. L., Fiorello, T., & Gornbein, J. (1996). The spectrum of behavioral changes in Alzheimer's disease. *Neurology, 46,* 130–135.

Mountjoy, C. Q. (1986). Correlations between neuropathological and neurochemical changes. *British Medical Bulletin, 42,* 81–85.

Ott, B. R., Tate, C. A., Gordon, N. M., & Heindel, W. C. (1996). Gender differences in the behavioral manifestations of Alzheimer's disease. *Journal of the American Geriatrics Society, 44,* 583–587.

Phillips, L., & Van Ort, S. (1993). Measurement of mealtime interactions among persons with dementing disorders. *Journal of Nursing Measurement, 1,* 41–55.

Rantz, M. J., & McShane, R. E. (1995). Nursing interventions for chronically confused nursing home residents. *Geriatric Nursing, 16,* 22–27.

Robichaud, L., Hebert, R., & Desrosiers, J. (1994). Efficacy of a sensory integration program on behaviors of inpatients with dementia. *American Journal of Occupational Therapy, 48,* 355–360.

Ryden, M. B., Bossenmaier, M., & McLachlan, C. (1991). Aggressive behavior in cognitively impaired nursing home residents. *Research in Nursing and Health, 14,* 87–95.

Ryden, M. B., & Feldt, K. S. (1992). Goal-directed care: Caring for aggressive nursing home residents with dementia. *Journal of Gerontological Nursing, 18,* 35–42.

Shea, C. (1996, August 17). Psychologists degate accuracy of "significance test". *Chronicle of Higher Education,* pp. 14, 17.

Sloane, P. D., Rader, J., Barrick, A.-L., Hoeffer, B., Dwyer, S., McKenzie, D., Lavelle, M., Buckwalter, K., Arrington, L., & Pruitt, T. (1995). Bathing persons with dementia. *Gerontologist, 35,* 672–678.

Snyder, M., Egan, E. C., & Burns, K. R. (1995a). Interventions for decreasing agitation behaviors in persons with dementia. *Journal of Gerontological Nursing, 21*(7), 34–40.

Snyder, M., Egan, E. C., & Burns, K. R. (1995b). Efficacy of hand massage in decreasing agitated behaviors associated with care activities in persons with dementia. *Geriatric Nursing, 16,* 60–63.

Tabloski, T. A., McKinnon-Howe, L., & Remington, R. (1995). Effect of calming music on level of agitation in cognitively impaired nursing home residents. *Journal of Alzheimer's Care and Related Disorder Research, 10*(1), 10–15.

Teri, L., & Logsdon, R. G. (1991). Identifying pleasant activities for Alzheimer's disease patients: The pleasant events schedule-AD. *Gerontologist, 31*(1), 124–127.

Teri, L., Rabins, P., Whitehouse, P., Berg, L., Reisberg, B., Sunderland, T., Eichelman, B., & Philps, C. (1992). Management of behavior disturbance in Alzheimer disease: Current knowledge and future directions. *Alzheimer's Disease and Associated Disorders, 6*(2), 77–88.

Tripp-Reimer, T., Woodworth, G., McCloskey, J. C., & Bulechek, G. (1996). The dimensional structure of nursing interventions. *Nursing Research, 45,* 10–17.

Van Ort, S., & Phillips, L. R. (1995). Nursing interventions to promote functional feeding. *Journal of Gerontological Nursing, 21*(10), 6–14.

Vogelpohl, T. S., Beck, C. K., Heacock, P., & Mercer, S. O. (1996). "I can do it": Dressing: Promoting independence through individualized strategies. *Journal of Gerontological Nursing, 22*(3), 39–42.

Volicer, L. (1993). Alzheimer's disease: Course, management, and the hospice approach. *Nursing Home Medicine, 1*(5), 31–37.

Volicer, L., Hurley, A. C., & Mahoney, E. (1995). Management of behavioral symptoms of dementia. *Nursing Home Medicine, 12*(3), 300–306.

Volicer, L., Rheaume, Y., & Cyr, D. (1994). Treatment of depression in advanced Alzheimer's disease using sertraline. *Journal of Geriatric Psychiatry and Neurology, 7,* 227–229.

Watkins, P. B., Zimmerman, H. J., Knapp, M. J., Gracon, S. I., & Lewis, K. W. (1994). Hepatotoxic effects of tacrine administration in patients with Alzheimer's disease. *Journal of the American Medical Association, 271,* 992–998.

Zimmer, J. G., Watson, N., & Treat, A. (1984). Behavioral problems amongpatients in skilled nursing facilities. *American Journal of Public Health, 74,* 1118–1121.

CHAPTER FIVE

Quality of Life in Late-Stage Dementia

Sandy C. Burgener

P ersons with Alzheimer's disease (AD) have received a great deal of attention from the research community, with the majority of research directed at the study of the progression of AD; identification of dysfunctional behaviors; behavioral control through pharmacological, environmental, and social interventions; and management of the disease process (Duffy, Hepburn, Christensen, & Brugge-Wiger, 1989; Lyman, 1989). However, as Lawton (1995) and Cotrell and Schulz (1993) explicated, this approach is limited because of the lack of attention given to understanding of positive patient outcomes. Identification of specific patient needs and other factors that facilitate positive patient outcomes is a necessary precursor to identifying additional variables for assessment and subsequent intervention development. Facilitating positive patient outcomes, although a worthwhile outcome in itself, also has the potential of influencing other aspects of this devastating disease process. For example, recent studies have supported the relationship between patient and caregiver behaviors, suggesting that more positive patient behaviors may result in a more positive caregiving experience (Burgener, Jirovec, Murrell, & Barton, 1992; Meddaugh, 1990). Considering the wealth of research identifying the influence of difficult patient behaviors on caregiver burden, interventions designed to increase positive patient outcomes, reflecting increased patient quality of life (QOL), should decrease caregiver burden.

Lawton (1995) described the "stripping of personhood" that is common with AD patients and the resulting demoralizing effect this has on both institutional and family caregivers. This lack of attention to the patient's personhood robs the family caregiver of a previously valued relationship as well. Lawton suggests that attention to the AD patient's personal states, reflected in quality-of-life dimensions, can increase maintenance of the patient's personhood, provide positive feedback for caregivers, and enrich the total caregiving experience. Additionally, interventions designed to increase positive patient outcomes should decrease the prevalence of depressive disorders in AD patients, found to occur in as many as 87% of AD patients (Merriam, Aronson, Gaston, Wey, & Katz, 1988; Pearson, Teri, Reifler, & Raskind, 1989). Interventions designed to decrease depressive disorders have the potential to decrease the costs of care and, importantly, increase the patient's quality of life. Exploration of patient quality of life, then, even in later disease stages, holds promise for identifying interventions to facilitate positive outcomes for both the AD patient and the caregiver while focusing on the positive rather than the negative aspects of the disease consequences.

As noted by Stoll (1977), the concept of quality of life has particular relevance for persons with chronic diseases, such as irreversible dementia, due to the emphasis on palliation or symptom control rather than cure. For older adults who are often afflicted by chronic illnesses, this concept has taken on new importance and has become a priority for researchers during recent years (Butler, 1992). Although this concept may at first appear to be straightforward, multiple definitions exist for quality of life, making a consensus regarding operationalization difficult at best. Applying this concept with patients with AD, especially patients in the later disease stages, presents even more challenges as definition and measurement of the concept must be examined in relation to the losses and functional constraints that are inevitable as dementia progresses. To examine and, one hopes, to clarify this concept within the context of care of the dementia patient during the later disease stages, quality-of-life definitions will be given, with particular emphasis on Lawton's (1995) well-developed conceptualization of quality of life in the AD patient. The empirical basis for application of this concept will then be explored, describing interventions specific to care of the late-stage AD patient. Finally, issues regarding measurement of quality of life will be discussed. The intent of this chapter is to provide caregivers, both in home and institutional settings, with an objective basis from which to design care interventions, while focusing results of care on positive patient outcomes reflecting improved patient quality of life.

CHARACTERISTICS OF LATE-STAGE DEMENTIA

The challenge of identifying interventions to achieve patient quality of life becomes evident when the multiple effects of the disease are reviewed. Patient characteristics and abilities have been found to consistently change across the disease process (Hughes, Berg, Danziger, Cohen, & Martin, 1982). As patients progress from the middle to late disease stages, behavior is marked by functional losses, including gradual loss of ability to dress, bathe, and eat independently. Generally, all ability to perform instrumental activities of daily living (e.g., ability to use the telephone, shop, prepare meals, transport oneself independently, do housework, take medication, and manage finances) are lost as patients move from the middle to late disease stages. The later disease stages are identified by diminished ability to perform basic self-care tasks, incontinence of bowel and bladder, and loss of self-feeding ability (DeJong, Osterlund, & Roy, 1989). In very late disease stages, verbal communication becomes increasingly impaired, with many patients becoming totally incoherent or mute. Patients gradually lose their ability to ambulate independently, requiring the use of supportive devices and caregiver assistance. The final disease stages are characterized by the need for total assistance with care, immobility, and decreased ability to swallow, requiring use of diet modification or assistive devices for feeding. These progressive changes in patient functioning mark late-stage AD and present challenges to caregivers to define positive approaches to care to ensure the patient's quality of life.

THEORETICAL BASIS FOR QUALITY OF LIFE

Multiple definitions of quality of life are found in the literature, with a common theme being a "degree of satisfaction with perceived present life circumstances" (Young & Longman, 1983). Based on studies with healthy individuals, Campbell, Converse, and Rodgers (1976) described quality of life in broad terms, including satisfaction with marriage, family life, friendships, standard of living, housing, finances, and religion. Satisfaction within this model is viewed as a subjective evaluation of the attributes of each quality-of-life domain, reflecting the discrepancy between the individual's aspirations and reality. Ferrans and Powers (1985) described quality of life similarly, although their view of quality of life evolved from multiple studies of patients with chronic illnesses, such as renal impairment. Quality-of-life components within this model include a person's subjective opinion regarding life satisfaction; physical health; mood or affect; relationships such as friendships, marriage, and family; life goals; environmental status such as housing, neighborhood, city, and nation; self-esteem; and perceptions of stress related to disease treatments. Simpler views of quality of life are found, however, with Cohen (1982), suggesting quality of life can be judged by the extent to which an individual is facilitated or hindered in his or her ability to live according to plan. Inherent in the notion of fulfillment of a "plan" is the concept of goal fulfillment at different points in a person's life. Goal obtainment can be hindered by illnesses or medical or nursing treatments, reflecting the impact of disease on quality of life.

Although definitions of quality of life are varied, most definitions include an inherent subjective evaluation of various aspects of one's present situation in relation to a personalized desired outcome. This requirement of a subjective evaluation makes application of most quality-of-life models inappropriate for the dementia patient, as subjective evaluation is often not possible or valid, especially in the later disease stages. Only one quality-of-life model has been developed specifically for persons with irreversible dementia, the quality-of-life perspective developed and tested by Lawton (1995). Due to the inherent problems in application of other quality-of-life models and the specificity of Lawton's view for this population, this model was chosen to guide the design of interventions affecting quality-of-life outcomes for late-stage AD patients.

Lawton's (1995) formulation of "the good life" includes four sectors or domains, displayed in Figure 5.1. These four domains include (1) psychological well-being, consisting of the person's affective states, including anxiety, depression, agitation, and positive affective states; (2) behavioral competence, including physical health, functional ability, and cognition, along with the more complex domains of time use and social behavior; (3) the objective environment, consisting of structured events and the architectural features of the environment; and (4) perceived quality of life.

Lawton's (1995) conceptualization of quality of life contains one domain that requires subjective evaluation, the perceived quality-of-life domain. As AD patients in later disease stages may not provide reliable information regarding subjective experiences, this particular domain would not always be applicable with this patient population. The objective environment domain, although often not within the direct influence of the AD patient, may be affected by caregivers, providing some direction for environmental interventions. Two quality-of-life domains, however, psychological well-being and behavioral competence, are reflected by individual patient factors and behaviors and may be amenable to interventions directed to positive patient outcomes. Positive and negative

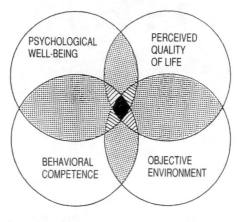

FIGURE 5.1   Quality-of-life dimensions.

From M. P. Lawton, 1983, *The Gerontologist, 23,* p. 355. Copyright 1983 by the Gerontological Society of America. Reproduced with permission.

affect, representing psychological well-being, are reflected in behaviors available for assessment by an objective observer. The person-centered abilities (physical, functional, and cognitive) inherent in the behavioral competence domain are readily available for assessment, along with the patient's time use and social behaviors. Lawton (1995) stated that quality of life is an appropriate organizing framework for AD patients, not only because of the ability to operationalize the major concepts with this population, but because of the relevance for both the patient and caregiver.

APPLICATION OF QUALITY-OF-LIFE DOMAINS

Lawton's (1995) conceptualization of quality of life serves as an appropriate basis from which to examine care issues for the AD patient. Using the three QOL components (psychological well-being, behavioral competence, and objective environment) applicable with late-stage AD patients, direction for person-centered care designed to maintain or improve quality of life becomes more evident. Each of the three components applicable to this patient population will be reviewed, providing caregivers with a theoretically driven and empirically supported basis from which to design effective care approaches.

PSYCHOLOGICAL WELL-BEING

Positive and negative affective states are the two major dimensions of psychological well-being. Interventions designed to increase positive affective states and decrease negative affective states will result in higher levels of psychological well-being. Activities and experiences available during the early stages of AD that positively impact on positive outcomes are no longer possible for patients in the later disease stages (DeJong, Osterlund, & Roy, 1989). Loss of autonomy, decreased interest in others and the external environment, impaired communication, and increased dependency on caregivers are changes that limit the interventions available to improve the patient's psychological well-being. However, other experiences still available to the late-stage AD patient that may impact on psychological well-being include pain or comfort experiences, need for positive stimulation (interpersonal and environmental), individualized touch experiences, amelioration of depressive states, and spiritual support.

Pain and Comfort States

Assessment of pain and comfort states in the late-stage AD patient has been a long-neglected area of concern. The assessment and treatment of discomfort and pain is very important and has become a focus for clinical research in recent years (Hurley, Volicer, Hanrahan, Houde, & Volicer, 1992; Parmalee, Smith, & Katz, 1993; Sengstaken & King, 1993). Sengstaken and King (1993) found that while chronic pain was common among nursing home residents, in contrast to communicative residents, noncommunicative residents were less likely to be identified by physicians as experiencing pain. Because verbal communication is significantly impaired in the late-stage AD patient, appropriate identification of pain expression can often be overlooked. Parmalee et al. (1993) examined observations of pain expressions in institutionalized patients and found that cognitively impaired patients report less intense pain and fewer localized complaints than do cognitively intact patients, especially at back and joint sites.

Expressions of pain have been observed consistently in AD patients, including late-stage patients, and entail grimacing and other specific facial expressions, verbal outbursts, increased restlessness and movement, and increased agitation (Hurley et al., 1992; Jansson, Norberg, Sandman, Athlin, & Asplund, 1993). These types of behaviors are often interpreted as disturbed, previously attributed to external factors and neurological pathology. Measures to assess expressions of discomfort are now available for use by caregivers, allowing for a more meaningful interpretation of disturbed behaviors and more appropriate treatment of discomfort states (Hurley et al., 1992). Education for both institutional and family caregivers is necessary to increase the understanding of the AD patient's expression of pain and utilization of available pain assessment tools, facilitating the appropriate interpretation of behavior and treatment of discomfort. Decreased discomfort states in the AD patient initially have been shown to increase the patient's positive affect, thus improving psychological well-being.

Behavioral Disturbance

Although loss of verbal communication ability during the later disease stages makes evaluation of the effect of interpersonal contact difficult at best, some studies suggest that AD patients remain responsive to positive interpersonal contacts and environmental stimulation (Albert, Cohen, & Koff, 1991; Burgener et al., 1992; Clair & Bernstein, 1990; Jansson et al., 1993; Smith, 1990; Wright, 1991). Albert et al. (1991) found no differences in AD patients at mild to moderate disease stages compared to persons without dementia in the ability to perceive emotions in the facial expressions of others, when outcomes were adjusted for degree of perceptual impairment. These findings are supported by a study by Burgener et al. (1990) in which significant correlations were found between the caregivers' smiling behaviors and the patient's calm/functional behaviors. In fact, the caregivers' smiling behaviors were found to be the most consistent predictors of functional patient behaviors. Other caregiver behaviors found to be related to calm/functional patient behaviors included use of a relaxed, flexible caregiver approach, attending to the patient's comfort, and use of distraction through small talk and social behaviors. Wright (1991), in her study of the effects of dementia on the marital relationship, found that patients, even in the later disease stages, responded positively to close spousal contacts characterized by interpersonal warmth.

These collective findings suggest that interventions to enhance positive interpersonal contacts will result in improved behavioral and affective outcomes for the AD patient. Personal contacts with the patient and caregiving experiences may be facilitated when institutional and family caregivers are aware of their own facial expressions and general approach to the patient. Using positive interpersonal behaviors such as a smiling expression, a relaxed and flexible approach, a gentle tone of voice, and an interpersonal, rather than task, orientation to the contact, should result in more positive patient behaviors and affect. This may require that caregivers become more aware of their own facial expressions and tone of voice, with deliberate use of smiling behaviors and a soft, gentle tone of voice, especially during stressful caregiving tasks, such as bathing and dressing. A relaxed, flexible approach may require the caregiver to resist rushing the patient through care tasks. A relaxed approach is facilitated by allowing adequate time to complete caregiving tasks and being willing to postpone or reschedule appointment times or other tasks if the caregiving episode requires more time than planned. Rushing the patient and remaining inflexible often results in a more resistive patient response, eliciting frustration for both patient and caregiver. Being more personal, even while completing a task, requires that the caregiver attend to the person rather than the task. A personal approach may include talking with the patient about his or her past, commenting on positive patient responses, or focusing on things in the environment known to be valued by the patient, such as family pictures. These combined caregiver behaviors may facilitate completion of a caregiving task by facilitating positive patient behaviors.

Individualized Touch Experiences

Although use of touch has been supported in the research literature as a positive interpersonal behavior with older adults (Hollinger, 1986; Langland & Panicucci, 1982), more recent studies have begun to raise questions about the positive effects of touch with late-stage dementia patients. Burgener (1989), in her study of institutionalized AD patients, found higher levels of functional patient behaviors when no touch was used in a caregiver/patient contact. In a later study, Burgener et al. (1992) observed varying patient responses to touch, with some patients responding positively to the use of interpersonal touch, whereas other patients avoided touch when possible. One patient became so upset when touched that his family consented to his participation in the study only if the researchers agreed he would not be touched during the study procedures. This patient spent much of his time with his arms crossed over his chest to protect himself from touch. Cohen-Mansfield and colleagues (Cohen-Mansfield, Werner, & Marx, 1990; Marx, Werner, & Cohen-Mansfield, 1989) found higher levels of screaming behaviors when touch was included as part of a caregiver/patient contact. Ryden, Bossemaier, and McAlchlan (1991) reported similar findings, with higher levels of agitated behaviors occurring with the presence of caregiver touch in institutional settings. In a contrasting case study report of four institutionalized AD patients in advanced disease stages, Jansson et al. (1993) reported more relaxed facial expressions and smiling behaviors in one patient when the caregiver caressed the patient's cheek with her hand. Because many of the AD patients in institutional settings are in the later disease stages, these findings suggest the effects of touch with institutionalized patients are varied and need to be evaluated individually with each patient and that touch cannot be assumed to consistently result in a positive patient experience.

It is important to note, however, that most studies of touch with AD patients have occurred in institutional settings with paid caregivers rather than family members. Wright (1991), in her study of the patient/ caregiver marital relationship in the home setting, found that AD patients, even in advanced disease stages, responded positively to touch by the spousal caregiver. It may be that a variety of factors that mediate the patient's responses to touch have not been systematically studied, such as the quality and type of relationship between the AD patient and caregiver, the type of touch used (comfort or interpersonal touch rather than procedural touch), the patient's level of agitation prior to the touch experience, and the patient's prior experiences with and attitudes toward touch. Although a great deal remains to be learned concerning the effects of touch and the AD patient, findings to date assist in alerting caregivers to the possible variety of patient responses. Institutional caregivers especially need to observe patients individually for positive or negative touch responses. As many of the studies have included patients at advanced disease stages, the importance of evaluating individual responses in patients with late-stage AD is well supported. Interpersonal touch may be a caregiver behavior that facilitates psychological well-being in some advanced AD patients, but not in others. A systematic evaluation of the effects of touch should be completed prior to inclusion of this interpersonal behavior into a caregiving routine. An individualized approach to the inclusion of touch can then be implemented, increasing the likelihood that patient/caregiver contacts will produce positive outcomes.

Spiritual Support

Although neglected in the research literature, spiritual support for the patient with advanced AD may provide a source of peace and comfort facilitative of positive patient states. In two related research reports, Burgener and colleagues (Burgener & Chiverton, 1994; Burgener, Shimer, & Murrell, 1993) reported findings concerning the responsiveness of patients to contacts concerned with understanding and meeting the patient's spiritual needs. In semi-structured interviews conducted in institutional settings with AD patients at mid- and late-disease stages, Burgener et al. (1993) reported the unexpected responsiveness of patients to questions concerning their spiritual needs. Patients often described how they continued to pray and read the Bible (although it is understood that comprehension is quite limited). The meaningfulness of prayer was especially evident, as some patients consistently described the content of their prayers, noting both in verbal and nonverbal expression the comfort they received from prayer. Jansson et al. (1993) found that sacred music produced an especially profound response in a patient with advanced AD. Results from a questionnaire assessing the need for spiritual support for family caregivers indicated that caregivers are often equally or even more concerned for spiritual support for patients (Burgener, 1994). One caregiver vividly described the neglect of the religious community for her mother, having written her off as a "victim" or "nonperson" once the dementia diagnosis was received. One caregiver reported that the only time his wife was verbally responsive was during church services, when she would recite familiar scriptures and sing hymns.

Although the real effects of spiritual support for the AD patient are difficult to assess, especially during the later disease stages, some evidence exists for the continued benefits of spiritual care. As religious experiences are a significant factor in contributing to psychological well-being for older nondemented persons, considering the enduring nature of the spiritual aspects of the person, it is quite possible that spiritual care of AD patients would positively impact on their psychological well-being as well. Interventions designed to facilitate spiritual care may be easy to implement, including planned prayer time, reading of familiar or comforting Bible passages, and visits from familiar clergy or religious associates. Especially if the AD patient had been active in religious activities prior to the disease, opportunities for these activities may provide fulfillment, considering the multiple losses inherent throughout the disease.

Treatment of Depressive States

Treatment of depressive disorders may be important to improve the psychological well-being of the late-stage AD patient. Although several studies have reported depression rates to be much higher (33% to 87%) in mildly impaired AD patients compared to severely impaired patients (12%), depression continues to be observed in this group (Merriam et al., 1988; Reifler, Larson, & Hanley, 1982). Reifler and Larson (1989) made the distinction between depression as a cause of dementia and depression as a complication of dementia, emphasizing that depression in AD is not solely an emotional disorder on which dementia is superimposed. They proposed that AD patients become increasingly depressed as they are faced with numerous losses, failure in self-care and functional ability, and loss of energy and interest in life. Furthermore, they found that psychological interventions were an important addition to pharmacological treatment, evidenced by the effectiveness of the placebo treatment in antidepressant clinical trials. Late-stage AD patients may benefit from continued assessment for depression, with psychological intervention remaining a treatment option. In support of the observations by Reifler and Larson concerning the effectiveness of psychological interventions, Burgener et al. (1993) found that even advanced AD patients seemed relieved to have someone talk with them about their emotional responses and impact of the disease on their life, especially if the focus of the intervention included positive aspects of coping with losses, rather than centering on the devastating effects of the disease. Attention to and treatment of depressive disorders in advanced AD patients has the potential to improve patient quality of life. A summary of specific dimensions of psychological well-being, including an overview of suggested interventions, is found in Table 5.1.

OBJECTIVE ENVIRONMENT

Various aspects of the patient's objective environment are included in Lawton's (1995) model as being relevant to quality of life. The environmental structure, including architectural features, are environmental aspects applicable to AD patients early in the disease process. As AD progresses and mobility diminishes, architectural features may be less important to the patient, whereas structure and other environmental aspects become more relevant. With disease progression, however, AD patients become less able to exert direct control over their environment, with caregivers becoming largely responsible for environmental quality. Personal aspects of the environment, such as friends, family pets, and familiar housing and neighborhoods, may remain important and comforting to AD patients in advanced disease stages, although subjective patient responses to these environmental aspects are often difficult to assess. The environmental factors that will be examined relevant to care of advanced AD patients that can be directly influenced by caregivers include use of music, structured care routines, facilitation of nonverbal communication, and interventions to facilitate a low-stimulus environment.

Use of Music

One environmental stimulation reported to increase positive affective and behavioral responses in late-stage AD patients is the use of music (Clair

TABLE 5.1   Summary of Quality-of-Life Domain: Psychological Well-Being

Patient experience	Intervention
Pain and comfort states	• Observe nonverbal pain expressions • Educate caregivers regarding patient's expressions of pain • Integrate pain assessment into caregiving routine
Positive stimulation	• Use positive facial expressions (smiling) and a calm tone of voice • Attend to patient when interacting • Remain flexible when giving care • Use distraction if patient becomes agitated • Maintain previous interpersonal behavior patterns as long as possible
Individual touch experiences	• Observe verbal and nonverbal responses to touch • Use procedural touch cautiously • Individualize use of touch based on patient response
Spiritual support	• Assess previous religious behaviors • Introduce planned spiritual support experiences, if appropriate, such as use of religious music, prayer, Bible readings, contact with clergy
Depressive states	• Assess for depression or sadness • Attempt to discuss the patient's feelings with him or her • Seek treatment if depression persists

& Bernstein, 1990; Jansson et al., 1993; Smith, 1990). In reporting responses to music experiences with two severely regressed AD patients, Norberg, Melin, and Asplund (1986) found that the patients responded more positively to music than to touch and object presentations. In a later study, Jansson et al. (1993) found facial expression to change in advanced AD patients when soft music was included in the environment, changing from disgust or anxiety to a calmer expression. Moaning behaviors were also reported to stop when music was introduced into the environment.

Smith (1990) reported the positive effects of music therapy to include stimulation, increased movement and word recall, and patient comfort. She concluded that music provides the AD patient with familiar and comforting stimulation while tapping the speech centers responsible for automatic language, possibly increasing verbal responses. Smith further suggested that music therapy provides caregivers, who often feel helpless during later disease stages, with a readily available intervention that may provide comfort to both patient and caregiver.

Incorporating soft music, especially music that was appreciated by the patient prior to the onset of dementia, may provide patients with advanced AD the opportunity for positive and familiar stimulation. The comforting effects of music have been observed by family caregivers in the home setting, easing the tension in often difficult situations, such as during eating and dressing tasks. Although music may not facilitate positive affective states in all patients, the use of calming music is an easy-to-implement intervention that may provide positive benefits for both patients and caregivers.

Standardized Care Routines

The maintenance of structured care routines facilitates continued patient involvement in care and decreased patient frustration (Burgener et al., 1992; Hall, Kirschling, & Todd, 1986). As memory and functional ability decline, purposeful activity becomes increasingly difficult for AD patients. Patients in advanced disease stages become more impaired in their ability to initiate meaningful behaviors, relying more on routinized behavioral responses and environmental cues. In both the home and institutional settings, caregivers have reported the benefits of keeping the patient's routine as consistent as possible. Following a familiar pattern of care prevents the patient from having to respond to change, promoting familiarity and more automatic responses. Because facilitation of patient self-care has been associated with calmer, more functional patient behaviors (Burgener et al., 1992; Teri, Borson, Kiyak, & Yamagishi, 1989), the facilitation of automatic responses and self-care in late-stage AD patients may result in positive patient outcomes.

Facilitation of Nonverbal Communication

The patient's ability to communicate verbally becomes dramatically impaired in the later stages of AD. Patients have been observed becoming increasingly agitated and frustrated as their verbal ability to respond to questions and commands becomes nonexistent. Nonverbal communication is often the only mechanism that can be used to obtain information regarding the patient's internal states. To decrease the patient's frustration in interacting with others and to improve the interpretation of patient needs, caregivers and patients may both benefit from the incorporation of nonverbal communication mechanisms into care. Jansson et al. (1993) described the caregivers' ability to meaningfully interpret the facial expressions of severely demented patients. They concluded that patients in advanced disease stages are capable of continuing personal experiences and of communicating these experiences to caregivers. Caregivers who are attentive to a patient's facial expressions may use the interpretation of these expressions to provide care that more appropriately meets the patient's needs. Easy-to-use devices, such as communication boards, have been found to facilitate care in both home and institutional settings (Burgener, Bakas, Murray, Dunahee, & Barton, in press). Patients in advanced AD stages are often able to point to an appropriate picture to convey information to the caregiver. Communication boards require little physical movement by the patient and can be keep at the patient's bedside to facilitate use.

Caregivers can also incorporate the use of hand movements and gestures into their care routines to facilitate patient understanding and response to requests. Although the patient may not be able to understand a verbal request, accompanying the request with the movement that demonstrates an appropriate response will increase the patient's understanding. These simple interventions and attention to a patient's nonverbal expressions may decrease the frustration often present during patient/caregiver interactions when verbal communication is primarily utilized to convey meanings. Improved communication and accurate interpretation of the patient's nonverbal expressions will facilitate appropriate responses, meeting patient needs.

Low-Stimulus Environment

One additional environmental mechanism to facilitate patient quality of life is maintenance of a low-stimulus environment (Hall & Buckwalter, 1987; Hall et al., 1986). As patient abilities diminish, environmental stimulation or "noise" becomes increasingly difficult to interpret, often precipitating catastrophic reactions, anxiety, or withdrawal. A low-stimulus environment is characterized by reduction in extraneous noise (e.g., telephones, loud talking, or dishes clanging), reduction of crowding or unfamiliar persons (usually no more than 3 to 4 persons in a room), and minimal use of misleading or distracting stimuli (e.g., mirrors or easily misinterpreted artwork) (Hall et al., 1986). Although a totally quiet environment may not present enough stimulation for patients at advanced disease stages, positive, calming environmental stimuli should be the goal of care. A balance between adequate stimulation to promote patient alertness while satisfying the need for sensory input and an overly stimulating environment that increases confusion and anxiety needs to be maintained. Modification of the environment through attention to and elimination or modification of high-stimulus activities can result in calmer, more purposeful patient involvement. Interventions facilitating patient quality of life through the objective environment are summarized in Table 5.2.

BEHAVIORAL COMPTENCE

The third component or domain of quality of life relevant to the late-stage AD patient is behavioral competence. Lawton (1995) conceptualized behavioral competence as including health, functional health, cognition, time use, and social behavior. Aspects of each behavioral competence component are organized from complex to simple, with less

TABLE 5.2   Summary of Quality-of-Life Domains: Objective Environment

Environmental modification	Intervention
Use of music	• Assess for individual responses to music • Use soft music intermittently, especially during difficult situations
Structural care routine	• Follow familiar pattern of care • Build care pattern around "routinized" behaviors
Facilitation of nonverbal communication	• Accompany verbal requests with nonverbal cues • Use communication board or other visual aids • Observe for patient's nonverbal cues
Low-stimulus environment	• Reduce extraneous noise • Reduce crowding and unfamiliar persons or objects in a room • Avoid misleading or distracting stimuli (such as mirrors)

complex aspects of behavioral competence being more accessible to the AD patient (see Figure 5.2).

Health

Health concerns are certainly relevant to the patient's quality of life; however, health aspects of care as defined within Lawton's (1995) model (physical aspects of the person) are generally managed by a supervising physician rather than a caregiver. Additionally, aggressive management of physical problems and disease during the very late stages of AD continue to be challenged, with the focus of care often being on comfort, representing a palliative care approach. This type of approach has been shown to significantly decrease the costs of patient care, while being associated with less patient discomfort (Volicer et al., 1994). As a palliative care approach becomes accepted as the standard of care for late-stage AD patients, the emphasis on aggressive treatment for physical disorders may diminish (Rhymes, 1994). This shifting emphasis makes recommendations regarding appropriate care approaches for treatment of physical health disorders more tenuous. However, although limited

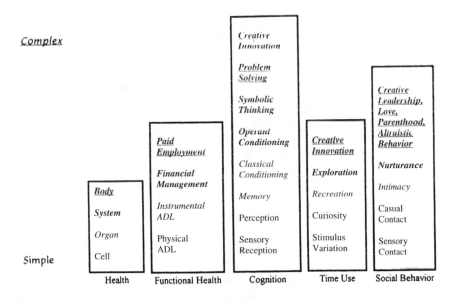

FIGURE 5.2   Hierarchy of behavioral competence.

From M. P. Lawton, 1983, *The Gerontologist, 23,* p. 355. Copyright 1983 by the Gerontological Society of America. Reproduced with permission.

by the patient's deteriorating function during later disease stages, interventions may be designed to facilitate quality of life outcomes with an emphasis on patient comfort.

Functional Health

During late-stage AD, aspects of functional health that remain available to the patient include only components of functional activities of daily living. Instrumental activities of daily living are no longer possible for the AD patient, with impairment being evident in many functional ADL behaviors as well. Because consistent relationships between the maintenance of self-care ability and functional patient behaviors are now being reported in the research literature, evidence is growing for the positive benefits of facilitating patient function in ADLs and self-care within the functional limitations of the late-stage AD patient (Burgener et al., 1992; Teri et al., 1989). Simplifying and breaking down tasks is one approach to facilitating the patient's functional self-care. Patients in advanced AD stages will not be able to complete a bathing or dressing task. However, they may be able to complete one small part of the task. In an observational study of patient responses during care procedures, Burgener et al. (1992) consistently noted calmer, more functional patient responses when patients were allowed to participate in care, even in a small way. One patient was observed becoming increasingly agitated during a bathing procedure. When the caregiver gave the patient a washcloth and allowed her to wash her face, the patient became immediately calmer and involved with the washing task. Patients with marked functional losses are often able to do very simple tasks, providing them with the opportunity to maintain some degree of functional ability, while preserving some sense of autonomy and personhood. Simplifying tasks and encouraging some degree of self-care has the added benefit of increasing patients' involvement in external events, preventing them from totally becoming a passive observer.

Simple interventions can be instituted to promote urinary and bowel continence during later disease stages. Providing a patient with cues for toileting, such as motion detector lights in bathrooms that light up automatically when the patient passes, will remind the patient where the bathroom is located and that toileting may be needed. Observation of other patient cues that toileting needs to occur, such as increased restlessness and agitation, will help prevent an incontinent episode. Although simplification of tasks and interventions to facilitate toileting behaviors may require creativity and some environmental adaptation, the outcomes of maintenance of optimal patient functioning, increased involvement in external events, and a sense of autonomy will justify the resources expended to facilitate patient functioning.

Cognition

Within the cognitive dimension, interventions utilized at earlier disease stages to promote or facilitate cognitive functioning are often not as effective or appropriate in later disease stages. Group interactions, structured recreational activities, and reminiscence therapy are often not possible or meaningful as the patient's disease progresses. As communication ability and mental alertness diminish, interventions described earlier to promote nonverbal communication may be useful resources to provide cognitive and sensory stimulation. Aspects of long-term memory may also be accessed through identification of the patient's past predominant skills and knowledge. AD patients, even in advanced stages of the disease, have been observed to retain predominant skills from previous, productive stages of their lives. During interviews with advanced AD patients, Burgener et al. (1992) learned that one patient had taught and spoken five languages during most of her adult years. After praising the patient on her past accomplishments, the patient then answered each of the researcher's questions in all five languages, making evident her retention of her language skills. Assessment of previous abilities and a focus on the retention of skills not only promotes cognitive functioning, but focuses care on the patient's abilities, rather than disabilities. Individualizing activities and interactions, based on the patient's previous predominant knowledge and skills, allows for a more meaningful use of time, while promoting cognitive function. Sensory stimulation, through use of environmental aids such as music, interpersonal or calming touch, and audiotapes of familiar persons, may also increase sensory reception, positively influencing cognitive stimulation and quality of life, as posited in Lawton's (1995) model.

Time Use and Social Behavior

The time-use and social-behavior dimensions of behavioral competence can be considered together, as the quality and quantity of social behavior directly influence the patient's use of time. Also, as the disease progresses, the patient loses the ability to control much of his or her time use, with caregivers and significant others contributing more to how the patient's time is structured. Maintaining past meaningful relationships especially becomes difficult as AD progresses. Family members and friends are often heard to say, "He/she doesn't even know who I am anymore, so there is no need to visit." Although patients often cannot correctly call a person by name or express their thoughts and feelings, evidence does exist for continued meaningful subjective experiences (Buckwalter et al., 1995; Burgener, et al., 1993; Jansson et al., 1993).

Loneliness is often evident in both facial expression and remaining verbal expression, with some patients becoming more animated and involved when talking about positive and familiar past experiences (Burgener et al., 1993). The inability to correctly call a family member or past acquaintance by name does not necessarily indicate the person is not familiar to the patient in other ways. Patients have often been observed to be calmer and more content following a visit by a familiar person, providing some indication of the meaningfulness of the visit and the positive use of the patient's time.

Even in late disease stages, patients express a need for "connecting with others," often observed as "calling out" or reaching for others. The continued support and expressions of caring from family and friends have the potential to positively affect a patient's social behavior, decreasing the patient's need to call out to others. Planned visits from family members and past acquaintances can help fill empty or lonely parts of the patient's day, providing the opportunity for meaningful sensory experiences. Caregivers can assist others in understanding that the lack of meaningful verbal response does not necessarily indicate the patient is not aware of or benefiting from the contact. As Wright (1991) noted in her study of the AD patient's marital relationship, continuing support and contact with family and loved ones can provide the quality of interaction necessary to facilitate the patient's quality of life. Table 5.3 summarizes interventions to assist meeting the patient's behavioral competence needs.

MEASUREMENT ISSUES IN ASSESSING QUALITY-OF-LIFE OUTCOMES

Although previously considered to be the proverbial "slippery noodle" in research with AD patients, progress has been made in recent years in the definition and measurement of quality-of-life outcomes with AD patients. Measurement issues are complicated somewhat with late-stage AD patients, however, due to the inability to consistently obtain meaningful verbal patient responses, posing a unique problem in defining outcome measures in accordance with the patient's perspective. As elucidated by Burgener and Chiverton (1994), positive outcomes have

TABLE 5.3   Summary of Quality-of-Life Domains: Behavioral Competence

Patient competence	Intervention
1. Health	• Provide palliative care interventions
2. Functional Health	• Simplify tasks to facilitate patient participation and self-care • Provide cues for toileting • Observe patient for signs of need to toilet
3. Cognition	• Assess for past predominant skills • Focus activities around retained skills • Provide familiar sensory stimulation
4. Time Use and Social Behavior	• Assist family/friends in understanding the patient's need for contact • Encourage visiting by close family members/friends

previously been defined from the caregiver's perspective of what is positive, reflecting a benefit more for the caregiver than the patient. For example, caregivers often define decreased wandering as being a positive patient outcome, when in fact no evidence exists for decreased wandering as being positive for the patient. Wandering may be troublesome or intolerable for the caregiver, but may actually be soothing to the patient as a means for stimulation and completing repetitive behaviors. The challenge for measuring quality of life outcomes for advanced AD patients then becomes the development and utilization of objective measures representing dimensions truly reflective of positive *patient* outcomes.

Lawton's (1995) quality-of-life model becomes especially helpful in defining appropriate outcome measures by defining components of QOL specifically relevant to the AD patient. In his article, Lawton described both new and well-established measures appropriate for operationalizing QOL components throughout the patient's disease process. The instruments described here, then, are limited to those instruments that are both most applicable to a patient in the later stages of AD and measure aspects of the patient's condition considered to be difficult to assess objectively, such as affect, discomfort, and general well-being.

PROGRESSIVE DETERIORATION SCALE

DeJong et al. (1989) described the development of the quality-of-life measure, the Progressive Deterioration Scale. This bipolar scale contains 27 items and is based on the same categories as the Global Deterioration Scale (Reisberg, Ferris, deLeon, & Crook, 1982), consisting of cognitive, ADL, incremental activities of daily living (IADL), and social behavior items. The scale was originally developed following open-ended interviews with AD patients' caregivers concerning their perceptions of how each patient's quality of life was affected by the disease process. The initial instrument was then further tested for validity and reliability with patients at varying stages of the disease process, including late-stage patients. Validity for the scale was supported by correlations with the Progressive Deterioration Scale and through its ability to distinguish between non-AD elders and AD patients with 95% accuracy. The scale was found to be useful in measuring QOL in late-stage AD patients, providing an objective indicator of overall QOL. The bipolar scale was relatively easy to administer, taking only approximately 10 to 15 minutes to complete. Although the scale does measure a relatively new domain, positive social behavior, the scale neglects to measure additional aspects of quality of life, such as affect, indicating one limitation of the measure as a comprehensive QOL indicator.

DISCOMFORT SCALE

A second measure that provides an indicator of the advanced AD patient's psychological well-being is the Discomfort Scale (Hurley et al., 1992). The scale contains nine behavioral descriptors rated on a 4-point, Likert-type scale from "no behavior exhibited" to "extensive behavior exhibited." Nine nurse experts reviewed the Discomfort Scale items for relevance, resulting in support for the scale's content validity and internal consistency. Factor analysis procedures revealed four categories of behavior embedded within the instrument: physical signs, vocalizations, facial expressions, and body language. The instrument's reliability with institutionalized, advanced dementia patients has received initial support. Ratings are made by an observer over a 5-minute period. One limitation of the Discomfort Scale is its emphasis on negative emotional states, thus not reflecting the range of emotional states possible in advanced AD patients.

CORNELL SCALE FOR DEPRESSION IN DEMENTIA

Another measure to operationalize psychological well-being in late-stage AD patients is the Cornell Scale for Depression in Dementia (CSDD) (Alexopoulos, Abrams, Young, & Shamoian, 1988). The CSDD is a 19-item instrument administered by a trained researcher or clinician. Items are rated on a four-choice response format: a = "unable to evaluate," 1 = "absent," 2 = "mild or intermittent," and 2 = "severe." The 19 items reflect five aspects of the patient's affective state: mood-related signs, behavioral disturbances, physical signs, cyclic functions, and ideational disturbances. Each item is rated by the caregiver and the clinician through an interview with the patient. If significant discrepancies appear in the ratings, the clinician interviews the caregiver to clarify the reason for the disagreement. Total administration time is approximately 30 minutes. The CSDD's reliability has been well supported with patients at various stages in the disease process. Internal consistency was also found to be adequate. Its validity was supported through its ability to distinguish demented patients with no depression, minor depression, probably major depression, and definite major depression in both hospitalized patients and nursing home residents. The scale provides an appropriate indicator of depressive states in advanced AD patients, making available meaningful interpretations of a patient's negative affect.

PSYCHOLOGICAL WELL-BEING IN COGNITIVELY IMPAIRED PERSONS

One newly developed, more global measure of well-being is the Psychological Well-Being in Cognitively Impaired Persons (PWB-CIP) measure. The PWB-CIP is a 16-item, observer-rated instrument developed specifically for use with AD patients at various stages of the disease process. It is based on the extensive work of Andrews and Withey (1976) on the measurement of well-being and the work of Lawton (1983, 1995) defining psychological well-being as consisting of positive and negative affect. The PWB-CIP represents positive and negative affective states and congruence between desired and attained goals, represented by congruence with the environment, which was described by Lawton (1983) as being central to psychological well-being. Additional items include the patient's ability to maintain interest in the environment. Half of the items represent a positive state of psychological well-being and the other half reflect a negative state of psychological well-being, with one additional item providing a global assessment of the patient's overall psychological well-being. The observer rates each item on a scale from 1 (never) to 4 (frequently), indicating how often the response or behavior was observed during the last 24 hours. A total PWB-CIP score is obtained by adding item ratings, with negative items being reverse-scored. Initial testing of the PWB-CIP's content validity is being carried out with national nursing experts in care of AD patients, with initial content validity scores being acceptable. The scale has been used by the nursing staff on one AD specialty unit and found to be an easy-to-administer indicator of a patient's general psychological well-being. Continued testing of the PWB-CIP is currently being carried out.

IMPLICATIONS FOR CARE OF ADVANCED AD PATIENTS

Caregivers in both home and institutional settings are often reported to feel helpless when designing effective care for AD patients in advanced disease stages. As a patient's cognitive, physical, and functional abilities deteriorate, caregivers often are at a loss to define positive ways to help maintain quality of life. Lawton's (1995) conceptualization of quality of life in AD patients appropriately defines QOL components within the reality of progressive dementia. Defining aspects of the person and environment relevant to quality of life with this population facilitates the development of interventions designed specifically to improve the overall condition of advanced AD patients. Although inherent in this discussion is the knowledge that all interventions will not be equally effective with all patients, providing both institutional and family caregivers with a variety of potential interventions increases the likelihood that effective approaches to care can be designed for individual patients. Although the universal nature of disease progression has been well documented, the unique abilities and characteristics of each AD patient make manifestation of the effects of AD unique for each person. While this uniqueness in patient responses makes global care recommendations difficult, becoming knowledgeable about and utilizing a variety of interventions will increase the likelihood that an effective care approach can be developed. Finding effective ways to increase the patient's quality of life, especially during the very limiting end stages of the disease, has the potential to significantly decrease the caregiver's frustration and feelings of helplessness.

Although continued study is necessary to explore some specific mechanisms to increase patient quality of life, such as assessment and treatment of discomfort and the effects of spiritual support on the patient, initial empirical support has been obtained for many of the suggested interventions. The development, testing, and application of interventions within this framework hold the potential of impacting positively on patient quality of life during the late stages of AD, an important outcome to both patients and caregivers.

REFERENCES

Albert, M. S., Cohen, C., & Koff, E. (1991). Perception of affect in patients with dementia of the Alzheimer's type. *Archives of Neurology, 48,* 791–795.

Alexopoulos, G. S., Abrams, R. C., Young, R. C., & Shamoian, C. A. (1988). Cornell scale for depression in dementia. *Biological Psychiatry, 23,* 271–284.

Andrews, F. M., & Withey, S. B. (1976). *Social indicators of well-being.* New York: Plenum Press.

Buckwalter, K. C., Gerdner, L. A., Hall, G. R., Stolley, J. M., Kudart, P., & Ridgeway, S. (in press). Shining through: The humor and individuality of persons with Alzheimer's disease. *Journal of Gerontological Nursing, 21*(3), 11–16.

Burgener, S. (1989). *Communicating with residents with Alzheimer's dementia: A study of nurse/resident interactive behavior.* Unpublished doctoral dissertation, Wayne State University, Detroit.

Burgener, S. C. (1994). Caregiver religiosity and well-being in dealing with Alzheimer's dementia. *Journal of Religion and Health, 33,* 175–189.

Burgener, S. C., Bakas, T., Murray, C., Dunahee, J. A., & Barton, D. (in press). Effective caregiving approaches with Alzheimer's patients. *Geriatric Nursing.*

Burgener, S. C., & Chiverton, P. (1994). Conceptualizing psychological well being in cognitively impaired older persons. Image: Journal of Nursing Scholarship. 24, 209–213.

Burgener, S., Jirovec, M., Murrell, L., & Barton, D. (1992). Caregiver and environmental variables related to difficult behaviors in institutionalized, demented elderly persons. *Journal of Gerontology, 47,* P242–P249.

Burgener, S., Shimer, R., & Murrell, L. (1993). Expressions of individuality in cognitively impaired elders: The need for individual assessment and approaches to care. *Journal of Gerontological Nursing, 19*(4), 13–22.

Butler, R. N. (1992). Quality of life: Can it be an endpoint? How can it be measured? *American Journal of Clinical Nutrition, 55,* 1267S–1270S.

Campbell, A., Converse, P., & Rodgers, W. (1976). *The quality of American life.* New York: Russell Sage Foundation.

Clair, A. A., & Bernstein, B. (1990). A preliminary study of music therapy programming for severely regressed persons with Alzheimer's-type dementia. *The Journal of Applied Gerontology, 9,* 299–311.

Cohen, C. (1982). On the quality of life: Some philosophical reflections. *Circulation, 66,* 111–129.

Cohen-Mansfield, J., Werner, P., & Marx, M. S. (1990). Screaming in nursing home residents. *Journal of the American Geriatrics Society, 38,* 785–792.

Cotrell, V., & Schulz, R. (1993). The perspective of the patient with Alzheimer's disease: A neglected dimension of dementia research. *Gerontologist, 33,* 305–311.

DeJong, R., Osterlund, O. W., & Roy, G. W. (1989). Measurement of quality-of-life changes in patients with Alzheimer's disease. *Clinical Therapeutics, 11,* 545–554.

Duffy, L. M., Hepburn, K., Christensen, R., & Brugge-Wiger, P. (1989). A research agenda in care for patients with Alzheimer's disease. *Image: Journal of Nursing Scholarship, 21,* 254–257.

Ferrans, C. E., & Powers, M. J. (1985). Quality of life index: Development and psychometric properties. *Advances in Nursing Science, 6,* 15–24.

Hall, G. R., & Buckwalter, K. B. (1987). Progressively lowered stress threshold: A conceptual model for care of adults with Alzheimer's dementia. *Archives of Psychiatric Nursing, 1,* 399–406.

Hall, G., Kirschling, M. V., & Todd, S. (1986). Sheltered freedom: An Alzheimer's unit in an ICF. *Geriatric Nursing, 8*(3), 132–137.

Hollinger, L. M. (1986). Communicating with the elderly. *Journal of Gerontological Nursing, 12,* 9–13.

Hughes, C. P., Berg L., Danziger, W. L., Cohen, L. A., & Martin, R. L. (1982). A new clinical scale for staging of dementia. *British Journal of Psychiatry, 140,* 566–572.

Hurley, A. C., Volicer, B. J., Hanrahan, P. A., Houde, S., & Volicer, L. (1992). Assessment of discomfort in advanced Alzheimer patients. *Research in Nursing and Health, 15,* 369–377.

Jansson, L., Norberg, A., Sandman, P. O., Athlin, E., & Asplund, K. (1993). Interpreting facial expressions in patients in the terminal stage of the Alzheimer's disease. *Omega, 26,* 309–324.

Langland, R. M., & Panicucci, C. L. (1982). Effects of touch on communication with elderly confused clients. *Journal of Gerontological Nursing, 11,* 10–14.

Lawton, M. P. (1983). The dimensions of well being. *Experimental Aging Research, 9,* 65–72.

Lawton M. P. (1995). Quality of life in Alzheimer's disease. *Alzheimer's Disease and Associated Disorders, 8*(Suppl. 3), 138–150.

Lyman, K. (1989). Bringing the social back in: A critique of the biomedicalization of dementia. *Gerontologist, 29,* 597–605.

Marx, M. S., Werner, P., & Cohen-Mansfield, J. (1989). Agitation and touch in the nursing home. *Psychological Reports, 64,* 1019–1026.

Meddaugh, D. I. (1990). Reactance: Understanding aggressive behavior in long-term care. *Journal of Psychosocial Reports, 28,* 28–33.

Merriam, A. E., Aronson, M. K., Gaston, P., Wey, S. L., & Katz, I. (1988). The psychiatric symptoms of Alzheimer's disease. *Journal of the American Geriatrics Society, 36,* 7–12.

Norberg, A., Melin, E., & Asplund, K. (1986). Reactions to music, touch, and object presentation in the final stage of dementia: An exploratory study. *International Journal of Nursing Studies, 23,* 315–323.

Parmalee, P. A., Smith, B., & Katz, I. R. (1993). Pain complaints and cognitive status among elderly institution residents. *Journal of the American Geriatrics Society, 41,* 517–522.

Pearson, J. L., Teri, L., Reifler, B. V., & Raskind, M. A. (1989). Functional status and cognitive impairment in Alzheimer's patients with and without depression. *Journal of the American Geriatrics Society, 37,* 1117–1121.

Reifler, B. V., & Larson, E. (1989). Excess disability in dementia of the Alzheimer's types. In Light, E. & Leibowitz, B. (Eds.) *Alzheimer's disease treatment and family stress: Directions for research* (pp. 363–382). Rockville, MD: National Institute of Mental Health.

Reifler, B. V., Larson, E., & Hanley, R. (1982). Coexistence of cognitive impairment and depression in geriatric outpatients. *American Journal of Psychiatry, 139,* 623–626.

Reisberg, B., Ferris, S. H., deLeon, M. J., & Crook, T. (1982). The Global Deterioration Scale (GDS): An instrument for assessment of primary degenerative dementia. *American Journal of Psychiatry, 139,* 1136–1139.

Rhymes, J. A. (1994). Nonaggressive management of the illnesses of severely demented patients: An ethical justification. *Journal of the American Geriatrics Society, 42,* 686–687.

Ryden, M. B., Bossemaier, M., & McAlchlan, C. (1991). Aggressive behavior in cognitively impaired nursing home residents. *Research in Nursing and Health, 14,* 87–95.

Sengstaken, E. A., & King, S. A. (1993). The problems of pain and its detection among geriatric nursing home residents. *Journal of the American Geriatrics Society, 11,* 541–544

Smith, S. (1990). The unique power of music therapy benefits in Alzheimer's patients. *Activities, Adaptation, and Aging, 14,* 59–63.

Stoll B. (1977). *Breast cancer management.* London: Heinemann.

Teri, L., Borson, S., Kiyak, A., & Yamagishi, M. (1989). Behavioral disturbance, cognitive dysfunction, and functional skill: Prevalence and relationship in Alzheimer's disease. *Journal of the American Geriatrics Society, 37,* 109–116.

Volicer, L., Collard, A., Hurley, A., Bishop, C., Kern, D., & Karon, S. (1994). Impact of special care unit for patients with advanced Alzheimer's disease on patients' discomfort and costs. *Journal of the American Geriatrics Society, 42,* 597–603.

Wright, L. (1991). The impact of Alzheimer's disease on the marital relationship. *Gerontologist, 31,* 224–237.

Young, K. J., & Longman, A. J. (1983). Quality of life and persons with melanoma: A pilot study. *Cancer Nursing, 6,* 219–225.

PART TWO

Ethical Issues

The Moral Basis for Limiting Treatment: Hospice Care and Advanced Progressive Dementia

Stephen G. Post and Peter J. Whitehouse

As mentioned in the introduction, the modern hospice movement began in the late 1960s from a moral imperative to meet the needs of those terminally ill and close to death. Hospice care is morally shaped by the principle of beneficence in serving the needs of the dying, by "do no harm" in precluding burdensome treatments, and by autonomy in respecting the choices of patients. There are few better examples of implemented beneficence than the well-known St. Christopher's Hospital in London, established in 1966 by Cicely Saunders, M.D. (Stoddard, 1990). The British success, coupled with the research of Elisabeth Kübler-Ross on the experience of dying people (Kübler-Ross, 1969), gave rise to the American hospice movement in the mid 1970s. There are now several thousand hospices and many more hospice services in the United States addressing the needs of predominantly cancer patients and, in much lower numbers, AIDS and cardiac patients. With exceptions, Alzheimer patients have been denied access to hospice care in the past, although this is changing.

Denial of access, however, can be misunderstood. Hospice care is not best defined as a locus, since such care can be provided in hospitals, residences, and nursing homes as well as in hospice centers. In selecting hospice care, a person decides on a philosophy of care emphasizing comfort and quality of life in contrast to life prolongation except as a side effect of palliative treatments. This philosophy can be chosen and implemented in a wide variety of settings, usually with the help of a hospice team. The hospice model provides a liberation from aggressive medical technologies that too often hold people captive or undermine dignity. The hospice philosophy rests on the commitment to removing suffering rather than removing the sufferer, and is therefore to be contrasted with assisted suicide and euthanasia.

People with end-stage Alzheimer's disease (AD) or other progressive dementias have not readily fit the hospice mold for several reasons. First, such a person will ordinarily lack the decision-making competence to select hospice care except precedently by advance directive and will have less cognitive capacity in such a setting than will most cancer patients. Second, many hospices only admit patients who are likely to die within 6 months. Medicare still requires this as a condition for payment, although this policy may be revised. A new model predicts the likelihood of dying within 6 months following the onset of a fever in people with advanced Alzheimer's disease. Used in combination with clinical judgment, this can indicate patients for Medicare hospice coverage under current restriction (Volicer et al., 1993). Finally, hospice care is renowned for effective pain management through a combination of therapies. Patients with end-stage AD often are thought to be free from pain, in contrast to cancer patients. But there is more pain and discomfort in these patients than might otherwise be supposed, and there are ways in which they can be made more comfortable by properly trained hospice personnel familiar with AD.

A hospice approach is increasingly considered highly appropriate for the care of people with advanced dementia (Fabiszewski, Volicer, & Volicer, 1990). A significant majority of physicians (61%) affiliated with the American Geriatrics Society, as well as of family caregivers (71%) associated with the Alzheimer's Association, favor hospice care in cases of end-stage dementia (Luchins & Hanrahan, 1993). For many people with severe dementia who lack insight into their surroundings and the intentions of others, aggressive medical interventions can be interpreted as torturous, violating the principle of "do no harm" (Rango, 1985).

In this chapter, we place the hospice option for end-stage AD patients in the context of two moral debates, that is, the distinction between killing and letting die, and the moral significance of quality of life with regard to treatment limitations. Although our discussion of the first debate inevitably addresses the problem of pain, it is directly applicable to the added problem of diminished mental capacity typical of progressive dementia. A final section discusses clinical ethics and hospice care for end-stage AD patients. Throughout, we attempt to constructively connect literature in hospice ethics and dementia ethics.

THE MORAL DISTINCTION BETWEEN KILLING AND LETTING DIE

Hospice care calls a halt to the momentum of invasive technologies, although it is on the cutting edge of advances in palliative care. This resistance to the grip of technologies disturbs medical vitalists, who would do everything that can be done to keep alive even the smallest fraction of human life no matter how neurologically devastated. It also disturbs those holding to the characteristically American assumption that anything but the most technologically aggressive treatment is a step down from the "best" medical care.

From the opposite side, proponents of assisted suicide or mercy killing are critical of hospice care for not going far enough in those cases where comfort cannot be accomplished without the loss of mental lucidity. They argue that hospice rejection of assisted suicide fails to serve the needs of some patients.

Both vitalists and proponents of assisted suicide, then, believe that hospice care is problematic. For the vitalist, hospice care errs in accepting death, whereas for suicide proponents it errs in not accepting killing. We think, however, that hospice care offers the right options for those with end-stage AD. To keep a patient with advanced dementia comfortable requires neither causing death by human hands nor striving for prolongation. Euthanasia (mercy killing) is not a desirable option because of the possibilities for abuse, and because it confuses the identity of the physician as healer (Kass, 1985). One example of such abuse involves four Austrian nursing aides, who allegedly killed 49 elderly demented residents in a long-term care setting (Protzman, 1989). One aide was quoted by police as saying, "The ones who got on my nerves were dispatched directly to a free bed with the Lord."

Although treatment refusal or withdrawal was deeply controversial in the 1970s, it is now commonplace. This dramatic sea of change in American medical ethics is partly due to paradigm cases such as that of Karen Ann Quinlin (*In re Quinlan,* 1975), in which removal of ventilator support was first legally permitted, and also to ground gained by hospice philosophy. Hospice care has resisted the further move to suicide and mercy killing because good hospice care eliminates the need for these options in almost all cases. In addition, removal of the sufferer by killing would remove the need for such care, or so what we shall call the "incompatibility thesis" would suggest.

INCOMPATIBILITY

The incompatibility thesis states that where health care systems do not already provide adequate hospice care, legalization of assisted suicide or voluntary euthanasia may preempt development of such care. The thesis has at least surface plausibility. After all, if the removal of the sufferer is legal, where is the impetus for the development of alternative approaches to the problem of pain or diminished quality of life in dementia? Over the last century, the prohibition on assisted suicide and voluntary euthanasia has formed the cultural background necessary for biomedical advances in hospice care and, to an extent, for good long-term care. This background ought not to be easily reversed.

Incompatibility has been a minor premise of some arguments against assisted suicide and euthanasia. But it is seldom afforded centrality because advocates for these practices tend to provide an analysis focused on individual rights. Moreover, giving credence to incompatibility suggests a sacrifice of the immediate freedom of individuals to request assisted death, thereby holding them in the grip of a concern about the hypothetical future health care system.

Critics of incompatibility can argue by analogy that acceptance of the right to withdraw or withhold life-sustaining therapy did not preclude the development of new and more advanced therapies; indeed, these technologies continue to develop at a fast pace and resources are invested in them. Nor has preventive care diminished support for basic research and high-technology management of various illnesses. Therefore, it is mistaken to assert simplistically that legalization of assisted suicide and euthanasia will hamper development of comfort care. It will be important to observe the Netherlands, where interest in hospice care may or may not be compromised by the availability of assisted suicide and euthanasia.

It may also be argued that in any case, the incompatibility thesis is dependent on contextual factors, including political and cultural pressures, the interests of researchers, and the activism of patients, risk groups, and family members. For example, were preemptive assisted suicide for people with progressive dementia legalized, it is likely that advocacy groups such as the Alzheimer's Association would still press for better long-term care and basic research.

It is not possible to prove or disprove the incompatibility thesis because it remains hypothetical. But cautious observers—including the authors of this chapter—would prefer the development of more hospice care support and facilities for people with AD to the quicker and cheaper option of senicide (Post, 1990). There are some within the hospice movement who would be willing to add assisted suicide as an option, but for people with late-stage AD, assisted suicide is impossible. The more cautious will emphasize that what progress has been made to date in comfort care and advanced palliative technology is due to the grip of prohibition. Susan M. Wolf, for example, stated: "It is not a new claim that rejecting euthanasia has forced us, and continues to force us, on how to supply palliative care and pain relief expertly" (Wolf, 1989, p. 15). This rejection has spurred biomedicine to develop the palliative and hospice care that, if properly applied, can usually make an otherwise intolerable dying tolerable.

Translated into health care policy, because the U.S. health care system has not adequately attended to the art of hospice care, the incompatibility thesis indicates that states should proceed with great care, if at all, with referendums on assisted suicide or voluntary euthanasia (Cleeland et al, 1994).

If assisted suicide or voluntary euthanasia is implemented in the absence of a fully adequate comfort care system, the following may occur: (1) funds may be diverted from hospice care; (2) the training of physicians, nurses, and others may be undermined; and (3) research in comfort care may be cut back.

HOSPICE VIEWS

Hospice opposition to assisted suicide and euthanasia may be criticized as somewhat of a dogmatic orthodoxy that palliation and comfort care are the best roads to death, and that all else is heresy. Hospice workers appear to be motivated by moral idealism, and their concern with incompatibility has an integrity grounded in the successful experience of comforting the dying. However, as more profit-making enterprises enter the hospice field, financial incentives may undermine orthodoxy.

Robert J. Miller wrote, "The basic principles of modern pain control have been developed out of the hospice experience" (Miller, 1992). He described the hospice movement's commitment to patient autonomy, which includes choices regarding the removal of artificial nutrition and hydration as well as any and all other treatments unrelated to palliation. However, this commitment exists within a context of an overriding choice for comfort rather than assisted suicide or euthanasia. Miller's survey of hospice staff (including nurses, physicians, administrators, social workers, and volunteers) indicates that only 5% favor assisted suicide, and only 1.5% favor mercy killing; 55% to 65% of respondents in public opinion surveys favor these options. Miller observed: "Those most in a position to see the daily degree of suffering of the dying, and most in a position to act on it [the nurses and doctors] were the least likely to agree to perform such acts" (p. 131). The major reason for this opposition was that it would "divert attention away from efforts to provide optimal palliation and more appropriate and compassionate terminal care (p. 131)." This concern with diversion can be identified with the incompatibility thesis.

David Cundiff is a representative hospice physician who has written against assisted suicide and voluntary euthanasia. Cundiff (1992) contrasted assisted suicide with the routine practices of treatment refusal or withdrawal upon request. He cited polls of cancer specialists indicating that requests for assisted suicide are very uncommon. Those requests that Cundiff himself heard stemmed from poor pain control and/ or inadequate psychosocial support. Those who made requests "almost always changed their minds once their physical symptoms [were] controlled and they [were] placed in a caring, supportive, hospice environment" (p. 87). Cundiff's thesis was that "vastly improved hospice training for health care professionals, along with better quality and greater availability of hospice services, can render the issues of euthanasia and assisted suicide essentially moot." Cundiff can be contrasted with Timothy E. Quill, another physician who has years of hospice experience and who represents a small but perhaps increasingly influential minority among hospice caregivers. Quill has evolved from an initial endorsement of assisted suicide unconcerned with incompatibility to a support for both assisted suicide and voluntary euthanasia that is clearly haunted by incompatibility. Writing influential guidelines on assisted suicide in 1992, Quill, Christine K. Cassel, and Diane E. Meier mentioned their concern for better palliation and comfort care, acknowledging that this care in almost all cases results in a tolerable death. They defended assisted suicide only so long as the alternatives have "at least been considered, and preferably have been tried" (Quill, Cassel, & Meier, 1992, p. 138).

In contrast, the major 1994 guidelines proposed for regulating "physician-assisted death," written by Quill and Meier, among others, elevated the incompatibility thesis. These differed from earlier guidelines by including support for euthanasia and for the inclusion of patients with other than terminal illnesses (e.g., patients with multiple sclerosis). Importantly for this discussion, comfort care is considered a required treatment before the "assisted death" option is allowed (Miller et al., 1994). Supreme moral authority is placed in "certified palliative-care consultants," who would be given the power to "override agreements by patients and physicians to undertake physician-assisted death"(Quill et al., 1992, p. 138). Palliative care committees would function to refine policy guidelines and promote good palliation, retrospectively monitor cases of physician-assisted death, and negotiate cases in which palliative-care consultants and patients and/or their primary care physicians are at odds.

Such a multilayered and complex process would serve to reduce hasty action and errors in judgment, although patient autonomy and the physician–patient dyad pay a heavy price to a new bureaucracy. The authors acknowledge that such cautious regulation goes far beyond the various initiatives being proposed in some states, and contrasts with policies in the Netherlands.

This considerable development between the 1992 (Quill, Cassel, & Meier, 1992) and the 1994 (Miller, Quill, Brody, Fletcher, Gostin, & Meier, 1994) guidelines indicates an evolution in Quill's thought. The movement from assisted suicide for the terminally ill requiring no efforts at comfort care to assisted death for the chronically debilitated and terminally ill with mandated comfort care is significant and cautious. In our view, the 1994 guidelines are preferable with regard to the use of comfort care. While palliative care committees would be cumbersome, the requirement of comfort care would have the effect of enhancing expertise regarding and resource commitment to palliative measures. An assisted death that exhausts all means of comfort care is more respectful of the sanctity of human life than one that does not.

Long-Term Care

While pain is usually controllable in the hospice context for cancer patients and others, what of those who face the loss of memory and perhaps of their self-identity? AD is a significant topic in the international debate over physician-assisted suicide. Even though hospice care is offered to some severely demented AD patients, preemptive assisted suicide in response to neurodegeneration is desired by some.

Reports consistently indicate that in the Netherlands, where assisted suicide and mercy killing are accepted, about 10% of requests come from patients with chronic degenerative neurological disorders, even though Netherlands health system provides ample palliative and long-term care (de Wachter, 1992). Margaret P. Battin wrote of progressive dementia: "This is the condition the Dutch call *entluistering,* the 'effacement' or complete eclipse of human personality, and for the Dutch, *entluistering* rather than pain is a primary reason for choices of [active] euthanasia" (Battin, 1992, p. 120). Battin herself made some defense of assisted suicide or mercy killing in cases of progressive dementia if requested by a living will or by personal directive.

In 1990, Dr. Jack Kevorkian assisted AD patient Janet Adkins in suicide. The 54-year-old member of the Hemlock Society was happily married with three grown sons, intellectually very active, and horrified by the prospects of decline. When her symptoms worsened, assisted suicide soon followed. While many would not accept such an early preemptive suicide as morally justifiable, it is also possible that many members of our society would prefer suicide to advanced dementia. People justifiably fear progressive neurodegenerative diseases that devastate selfhood (Post, 1993; Rohde, Peskind, & Raskind, 1995).

The incompatibility thesis is worthy of discussion in the context of dementia. It is hard to imagine that the availability of physician-assisted death would hinder research efforts to find a cure for AD. But should assisted suicide and euthanasia be legally permitted before good AD special care and hospice programs are developed to enable patients to better adapt to their incapacities? Despite the efforts of AD-advocacy groups, will society invest in expensive special care units and hospice designs for people with dementia when assisted suicide or voluntary euthanasia are already available and much cheaper? Possibly not.

QUALITY OF LIFE AND TREATMENT LIMITATIONS

What are the morally appropriate levels of life-extending medical treatment for patients in the advanced stages of progressive and eventually fatal dementia such as AD? The response to this question requires some general reference to "quality of life" or else a rejection of qualitative judgments in favor of a vitalistic philosophy demanding aggressive efforts to extend life no matter how poor its quality. Quality of life can be defined in terms of capacities to make judgments and solve problems; to remember recent events; to remember past events; to handle business, financial, and/or social affairs; to pursue hobbies and interests; to form and maintain relationships with others; to recognize close family members or friends; to experience emotions; to recognize oneself; to plan for the future; to eat; to control bladder and bowel; and to communicate through speech. The fact that all of these capacities may eventually be lost to severe dementia explains why people fear Alzheimer's disease as much as or more than terminal cancer or other diseases that leave self-identity intact.

There are valid cautions about using quality of life as an indicator of appropriate treatment levels. First, quality of life is partly contingent on the extent to which a supportive environment is created to enhance well-being; it is a self-fulfilling prophecy since quality of life is dependent in crucial ways on the attitudes and actions of caregivers. Second, a valid qualitative measure of a patient's internal experience is impossible; quality of life has a subjective aspect that no outward observer can fully assess. Finally, the assessment of poor quality of life might be misused to rid society of unproductive members.

Still, in clinical discussions with patients regarding treatment limitation, or with patient surrogates, reference to quality of life is not uncommon. This is especially so when AD reaches its end-stage.

It is due to a wide disparity of perspective regarding quality of life that within the medical community "consensus breaks down when the attempt is made to determine the nature of the therapeutic obligation to the demented patient, particularly with respect to life-sustaining treatment" (Rango, 1985). Volicer (1986) detected a lack of consensus among health care professionals regarding patients in the persistent vegetative state and in advanced dementia.

In a 1991 cross-national empirical study of physicians' attitudes toward life-extending treatment interventions in cases of elderly people with severe dementia, considerable disagreement was evident (Alemayehu et al., 1991). The authors prepared a questionnaire asking "What decisions would physicians make when confronted with a critically ill, demented elderly man?" They presented the case of an 82-year-old man with life-threatening gastrointestinal bleeding who 3 years earlier had been diagnosed by a neurologist as suffering from probable AD. The patient could not answer a simple question coherently but seemed to understand some simple commands. His behavior was agitated, he wandered, did not recognize his daughter, and had urinary incontinence. In seven countries, physicians in academic medical centers at family practice, internal medicine, and geriatric rounds were questioned about their views on treatment levels. The authors concluded that there is a wide variation of opinion both within and among countries. For example, only 6% of Australian physicians recommended treatment in a medical intensive care unit, whereas 32% of U.S. physicians did so. Conversely, 21% of Australian physicians chose supportive care, compared to only 3% of U.S. physicians. The variation that this study found is difficult to interpret.

The concept of quality of life is extremely complex because of the objective–subjective axis (external observations vs. internal self-perceptions) (Birren & Dieckmann, 1991; Walter & Shannon, 1990). Several philosophers have argued that as dementia progresses in severity, only supportive care is morally fitting. Brock (1988) asked, What health care and expenditure of resources on health care are owed on grounds of justice to the severely demented elderly? He concentrated on the effects of dementia such as the erosion of memory and other cognitive functions that "ultimately destroy personal identity." This loss implies, for Brock, that the "severely demented have lost an interest in treatment whose ultimate purpose is to prolong or sustain lives" (p. 89). They retain, however, an interest in comfort, so that a painful tumor might be removed for palliative reasons.

Callahan (1987) pointed out that for the patient who is severely demented, "On the one hand, he has lost his capacity for reason and usually—but not always—human interaction. On the other hand, there will be no clear ground for believing that the capacity to experience emotions has been lost" (p. 183). Callahan's conclusion is that "death need not be resisted."

As early as 1976, Robert Katzman wrote: "In focusing attention on the mortality associated with Alzheimer disease, our goal is not to find a way to prolong the life of severely demented persons . . . " (p. 217). Our concern is with the loss of relational capacity and self-identity, both critical determinants of quality of life. Since the severity of progressive dementia occurs on a continuum, there are morally significant thresholds such as when the patient becomes mute and lacks all interactive capacities or no longer recognizes loved ones. These thresholds will not be reached synchronously, but together represent an objective loss of relational potential. Loved ones will often state that the patient is "no longer there." When these points are arrived at, has the meaning and substance of human life deteriorated to the extent that the use of medical technologies for nonpalliative reasons becomes morally questionable? In neonatal intensive care units, infant life is saved in the hope that some capacity for interaction will emerge. In the case of advanced progressive dementia, there is no such hope.

A less relational view of quality of life might attribute higher value to the inner experiences of the self despite the fact of relational loss, or suggest that more self-identity may still be present in the patient than meets the eye. Patients with severe dementia can demonstrate underlying affective responses and some self-identity may remain. But in the profound and terminal stages, there is no discernible self-identity remaining. It is very unlikely that self-identity is maintained; the appearances of loss cannot be explained as a deterioration in communicative abilities alone.

Unaware of environment, mute, bedridden, incontinent of bladder and bowel, with unmeasurable intellectual functions, and with death inevitable, comfort care is often all that medicine should offer. Comfort care means palliation only; it excludes artificial nutrition and hydration, dialysis, and all other medical interventions unless necessary for the control of pain and discomfort. Some treatments, for example, antibiotics, can be intended for palliation and comfort care but will extend life as an unintended side effect. The principle of comfort care only should not be imposed on patients who still evidence a degree of relational capacity and self-identity (Arras, 1988).

END-STAGE AD AND HOSPICE CARE: CLINICAL ETHICS

In this section, we offer guidelines to clinicians for applying the principles discussed earlier to the actual care of patients and families. We review attitudes and knowledge necessary to provide excellent care for dying patients with dementia. The care of patients with dementia is complex, making interdisciplinary teams a common practice.

Some clinicians recognize that they have neither the skills nor the interest to care for these chronic diseases and arrange for appropriate referral to other professionals. With regard to caring for dying patients with or without dementia, clinicians must develop a sense of their own attitudes toward death and decide whether or not this is a clinical activity for them. A knowledge of the psychology of death, that is, how people construct models of death and the dying process and deal with death anxiety, is essential if a clinician is to care for patients dying with dementia (Kastenbaum, 1992). Outlines of educational curricula for the medical treatment of the care of the terminally ill have been published that allow clinicians to compare their own knowledge base with common standards of practice (Schonwetter & Robinson, 1994). Clinicians must develop a knowledge of social and cultural diversity in attitudes toward death, learn about policies that might affect their ability to provide care, and strive to be informed about the natural history of end-stage dementia and technology that can be associated with dying.

The first aspect of good care is early planning based on a well-established relationship with the family. A discussion of death should not be left until the dying process is well advanced, particularly in the case of the patient with dementia who may lose the ability to participate in a dialogue concerning planning later in the course of the illness. Advance directives should be discussed and prepared that communicate desires for and limitations on care at the end of life (Emmanuel & Emmanuel, 1989). Individuals should be identified who will make surrogate decisions if necessary (e.g., by creating a durable power of attorney). The clinician should be aware of some of the conceptual issues concerning the difficulties of having a mildly demented (or nondemented) self plan for care of a future severely demented self (Dresser & Whitehouse, 1994; Dworkin, 1993). The clinician must realize that advance directives have a mixed record of impact on the actual provision of care, especially when they are not made available to all clinicians at all sites caring for the patient.

Furthermore, it is important that family members participate in the process as much as is appropriate. When death approaches, it is not helpful to have distant family members unaware of any previous discussions enter into the dialogue to disrupt the agreed-upon ways of proceeding. The clinician should bring to the attention of family members educational material designed to help families consider these difficult issues of terminal care.

It is important that health care education associations provide information pointing out the clinical and moral rationale for hospice care in the end-stage of AD, thereby assuring families that the choice of this level of care is acceptable and reasonable. Hospice care is a pathway that should be widely sanctioned by advocacy groups and health care professionals. Clinicians should learn about the diverse factors influencing decision-making concerning the end of life. Individuals affected by AD may have different levels of knowledge and anxiety about death and dying; they may be informed by various religious and cultural traditions of the family that need to be considered. The clinician must be aware of policies in existence in different health care environments. For example, some nursing homes may have written or unwritten policies that limit choice. The patient and his or her family must inquire as to the policies and procedures followed in different institutions in which the patient may be placed. State and federal regulation can limit options in preparing for death (e.g., in the area of artificial nutrition and hydration).

Health Care Financing Administration rules determine who is eligible to receive reimbursement for hospice care through Medicare and may limit access to these services. These regulations are currently under review and may be broadened to be more sensitive to diseases that do not fit into the more traditional hospice-treated illnesses such as cancer. For patients with dementia, consideration is being given to determine a minimum magnitude of severity based on functional ability. To be eligible for hospice care, the patient may be required to exhibit incontinence, no functional speech, and no ability to ambulate, for example.

The clinician must be aware of the practical issues dealing with comfort care (Hurley, Volicer, Mahoney, & Volicer, 1993), which are discussed elsewhere in this volume. Knowledge is needed of alternative ways of feeding patients, of the often inappropriate use of physical restraints, and of drugs used to treat common life-ending conditions. The clinician must also remember that patients with dementia develop other illnesses later in life that may not be as thoroughly evaluated as in patients who are not demented. Particularly important for the clinician is the ability to assess the level of discomfort in advanced AD patients (Hurley et al., 1993), and to develop a sense of the quality of life of the patient.

As discussed earlier, some of the philosophies of hospice care are difficult to apply with AD patients. Many of the psychological interventions used in patients with other terminal diseases are based on the ability of the patient to communicate with his or her family and professional caregivers. To enhance the communication process with patients in mild to moderate stages of dementia, Rippich (1994) and colleagues developed the FOCUSED program. Such programs may be effective in hospice work.

A conceptual framework is needed to guide the process of dealing with the demented patient's psychological needs in the later stages of the disease. For example, the reality therapy has been the dominant overall approach to the treatment of patients with severe dementia in many long-term care facilities. With this approach, an attempt is made to orient the patient to the external world of the caregiver (i.e., making sure the patient is aware of the date, the weather, and the social life of the institution).

In contrast, the validation therapy (Feil, 1992) represents an alternative approach that may be useful for dealing with patients in advanced dementia. In the validation therapy, the clinician attempts to understand the world as seen through the eyes of the severely demented person. For example, if the patient believes that her parents are in fact still alive, as many do, then the clinician should deal with unresolved psychological issues in their past relationship and not be reminding the patient that her mother or father died long ago. Often, in demented patients their own world of the past has become their present.

In summary, the clinical ethics of caring for dying patients with dementia are complex and not for everyone. Clinicians need to decide whether they wish to participate in this challenging aspect of care or not. A broad understanding of dementia and its effects on patients and families, as well as of the ethical issues surrounding end-of-life care, contributes to the communication process that enhances good dying.

REFERENCES

Alemayehu, E., Molloy, D. W., Guyatt, G. H., Singer, J., Penington, G., Basile, J., Eisemann, M., Finucane, P., McMurdo, M., Powell, C., Zelmanowiez, A., Puxty, J., Power, C., Vitou, L., Levinson, S. A., Turpie, I. P. (1991). Variability inphysicians' decisions on caring for chronically ill elderly patients: An international study. *Canadian Medical Association Journal, 144,* 1133–1138.

Arras, J. (1988). The severely demented, minimally functional patient: An ethical analysis. *Journal of the American Geriatrics Society, 36,* 938–944.

Battin, M. P. (1992). Euthanasia in Alzheimer's disease? In R. H. Binstock, S. G. Post, P. J. Whitehouse (Eds.), *Dementia and aging: Ethics, values and policy choices* (pp. 118–137). Baltimore: Johns Hopkins University Press.

Birren, J. E., & Dieckmann, L. (1991). Concepts and content of quality of life in the later years: An overview. In J. E. Birren, C. R. Rowe, J. E. Lubben, & D. E. Deutchman (Eds.), The concept and measurement of quality of life in the frail elderly (pp. 344–360). New York: Academic Press.

Brock, D. W. (1988). Justice and the severely demented elderly. *Journal of Medicine and Philosophy, 13*(1), 73–99.

Callahan, D. (1987). *Setting limits: Medical goals in an aging society.* New York: Simon & Schuster.

Cleeland, C. S., Gonin, R., Hatfield, et al. (1994). Pain and its treatment in outpatients with metastatic cancer. *New England Journal of Medicine, 330,* 592–596.

Cundiff, D. (1992). *Euthanasia is not the answer: A hospice physician's view.* Totowa, NJ: Humana Press.

de Wachter, M. A. M. (1992). Euthanasia in the Netherlands. *Hastings Center Report, 22*(2), 23–30.

Dresser, R., & Whitehouse, P. J. (1994). The incompetent patient on the slippery slope. *Hastings Center Report, 24*(4), 6–12.

Dworkin, R. (1993). *Life's dominion.* New York: Vintage.

Emmanuel, L. L., & Emmanuel, E. J. (1989). The medical directive. *Journal of the American Medical Association, 261,* 3288–3293.

Fabiszewski, K. J., Volicer, B., & Volicer, L. (1990). Effect of antibiotic treatment on outcome of fevers in institutionalized Alzheimer patients. *Journal of the American Medical Association, 263,* 3168–3172.

Feil, N. (1992). *The Feil method.* Cleveland: Edward Feil Productions.

Hurley, A. C., Volicer, B. J., Hanarahan, P. A., Houde, S., & Volicer, L. (1992). Assessment of discomfort in advanced Alzheimer patients. *Research in Nursing and Health, 15,* 369–377.

Hurley, A. C., Volicer, B. J., Mahoney, M. A., & Volicer, L. (1993). Palliative fever management in Alzheimer patients: Quality plus fiscal responsibility. *Advances in Nursing Science, 16*(1), 21–32.

Kass, L. (1985). *Toward a more natural science: Biology and human affairs.* New York: Free Press.

Kastenbaum, R. (1992). *The psychology of death.* New York: Springer.

Katzman, R. (1976). The prevalence and malignancy of Alzheimer disease. *Archives of Neurology, 33*(4), 217–218.

Kübler-Ross, E. (1969). *On death and dying.* New York: Macmillan.

Luchins, D. J., & Hanrahan, P. (1993). What is the appropriate health care for end-stage dementia? *Journal of the American Geriatrics Society, 41,* 25–30.

Miller, F. G., Quill, T. E., Brody, H., Fletcher, J. C., Gostin, L. O., & Meier, D. E. (1994). Regulating physician-assisted death. *New England Journal of Medicine, 331,* 119–122.

Miller, R. J. (1992). Hospice care as an alternative to euthanasia. *Law, Medicine and Health Care, 20*(1–2), 127–132.

Post, S. G. (1990). Severely demented elderly people: A case against senicide. *Journal of the American Geriatrics Society, 38,* 715–718.

Post, S. G. (1993). Alzheimer disease and physician-assisted suicide. *Alzheimer Disease and Associated Disorders: An International Journal, 7,* 65–68.

Protzman, F. (1989, April 18). Killing of 49 elderly patients by nurse aids stuns Austria. *New York Times,* p. 1A.

In re Quinlan, 137 NJ. Super 227, 348 A2d, 801 [Ch. Dir.] 1976.

Quill, T. E., Cassel, C. K., & Meier, D. E. (1992). Care of the hopelessly ill: Proposed clinical criteria for physician-assisted suicide. *New England Journal of Medicine, 327,* 1380–1384.

Rango, N. (1985). The nursing home resident with dementia: Clinical care, ethics, and policy considerations. *Annals of Internal Medicine, 102,* 835–841.

Rippich, D. N. (1994). Functional communication with AD patients: A caregiver training program. *Alzheimer Disease and Associated Disorders: An International Journal, 8,* 95–109.

Rohde, K., Peskind, E. R., Raskind, M. A. (1995). Suicide in two patients with Alzheimer's disease. *Journal of the American Geriatrics Society, 43,* 187–189.

Schonwetter, R. S., & Robinson, B. E. (1994). Educational objectives for medical training in the care of the terminally ill. *Academic Medicine, 68,* 688–690.

Stoddard, S. (1990). Hospice: Approaching the 21st century. *American Journal of Hospice and Palliative Care, 7*(2), 27–30.

Volicer, B. J., Hurley, A., Fabiszewski, K. J., Montgomery, P., & Volicer, L. (1993) Predicting short-term survival for patients with advanced Alzheimer's disease. *Journal of the American Geriatrics Society, 41,* 535–540.

Volicer, L. (1986). Need for hospice approach to treatment of patients with advanced progressive dementia. *Journal of the American Geriatrics Society, 34,* 655–658.

Walter, J. J., & Shannon, T. A. (Eds.). (1990). *Quality of life: The new medical dilemma.* New York: Paulist Press.

Wolf, S. M. (1989). Holding the line on euthanasia. *Hastings Center Report, 19*(1), 13–15.

Palliative Care for Alzheimer Patients: Implications for Institutions, Caregivers, and Families

Mildred Z. Solomon and Bruce Jennings

F ew challenges facing the American health care system today are more difficult than those pertaining to the quality of care patients receive near the end of life. Too many patients die each year subject to invasive medical treatments they do not wish to receive; too many die in impersonal institutional settings cut off from family and friends; too many die in pain that could have been controlled (Principal Investigators for the SUPPORT Project, 1995; Solomon et al., 1993). However, of all the widely varying circumstances of terminal illness, no group of patients raises more ethically perplexing and emotionally troubling issues than those dying with Alzheimer's disease and other forms of advanced dementia.

As mentioned earlier, Alzheimer's is a progressive illness of devastating proportions that currently affects approximately 4 million persons in the United States and is expected to afflict 9 million by the year 2040 (Rice et al., 1993). In mid and late stages of the disease, dementia destroys memory, undermines neurologic behavior control mechanisms and linguistic communication, and affects personality. The condition disrupts the individual's ability to interact socially with others and to relate to oneself. In short, Alzheimer's attacks a person's most basic sense of identity.

Furthermore, care of Alzheimer patients places enormous stress on families as personal care, monitoring, and supervision requirements relentlessly increase. Wandering, fear of accident, incontinence, violent behavior, and other factors often overwhelm the caregiving capacities of families at home and lead to nursing home placement at some point during the course of the disease. In addition to the emotional consequences of the decisions that must be made in Alzheimer's care, families also often experience severe financial stress, which can be devastating. It is no exaggeration to say that Alzheimer's disease is an affliction that destroys the past, the present, and the future.

In Alzheimer's care, most key medical decisions must be made by family members or other surrogate decision makers, often with little explicit written or oral guidance from the patient when he or she still had capacity. This fact makes the care of patients dying with dementia particularly complex. Without an advance directive in place, family members have much less information to guide decision making and their rights and responsibilities can seem unclear. The situation is further complicated by the fact that health care professionals and paraprofessionals in long-term care settings often become like extra family for patients who have spent years in their care, and these caregivers too often face wrenching choices about how to serve the best interests of their patients. Moreover, the feelings of long-term caregivers and family members can conflict, adding even more uncertainty to an already ethically, legally, and psychologically complex decision-making process.

In addition to the impact this disease makes on persons with Alzheimer's disease, their families, and their caregivers, there are larger societal issues at stake as well. In the United States, the annual cost of caring for such patients has been estimated to be $100 billion (Rice et al., 1993). With the population aging and more individuals surviving well into their 80s, this figure will most likely double by the year 2040. This trend will have economic repercussions at all levels—societally, in terms of what health care services we will and will not be able to provide; organizationally, where fixed budgets will provide an incentive to reduce treatments perceived as marginally beneficial; and at the community level, where the financial consequences on families will be felt.

There is no societal obligation to provide expensive high-technology medicine if it offers no benefit and may in fact lead to a more protracted and painful period of suffering before death ensues than would otherwise have been the case. Yet decisions to terminate treatment should be based on the individual circumstances of a particular individual, not on the basis of generalized societal or organizational cost-cutting efforts. It is important, therefore, to be clear about the impulses that motivate decisions to forgo life-sustaining treatment among the demented.

Misplaced or overly generalized concerns about cost containment are not the only threat to a proper decision-making process. Demented patients in the advanced stages of Alzheimer's disease are a highly vulnerable group, susceptible to abuse and even abandonment. Although their sense of self may be threatened, dementing illness does not—and should not—diminish their moral claim to care and relief from suffering. Indeed, the very fact that so many people have a strong emotional reaction against "ever living like that" should make us more, not less, vigilant in scrutinizing biases and treatment decisions. As Stephen Post (1995) has argued, society's response to the needs of advanced Alzheimer patients is, in many ways, a test of its moral commitment to the old, the frail, and the vulnerable.

One enters, then, uncertain terrain where conflicting claims make it difficult to know how to proceed. Is it appropriate to forgo life-sustaining treatments for patients in the advanced stages of Alzheimer's? How can we be sure we are not further stigmatizing the demented, yet also protecting patients and loved ones from excessive suffering and a protracted and degrading death?

In this chapter, we argue that palliative and hospice care are appropriate treatment options for Alzheimer patients under certain conditions, and especially during the terminal phase of the disease when life-prolonging medical technology offers little meaningful benefit to the patient. We believe that hospice or hospice-like care should be available to Alzheimer patients in the end stage of the disease and that it *is* possible to move toward a palliative care model in ways that protect against potential abuses.

The chapter is divided into three parts. In the first section, we present a brief analysis of the ethical basis for making decisions to forgo life-sustaining treatments in Alzheimer patients, particularly those with end-stage dementia. In the second section, we call for greater attention to the full range of psychosocial and environmental needs of Alzheimer patients over the entire course of illness and argue for conceptualizing end-stage palliative care for these patients as one part of a single continuum of high-quality care. The final section of the chapter turns to the question of how the American health care system, and particularly long-term care facilities where most Alzheimer patients reside, might move toward a palliative model of care. We explore roles that institutions and professional caregivers can play to help make the envisioned shift from traditional, highly technologically oriented care near the end of life to comfort care.

ETHICAL BASIS FOR A PALLIATIVE CARE APPROACH

Many family members, health care professionals, and paraprofessional caregivers are hesitant to choose palliative care options for a loved one or patient, because they feel that doing so would somehow be ethically wrong. While sometimes misinformed or not well reasoned, such concerns are sincere. They must be addressed in a respectful, serious, and reasonable way.

Over the past 20 years an enormous body of law (both statutes and court opinions) (Meisel, 1989; National Center for State Courts, 1992) and professional opinion (American Dietetic Association, 1987; American Medical Association, 1992; American Nurses Association Task Force on the Nurse's Role in End of Life Decisions, 1992; President's Commission for the Study of Ethical Problems in Medicine and Biomedical and Behavioral Research, 1983; U.S. Congress, Office of Technology Assessment, 1987; Wanzer et al., 1984; Hastings Center, 1987) have clearly affirmed the right of the competent patient to refuse all forms of medical treatment, including life-sustaining medical treatment. Legally, this right is based on the "liberty interest" protected by the 14th Amendment to the U.S. Constitution, the right to privacy contained in many state constitutions, and the common law right to control what is done to one's own body; ethically, this right is based on the concepts of autonomy, self-determination, and respect for the individual as a being of moral worth.

Over time, these legal and ethical rights have been interpreted in ways that have a direct bearing on treatment decisions for demented patients. First, these rights survive the loss of mental capacity, and they may be exercised on a person's behalf by other, so-called surrogate decision makers. Second, the right to refuse life-sustaining medical treatment extends to all forms of medical intervention and technology, including artificial nutrition and hydration and antibiotic therapy for life-threatening infections, such as pneumonia, and urinary tract infections, which are often among the final illnesses Alzheimer patients experience before death.

Finally, the right to forgo treatment is not dependent on the patient's diagnosis, nor on the stage of the disease process, nor on the patient's life expectancy with or without the treatment. Some early state statutes authorizing the use of living wills contained wording that limited the use of these documents to the terminal phase of the patient's illness, but this restriction has been abandoned by more recent statutes on durable powers of attorney for health care, and the courts have generally not limited treatment refusals to patients expected to die in a short time. The patient's life expectancy and prognostic difficulties in establishing a "terminal condition"—matters that can be particularly problematic in Alzheimer's disease—are not central to decisions concerning the use of life-sustaining treatment. Instead, the key issues are the patient's own preferences and values and the balance of benefit and burden likely to be imposed by the treatment.

In keeping with this framework of ideas, the most desirable state of affairs for decision making in the context of advanced dementia is for the patient, while still in possession of the decision-making capacity, to make his or her wishes known by specifically designating an individual to serve as a surrogate decision maker and to talk with that person about personal values, religious beliefs, and specific wishes regarding medical treatment, if any. It is especially helpful for the patient to address his or her wishes concerning artificial nutrition and hydration, since this form of treatment is still the most sensitive and controversial issue in late-stage dementia. It is also clinically common as advanced dementia patients may lose their desire to receive food by mouth or their ability to swallow properly.

Unfortunately, however, advance planning and the use of explicit advance directives are the exception rather than the rule for patients with dementia and their families. Educational efforts to increase the use of advance directives are worthwhile and should continue, but they will probably never eliminate the need to handle cases in which decisions must be made by families for incompetent patients without such explicit guidance. The important point we wish to emphasize here is that in almost all states, family members have the legal authority and the moral right to make health care decisions for demented patients even without explicit written or oral advance directives. Surrogate decision makers can opt for conservative treatment plans, emphasizing palliative and comfort care measures and forgoing life-prolonging treatments such as artificial nutrition and hydration, hospitalization for intensive care, antibiotic therapy, and cardiopulmonary resuscitation.

Although family members and other surrogates clearly have the right to opt for palliative care for their loved ones, there is often a great deal of uncertainty about how to approach those decisions. What moral standards or guidance are available to them at such difficult moments? In keeping with the principle of respecting the patient's own identity as much as possible, surrogate decision makers should attempt to infer the patient's values and beliefs from what is known about the patient in the past. With advanced dementia, even when explicit statements by the patient are lacking, it is often possible reasonably to conclude that the person would choose comfort measures only rather than extended life prolongation given the diminished capacity to experience well-being and to engage in meaningful relationships with others, changes that are the natural outcomes of advanced dementia. On the other hand, a patient's religious and personal beliefs may have been such that prolonging life is of higher value than the quality of that life. In that case, it could be reasonable for a surrogate to conclude that life-sustaining measures, as well as necessary comfort measures, would be more in keeping with the patient's wishes.

In many instances, though, family members may simply feel uncertain about how their loved one would have wanted to proceed. In those cases, medical treatment should be based on the decision makers' sense of what would be in the patient's "best interests," a second well-established standard for surrogate decision making. Under these circumstances, it is not only permissible, but necessary, to compare what the condition of the patient is likely to be under one plan of care relative to another. Although life may be foreshortened under a palliative care plan, the ratio of benefits to burdens may be better for the patient with palliative care than with life-prolonging treatment; the option for palliative care—particularly high-quality palliative care delivered in an appropriate setting—may be best for the patient, all things considered. When that is the case, the palliative care option is a medically, ethically, and legally appropriate one for a family member or other surrogate to make.

Looking at the situation in this way may alleviate some of the ethical concerns family members and health care professionals have about choosing to forgo life-sustaining medical treatment in favor of palliative care. However, at least four specific concerns remain to be addressed directly. These are (1) concerns about "killing" the patient; (2) specific concerns about tube feeding; (3) negative attitudes about palliative care in general as a form of abandonment of the patient; and (4) concerns about safeguarding vulnerable persons from discrimination, abuse, and neglect.

Concerns About "Killing"

Many family members feel that not to "do everything possible" for the patient is tantamount to killing the patient. This belief is often accompanied by feelings of guilt, as if the family member actually wanted the patient to be dead. End-stage Alzheimer's disease is a particularly complex psychological challenge for family caregivers, many of whom may have provided emotionally draining and physically exhausting personal care to the patient for many years beforehand. Fantasies about the patient's death are not uncommon. Since decline and death can be foreseen well in advance, many family members go through a period of mourning long before the patient's physical demise and consider the end-stage patient to be in some sense "already gone," but in spite of this they may find themselves unable to let go of their caregiving role when seemingly called upon to do so by an overall change in treatment planning. Family members who have had various roles (or no role at all) in earlier caregiving often react differently to decisions to forgo life-sustaining treatment.

The key point to bear in mind is that it is the underlying disease process that brings about a patient's death, not the treatment planning decision per se. Family members are not required to use any and all available medical technology in a thoughtless, obligatory fashion, regardless of the patient's prior wishes or best interests. Moreover, decisions to pursue comfort care measures rather than life supports are guided by the intentions to respect the patient, to do what is best for him or her, and to preserve the patient's dignity as much as possible under the circumstances of an inevitable and foreseeable dying process.

CONCERNS ABOUT FORGOING MEDICALLY SUPPLIED FOOD AND FLUIDS

Many people have special feelings about providing food and water to helpless patients. For nearly all people, the act of providing sustenance symbolizes love and caring. Furthermore, there is a particular horror associated with the notion of watching someone starve to death. Since the decision to forgo artificial nutrition or hydration often arises in the final stages of Alzheimer's, and since palliative care plans would preclude the use of this technology to prolong life (although short-term hydration through IV lines may sometimes be used as a palliative measure), these perceptions can impede or undermine the decision to opt for palliation.

It is essential to recognize that in end-stage dementia, as in many other kinds of terminal conditions, the refusal of food by mouth and the loss of a desire to eat are a normal and natural part of the dying process. As the body's systems shut down near death, infusing fluids into the patient's system may actually increase discomfort rather than relieve it; retained fluid buildup can cause painful swelling, and since the dying patient is not actually experiencing feelings of hunger (as an otherwise healthy starving person would), this unpleasant sensation is not being alleviated by artificial nutrition and hydration either. As with artificial ventilation or any other form of life-sustaining technology, the treatment represented by artificial nutrition and hydration can sometimes be beneficial to the patient and sometimes unduly burdensome. Again, there is no moral or legal imperative to provide artificial nutrition and hydration no matter what. To forgo this type of treatment can be an act of loving kindness and virtue on the part of a family member; it certainly does not always or intrinsically signify malice or neglect.

MISPERCEPTIONS ABOUT HOSPICE AND PALLIATIVE CARE

Both the culture of medicine and nursing, and American society generally, contain a visceral reaction against passivity, and therefore both families and professional caregivers tend to denigrate decisions to forgo aggressive life-prolonging treatments as "giving up." Moreover, the notion of giving up on the patient is closely associated in many people's minds with the notion of abandonment. Consequently, hospice and palliative care are often misperceived as forms of "nontreatment," or as passive conditions in which everyone simply stands by and waits for death to come.

Yet nothing could be further from the truth. Even advanced dementia is typically not a state of unconsciousness or total lack of awareness of one's surroundings. It is not devoid of experience, and that experience can be enhanced by the nature, setting, and type of one's care. Hospice staff and palliative care professionals do not simply stand back and wait passively for death; they actively concern themselves with life and the experience of living near death.

In fact, as we will discuss below, palliative care in the final stages of an illness can have—and should have—the most continuity with earlier stages of caregiving for the patient with dementia. Far from representing an abrupt break with, or a turning away from, the goals of care physicians and families have pursued earlier, sometimes for many years, the palliative care option, based on respect, dignity, and the patient's best interests, can actually be the most natural extension of the life history of that care. On the contrary, aggressive, intensive, and highly technological medical treatment at the very end of life may more likely constitute a departure from past caregiving relationships and an abandonment of the goals and values that have sustained the relationship between patient and family through their long ordeal.

CONCERNS ABOUT DISCRIMINATION, ABUSE, AND NEGLECT

We believe that one of the best ways to protect against potential abuse is to locate the whole question of palliative care for Alzheimer patients within the larger realm of quality of care. As we have noted above, a fully ethical response to the dilemmas posed by Alzheimer's should recognize that a decision to use or forgo life supports is only one of many ethical choices families and caregivers confront over the course of caring for Alzheimer patients. An end-of-life decision about whether to hospitalize, to treat a pneumonia, to intubate—these should be seen as points akin to others that have arisen earlier in the course of the person's illness, including decisions about whether to remove driving privileges or how to structure the daily environment to allow for, or constrain, wandering.

Recognizing that end-of-life decisions are part of the whole trajectory of choices caregivers and families face over time is important for two reasons. First, this stance offers some protection against the potential abuses inherent in deciding to limit treatments for patients who can no longer speak for themselves. If we are confident that we have built the most caring and respectful environment for Alzheimer patients *through-out* the course of illness, then we have stronger ethical ground to stand on when it comes to terminating treatments. If, on the other hand, we have not been vigilant about designing optimal environments and systems of care for Alzheimer patients, then decisions to forgo treatments may well be criticized as one more example of the degree to which our society devalues nonproductive, frail, and demented elders. An ethically just response to the problem of Alzheimer's care will not simply ask, "When can we stop treatment?" but also "How can we ensure the greatest comfort and dignity for persons facing a progressive and inevitable assault on their selfhood?"

Furthermore, there is not only an ethical kinship between end-of-life dilemmas in Alzheimer's care and early or mid-stage dilemmas, but a conceptual kinship as well. It is to this connection, the relationship between quality of care in early and mid-stage Alzheimer care and the quality of care during end-stage illness, that we now turn.

QUALITY AND CONTINUITY OF CARE
THROUGH THE END OF LIFE

In her book *Day In, Day Out with Alzheimer's,* Karen Lyman (1993) points out that day care environments for early and mid-stage Alzheimer patients fall roughly into two types, what she calls the "medical model" and the "social model." She describes the characteristics of each, showing that they differ in terms of their expectations about client (or patient) behavior, in the props or furnishings used, in the conversational scripts between caregivers and clients, and in the ways in which space and time are organized.

Features of the medical model often symbolize an authoritarian rather than an exchange relationship with clients and are more focused on control rather than self-determination. Caregivers in the medical model are likely to attribute most behaviors to perceived stages of the disease rather than to the social conditions that might be shaping those behaviors. As Lyman (1993) puts it:

> Day-care providers often manage trouble in caregiving by relying upon . . . stereotypic lenses that filter the daily interpretations of "cognitive impairment" and "behavior problems." The result is a lack of recognition of the social context of many behaviors attributed to the course of the dementing illness. Yet I have observed that some people with dementia become "agitated" or "wander" when the program offers them little of interest, when they are anxious about being locked up, or they have had a misunderstanding or conflict with a caregiver. These are social factors that affect the ongoing experience of a dementing illness, aside from the course of the disease itself. (p. 159)

Overemphasis on "disease typifications" and disease progression can also encourage staff to overlook the profound effects that the architectural design may be having on Alzheimer patients' behavior, the quality of their care, and the stress their caregivers experience. Problems with facility design can make the difference between a program that meets patients' needs and one that does not. For example, highly visible, obtrusive barriers to prevent "wandering" can increase agitation, whereas secured outdoor walkways can provide an appropriate outlet for the person's need to walk.

In the medical model, caregivers are also more likely to attribute the naturally occurring differences that one should expect to see in any range of individuals to disease stage or disease progression instead. In contrast, day care programs based on a social rather than a medical model are more flexible, more individualized, and more likely to enhance self-determination and selfhood. However, in part because of their flexibility and less authoritarian stance, they tend to create greater stress for the caregivers who work there.

One particularly outstanding facility Lyman observed successfully combined many features found in medical settings with the tone and practices of a social model. The staff espoused and implemented a multidisciplinary team approach, in which psychosocial needs were emphasized and supported by medical activities:

> Valley [the fictional name of this facility] was unique in exhibiting little of the medical model in staff-client interactions, while the structure of the program included many features found in medical settings. Although two

registered nurses worked in the program, a social worker and an activity director served in prominent positions. Program goals focused in part on cognitive stimulation to "maintain functioning" of persons with dementia. But the primary goals were psychosocial: "to relieve anxiety" and to "engage" people in activity and in social interaction, to prevent "excess disabilities."

At Valley, both official goals and informal norms emphasized knowing the individual. As Jennifer the manager said, "I wish I knew more about these people's history, how much is the disease and how much is the person." Recording observations about their patients helped staff to answer this question and enabled them to support the self-identity of the client. (Lyman, 1993, pp. 152–153)

As in the more socially oriented models of day care arrangements, hospice-like care for late-stage Alzheimer patients distinguishes itself from traditional forms of care by focusing not only the patients' medical needs, but also on the person's and the family's psychological, social, and spiritual needs. It recognizes that an illness is different from a disease, and that attending to meaning and suffering is as important as striving to relieve physical pain or control an infection. Thus, a second part of our argument relates to the issue of overmedicalization in its many forms—both during the early and mid stages of Alzheimer's disease, as Lyman points out, and in the late stages of related dementia.

There are many benefits to seeing all these choices as points along a single continuum. Doing so not only suggests that family members and other close caregivers have earned society's trust and respect as surrogate decision makers. It also allows us to define the continuum of dementia care in a new way—not just as a series of disconnected medical "crises," but as a set of choices about how best to sustain meaning and dignity in the life of persons who are losing their memory, their self-identity, and ultimately their ability to relate to others. Moreover, if we define the choices that are inevitable during the progression of this illness only in medical terms, then we lose the opportunity to do all that is possible both for the person with Alzheimer's and for his or her family. Construed in a broader way, end-of-life problems can be seen as no different in kind from other problems caregivers and families have experienced over the years of the patients' decline—namely, how best to individualize care and maximize comfort and dignity.

Although he does not express his point in exactly this way, our argument is similar to one that Daniel Callahan has made (Callahan, 1995) in which he sets out standards for termination of life-sustaining treatments in patients in the advanced stages of dementia. Callahan says that his goal is to "develop some kind of compromise position, aiming to minimize further stigmatization of dementia while simultaneously reducing the widespread fear that the life of the demented will be unconscionably prolonged" (p. 28). His response is to suggest giving a "high priority to providing decent nursing and palliative care for demented patients but a much lower priority to the use of expensive medicine to prolong life" (p. 29).

He then presents three standards for terminating treatment in late-stage Alzheimer patients that are meant to protect this middle ground. The suggested standards offer criteria for terminating life supports that guard against "the hazard of treating the demented too aggressively," while simultaneously attempting to ensure that our dread of the disease does not further stigmatize Alzheimer patients or their families.

According to Callahan (1995), if there is (1) evidence of suffering or (2) the likelihood that medical interventions, while prolonging biological function, will enhance the odds of further deterioration and a poorer quality death, then any one of three standards for terminating treatment can be invoked:

> (1) No one should have to live longer in the advanced stages of dementia than he would have in a pre-technological era;
> (2) The likely deterioration in a late-stage demented patient should lead to a shift in the usual standard of treatment, that of stopping rather than continuing treatment;
> (3) There is as great an obligation to prevent a lingering, painful and degrading death as there is to promote health and life. (p. 30)

We agree with these standards. More specifically, we recommend that (1) Alzheimer patients' prior statements of preference should count as important, though not exclusive, pieces of information about patients' values and preferences; (2) family members should be recognized as the key decision makers; (3) health care professionals have an obligation to support patients' and families' wishes, even when the health care professionals may disagree with those preferences; but that (4) health care professionals also have an obligation to challenge family decisions that are manifestly unreasonable or motivated by a conflict of interest.

Assuming that, when these conditions are present, palliative care for demented patients is an appropriate goal, the central question now becomes "How do we establish these conditions?" What can health care institutions, particularly long-term care facilities, and health care professionals do to shift from the current practice, which offers high-technology medicine for demented patients at the end of life to comfort care and palliation?

VISION, LEADERSHIP, TEAM-BUILDING, AND STRATEGIES FOR CHANGE

Nursing home executives and administrators of long-term care facilities operate under many constraints, but they also have more power than they often realize. They can set the tone, the goals, and the expectations for the staff, families, and residents. If change is going to occur, those people who run long-term care facilities must be the ones to define the need for change and to mobilize their staff to achieve it. While these leaders must recognize the need for change, to be successful they will have to gather support from other leaders within the organization and in particular will need to pay attention to and court the collaboration of the directors of medicine and nursing. Only a team approach involving staff from across the disciplines will ultimately succeed.

However, it is important to acknowledge that sometimes efforts to bring about change must begin before the whole team is together and in sync. When the administration is behind an innovative effort, a handful of committed individuals can set the tone. But the process must be understood from the start as a process, beginning modestly at first perhaps, but relentlessly gaining more converts to the cause as it grows over time. We emphasize the word *process,* because it is a grave mistake to think that changes in health care can be achieved through a single intervention or "magic bullet." Health care services are complex sociological activities involving many players with different degrees of power interacting in entrenched and often unconscious patterns of behavior. Enabling these health care professionals to interact in new ways is something that must be planned for, instituted, and reinforced over time. While promoting change is difficult, there are some very concrete steps that nursing home leadership can take to begin the process. Below we briefly describe some of the most important strategies available to nursing home leaders who want to take on this challenge.

SEARCH FOR INNOVATIVE MODELS

It is impossible to plan for change unless one has a clear vision of the desired outcomes and good examples of the processes and procedures others have put in place to arrive successfully at those outcomes. While not numerous, there are fortunately some very promising examples of palliative care services that have been or could be adopted for end-stage Alzheimer patients. The Dementia Special Care Unit at the E. N. Rogers Memorial Veterans Hospital (Bedford, MA) (Hurley, Mahoney, & Volicer, 1995; Volicer et al., 1994; Volicer, Rheaume, Brown, Fabiszewski, & Brady,

1986) provides an excellent example of how a long-term care facility re-organized itself to offer five different levels of care for residents and pre-pared families to make decisions about which level of care was appro-priate for their loved ones. The Jewish Home and Hospital in New York City, a 1,600-bed skilled nursing facility, has developed an ethics consult team that helps families, professional staff, and paraprofessional care-givers make and manage decisions to use or forgo artificial nutrition and other kinds of medical technology in frail elders, many of whom are patients with advanced dementia (Chichin & Olson, 1995; Olson, Chichin, Meyers, Schulman, & Brennan, 1994; Olson et al., 1992).

The Cobble Hill Nursing Home in Brooklyn, New York, has developed an exemplary model of continuous care. Their philosophy for mid-stage Alzheimer patients is to treat behavior, not as something to be con-trolled, but rather as a language or a means of communication, the only way a demented person has for expressing his or her desires and needs. This focus, on coming to understand rather than control the individual, carries through to end-stage care at the institution, where a palliative care option is offered to families. Cobble Hill offers extensive staff edu-cation and support to help caregivers accept family decisions to termi-nate life supports. They have also developed links to hospice care, so that nursing home residents choosing this option can receive hospice care within the facility (T. Yang-Lewis, personal communication, January 5, 1996).

Other models have emerged directly from the hospice world. For example as described in chapter 14 of this volume, the Jacob Perlow Hospice at Beth Israel Medical Center in New York City has broadened its hospice services to provide hospice care at home for late-stage Alzheimer patients. This shift to the Alzheimer population moves hos-pice care beyond the traditional concept of care primarily for cancer patients to an expanded definition and understanding of what hospice care can be and the populations it can serve. Energetic and committed nursing home leaders ought to seek out their counterparts at these innovative institutions to learn more about what the leaders there have done so that they can adapt these new models of care for their own institutions.

Regardless of the particular models different institutions have devel-oped, a likely common theme is that they have created mechanisms to avoid transfer to the hospital when acute problems occur. Transfer to a hospital is one of the key forms of burden (translocation stress) on de-mented patients. In the Bedford VA study, it was also the single greatest factor contributing to the cost differential between the traditional and palliative units that Volicer et al. (1994) documented in their study.

Therefore, a central element in the shift to palliative care will be that long-term care facilities must set up the means to care for dying patients onsite, without transfer to a hospital.

PROVIDE PROFESSIONAL AND PARAPROFESSIONAL STAFF EDUCATION

To provide successful palliative care and avoid inappropriate transfer to a hospital, staff education needs to focus on (1) improving knowledge of what is and is not ethically and legally permissible; (2) developing the clinical skills necessary for providing adequate pain relief and appropriate comfort measures and psychosocial support to residents and family members; and (3) developing the communication skills that will ensure better coordination among the health care team and, most especially, between the professional caregivers and the family.

Knowledge of Ethics and Law

Unpublished empirical research we have conducted in a small number of nursing homes provides data that corroborate anecdotal observations about ethical and legal misunderstandings common among nursing home staff and particularly among long-term care nurses. There are, we believe, three important myths that a nursing home administration should address through multidisciplinary education. First, many long-term care nurses do not see a difference between forgoing life-sustaining medical treatments and assisting with a suicide; they are therefore prone to think that they would be doing something illegal and/or unethical if they were to accede to family wishes to terminate potentially life-prolonging medical interventions.

Second, many long-term care nurses and a significant portion of physicians think that it is illegal to provide adequate amounts of narcotics if those doses, while necessary for pain relief, might also depress respiration and hasten death. This opinion exists despite the fact that it has long been argued by authorities in ethics (e.g., Hastings Center, 1987) that it is immoral *not* to provide adequate pain relief, even if death is hastened, so long as all other means have been tried, the risks have been disclosed to family members who agree to the plan, and the intent of the caregivers is to relieve suffering rather than to kill. Furthermore, recent guidelines published by the Agency for Health Care Policy and Research state that worries about hastening death have been exaggerated and that when narcotics are titrated appropriately, respiratory depression can almost always be avoided or minimized (Jacox et al., 1994).

Third, as we discussed earlier in this chapter, there is considerable controversy surrounding the question of medically supplied food and fluids. Our data indicate that long-term care nurses are even more likely than hospital-based nurses to object to the withholding or withdrawal of artificial nutrition and hydration.

Nursing home leaders can address these educational needs by creating discussion groups. Written materials could be circulated in advance of a meeting or distributed at its conclusion. Discussion groups should allow for a mix of both personal reflections and substantive input about what has been written in the ethics and legal literature. Encouraging participants to discuss their views and compare them to what has been written in the literature moves the conversation beyond simple expression of personal feeling, however important that is. A more informed discussion involving the analysis of established ethical and legal guidelines enables staff members to evaluate their own practice in the light of those guidelines. Doing so in group meetings establishes that the administration of the institution wants the staff to engage together in more open planning and discussion of treatment options for the residents.

Special meetings should be designed for the paraprofessional staff members who provide so much of the hands-on care within nursing homes and therefore need to be clear about the ethical and legal underpinnings of a palliative care approach. The Jewish Home and Hospital in New York City has developed a helpful survey instrument to profile paraprofessionals' views on many issues germane to termination of treatment and develop staff education programs tailored to the needs identified by the survey (Chichin, Schulman, Harrington, Norwood, & Olson, 1995).

Clinical Skills in Pain Relief and Palliation

Education should focus not only on ethics and law, but also on gaining the clinical skills to offer the most restraint-free environment possible and later the best possible palliative care. If we are to take the concept of continuum of care seriously, nursing home leaders could make explicit to staff the link between reducing physical and chemical restraints and providing the most humanistic and sensible palliative care to patients in the end stages of the illness.

To improve palliation, long-term care nurses and physicians need to be educated on both pharmacologic and nonpharmacologic pain management and symptom control (e.g., what to do for symptoms of dry mouth and how to handle urinary tract infections when it has been decided that antibiotics will not be used). Again, discussion groups can be an adequate forum for raising these issues, but we have found that bringing in expert mentors, such as hospice nurses, to talk about and troubleshoot in particular cases can be a very effective means of helping staff members develop these skills.

Communication Skills

Not everyone can talk easily about death and dying or offer the emotional support families need when they are facing difficult decisions. Successful palliative care programs recognize this fact, and while they try to encourage all staff members to grow in their ability to talk with residents and families, some institutions have experimented with designating special ethics consult teams composed of staff members who are particularly gifted at this kind of conversation and support. Sometimes this role is filled by nurses, sometimes social workers, physicians, or paraprofessional staff. It is important not to overwhelm families with too many team members at once. Some institutions have a cadre of staff who meet together on an ad hoc basis to discuss particular cases, and they circulate responsibility for individual consults among individuals on the team, so that no one team member gets burned out. In addition to these ethics consult teams, there are other steps longterm care facilities can take to improve communication with families. In the next section, we briefly describe several mechanisms for "institutionalizing" good communication among patients, families, and staff.

ESTABLISH INSTITUTIONAL MECHANISMS FOR BETTER COMMUNICATION, ADVANCE CARE PLANNING, AND CONFLICT RESOLUTION

Explain the Institution's Mission and Approach to Residents (If Possible) and to Families upon Admission

It is both ethically and pragmatically wise to explain the philosophy of care at the institution to residents with decision-making capacity and to families upon admission. It is ethically necessary so that there is full disclosure of the options that residents and families will or will not have if they enter the facility. It is pragmatically wise, because the admissions process is the appropriate time to encourage advance planning and the execution of advance directives, if residents still have the capacity to execute such documents. And, even if residents no longer have this capacity, early and open acknowledgment that the institution is committed to the least restrictive environment and the broadest set of palliative care options for residents as they enter the final stages of their illness are important issues for families to understand. The key message should be that the family will be a full partner in assessing the resident's changing needs over time and that the staff will be committed to helping them assess what options are in their loved one's best interests over the course of his or her stay in that facility.

Establish Regular Ethics Rounds to Discuss Goals of Care Prospectively

One reason for most American health care institutions routinely providing all that technology has to offer is that clinicians respond in an ad hoc fashion to specific presenting clinical problems as they arise, rather than standing back and asking at a deeper level what the goals of care are for this patient, and what the likely future scenario is under various alternative treatment plans. There is no reason for nursing homes not to establish monthly ethics rounds, where these deeper questions may be asked on a routine basis. Developing a schedule for these rounds (i.e., structuring them as a routine part of practice) is also a useful device for motivating broader staff participation. Even staff members who have been reluctant to get involved in the shift to a palliative model of care will likely be motivated to attend rounds if they become an established occurrence. Thus, in addition to encouraging more staff involvement, ethics rounds create the opportunity for divergent views to be aired and provide a natural check on overly zealous or one-sided approaches to care decisions.

Establish Ethics Committees and Retrospective Case Review

It is essential both to protect a vulnerable population at risk of neglect and abuse and to ensure that Alzheimer patients do not find themselves entrapped in medical treatment that prolongs their suffering and dying to no benefit. We see nursing home ethics committees as an important conduit to strike this balance. Through retrospective case review, ethics committees can provide an internal check against both overtreatment and undertreatment. They are also an important way for minority views to be heard so that reasoned argument, not unreflective consensus, can prevail.

In addition, prospective ethics committee review is an important vehicle for scrutinizing cases in which staff members may have reasons to question the motives or appropriateness of surrogate decision makers. Most cases of disagreement between families and health care professionals can be resolved at the bedside. However, there may be instances where there are potential conflicts of interest between surrogates and residents and outside review by an ethics committee would be appropriate. This is especially the case in those instances where family members may be requesting termination of treatment for a resident who, though demented, may still obviously be enjoying life and may even be overtly expressing a preference to continue living.

Expect Conflict and Strong Differences in Values and Beliefs

Any institution determined to institute a strong palliative care program should expect conflict and strong differences in the values and beliefs not only between families and staff members but also among the staff as well. Sometimes these differences simply reflect differences between individuals; sometimes they are based on differences in professional roles; sometimes they reflect cultural differences on the meaning of family, death, dying, privacy, and identity. Successful programs are ones that do not ignore those differences; instead, they develop a cultural climate and specific mechanisms, such as ethics committees and monthly ethics rounds, for dealing with the differences in an overt and public manner.

It is often helpful for those who chair ethics committee meetings or conduct ethics rounds to seek out controversy explicitly by asking members of the floor staff or others involved in the case, "Does anyone disagree with this recommendation?" When disagreements do surface, the skillful facilitator will go further, asking for clarifications about why individuals hold the views they do. Probing for the reasons behind people's ideas signals that all views are to be taken seriously, can help clarify thinking, and often identifies areas of agreement amenable to those holding what had appeared at first to be intractable positions.

Provide Support Groups for Staff and Family Grief

One of the features that distinguishes nursing homes from other health care institutions is the length of time that many residents live there and the strength of bonds that develop between patients and their professional and paraprofessional caregivers. When a decision is made to terminate treatment, that decision reverberates throughout the staff, whose needs for support may be nearly as great as or, in some cases, greater than the family's (Chichin, 1995; Olson, 1995). If institutions are going to become more proactive in allowing residents and their families to forgo life-prolonging medical options, then they must also find ways to provide support for the grief that caring staff members are likely to feel when a well-known and much loved resident dies. This can be accomplished simply by providing time for staff members to come together to discuss their feelings, perhaps at a meeting facilitated by the hospital chaplain or social worker or by someone who knew the resident well. Sometimes, when staff feel that it was wrong to let the resident die, it can be helpful to point out that at times the greatest way to show love and respect is to honor the resident's wishes even when they conflict with one's own.

CONCLUSIONS

We have stressed the power that individual nursing home administrators have to create new institutional protocols and procedures, but it would be wrong to ignore the fact that individual facilities and their staff are also highly influenced by outside entities, including state and federal regulations aimed at protecting residents from abuse and neglect that can easily be misapplied in a palliative care context. Decisions not to transfer seriously ill nursing home residents and to allow them to die onsite cannot occur without coordination with state regulatory offices. In some cases, state regulations will need to be clarified so that a decision not to provide antibiotics for pneumonia or not to intubate for medically supplied nutrition, for example, will not be misconstrued as neglect. One particularly powerful way to deal with this would be for groups of nursing homes and hospitals within a given region to work together with state regulators to discuss necessary changes in regulations and/or state laws.

We have also strongly advocated for conceptualizing palliative care options under the larger rubric of quality of care for Alzheimer patients and urged that it be seen as part of the continuum of care, from early through mid to late stages of the disease. Moreover, we have based part of our ethical justification for a palliative care approach to end-stage dementia on two parallel appeals: one for the freedom to terminate treatments likely to be nonbenefical, the other for a societal commitment to offer the very best possible care to early and mid-stage Alzheimer patients. We have suggested that "very best care" ought to include attention to the physical features of the caregiving environment so that it can be the least restrictive and most autonomy-enhancing possible, and that these programs should attend to psychosocial needs as well as medical ones.

Nonetheless, we must acknowledge the magnitude of constraints operating against just such a vision. At the moment, there are few models available for the kind of seamless care envisioned, nor are there many examples of socially oriented Alzheimer programs. Perhaps the growth of managed care and the growing numbers of Medicare enrollees in such plans may provide an opportunity to explore the possibilities of creating more continuity across settings and more holistic care in the future. Yet there are few signs of progress in that direction, and our appeals may come down to a naive case of wishful thinking. On the other hand, committed administrators, physicians, nurses, social workers, and other leaders within the field of long-term care can play a vital role in bringing the realities of care for Alzheimer patients closer to these ideals.

ACKNOWLEDGMENTS

The authors wish to thank Karen Heller, Ph.D., for her background research during the preparation of this manuscript.

REFERENCES

American Dietetic Association. (1987). Issues in feeding the terminally ill adult. *Journal of the American Dietetic Association, 87,* 78–85.

American Medical Association. (1992). *Current opinions of the Council on Ethical and Judicial Affairs of the American Medical Association: Withholding or withdrawing life prolonging treatment.* Chicago: Author.

American Nurses Association Task Force on the Nurse's Role in End of Life Decisions. (1992). *Position statement on forgoing artificial nutrition and hydration.* Washington, DC: Author.

Callahan, D. (1995). Terminating life-sustaining treatment of the demented. *Hastings Center Report, 25*(6), 25–31.

Chichin, E. (1995). Treatment termination in long-term care: Implications for health care providers. In E. Olson, E. Chichin, & L. Libow (Eds.), *Controversies in ethics in long-term care* (pp. 29–42). New York: Springer.

Chichin, E., & Olson, E. (1995). Ethics consult teams in geriatric long-term care. *Cambridge Quarterly of Healthcare Ethics, 4*(2), 178–184.

Chichin, E. R., Schulman, E., Harrington, M., Norwood, J., & Olson, E. (1995). End-of-life treatment decisions in the nursing home: Ethics and the nursing assistant. In P. R. Katz, R. L. Kane, & M. D. Mezey (Eds.), *Quality care in geriatric settings* (pp. 116–129). New York: Springer.

Hastings Center. (1987). *Guidelines on the termination of life-sustaining treatment and the care of the dying.* Bloomington: Indiana University Press.

Hurley, A., Mahoney, M., & Volicer, L. (1995). Comfort care in end-stage dementia: What to do after deciding to do no more. In E. Olson, E. Chichin, & L. Libow (Eds.), *Controversies in ethics in long-term care* (pp. 73–90). New York: Springer.

Lyman, K. (1993). *Day in, day out with Alzheimer's care: Stress in caregiving relationships.* Philadelphia: Temple University Press.

Meisel, A. (1989). *The right to die.* New York: Wiley.

National Center for State Courts. (1992). *Decision making regarding life-sustaining medical treatment* (2nd ed.). Williamsburg, VA: National Center for State Courts.

Olson, E. (1995). Treatment termination in long-term care: What about the physician? What about the family? In E. Olson, E. Chichin, & L. Libow (Eds.), *Controversies in ethics in long-term care* (pp. 43–56). New York: Springer.

Olson, E., Chichin, E., Meyers, H., Schulman, E., & Brennan, F. (1994). Early experiences of an ethics consult team. *Journal of the American Geriatrics Society, 42*(4), 437–441.

Olson, E., Martico-Greenfield, T., Carlos, A., Jackson, R., Guilfoy, V., & Jennings, B. (1992). Ethics education in long-term care: *The Decisions Near the End of Life* program. *Journal of Health Administration Education, 10*(4), 612–622.

Post, S. (1995). *The moral challenge of Alzheimer's disease.* Baltimore: Johns Hopkins University Press.

President's Commission for the Study of Ethical Problems In Medicine and Biomedical and Behavioral Research. (1983). *Deciding to forgo life sustaining treatment: Ethical, medical, and legal issues in treatment decisions.* Washington, DC: U.S. Government Printing Office.

Principal Investigators for the SUPPORT Project. (1995). A controlled trial to improve care for seriously ill hospitalized patients: The study to understand prognoses and preferences for outcomes and risks of treatments (SUPPORT). *Journal of the American Medical Association, 274,* 1591–1598.

Rice, D. P., Fox, P. J., Max, W., Webber, P. A., Lindeman, D. A., Hauck, W. W., & Segura, E. (1993). The economic burden of Alzheimer's disease care. *Health Affairs, 12*(2), 164–176.

Solomon, M. Z., O'Donnell, L., Jennings, B., Guilfoy, V., Wolf, S., Nolan, K., Jackson, R., Koch-Weser, D., & Donnelley, S. (1993). Decisions near the end of life: Professional views on life-sustaining treatments. *American Journal of Public Health, 83,* 14–23.

U.S. Congress, Office of Technology Assessment. (1987). *Life-sustaining technologies and the elderly.* Washington, DC: U.S. Congress, Office of Technology Assessment.

Volicer, L., Collard, A., Hurley, A., Bishop, C., Kern, D., & Karon, S. (1994). Impact of special care unit for patients with advanced Alzheimer's disease on patients' discomfort and costs. *Journal of the American Geriatrics Society, 42,* 597–603.

Volicer, L., Rheaume, Y., Brown, J., Fabiszewski, K., & Brady, R. (1986). Hospice approach to the treatment of patients with advanced dementia of the Alzheimer type. *Journal of the American Medical Association, 256*(16), 2210–2213.

Wanzer, S. H., Adelstein, S. J., Cranford, R. E., Federman, D., Hook, E. D., Moertel, C. G., Safar, P., Stone, A., Taussig, H. B., & vanEys, J. (1984). The physician's responsibility toward hopelessly ill patients. *New England Journal of Medicine, 310,* 955–959.

Nursing Staff As Moral Agents

Ann C. Hurley, Sally A. MacDonald, Sara T. Fry, and Veronika F. Rempusheski

A moral agent acts for himself or herself, or in the place of another by the authority of that person, and does so by conforming to a standard of the "right behavior." Nurses are licensed professional caregivers whose actions as moral agents are grounded in professional codes and societal expectations. The moral basis of nursing is derived from the professional code of ethical conduct that offers general ethical principles to guide and evaluate nursing actions. The most fundamental of these principles is respect for individuals, but others include avoiding harm, doing good, respecting self-determination, keeping promises, and treating people fairly.

Caregiving activities are based on the exhortation to "let nature put the patient in the best condition," as taught by Nightingale (1946), and the role of the nurse, as articulated by Henderson (1977), "to assist the individual, sick or well, in the performance of those activities contributing to health or its recovery (or peaceful death) that he would perform unaided if he had the necessary strength, will or knowledge" (p. 4). The nursing profession is committed to the care and nurturing of sick and well people, individually and in groups.

This chapter takes the stance that clinical and ethical decision making are two inseparable components of moral agency in the nursing role, and that the nurse-patient-family relationship underlies this role in caring for patients with late-stage dementia. That is, nurse caregiving has a moral basis that is translated into all nursing actions planned and carried out for patients and their family members—the nurse is simultaneously a moral agent and a care provider. To be a moral agent requires the application of both ethical sensitivity and moral reasoning to caregiving activities. "Ethical sensitivity involves identifying the ethical aspects of a situation that affect the welfare of an individual," and "moral reasoning is the ability to determine what ought to be done in a particular situation" (Fry, 1994, p. 3).

The quotes given throughout this chapter were obtained during interviews with staff members at the Dementia Special Care Unit (DSCU) as part of research for *Reaching Consensus: The Process of Recommending Treatment Decisions for Alzheimer Patients* (Hurley, Volicer, Rempusheski, & Fry, 1995). They illustrate the moral agency of the nursing role in caring for patients with late-stage dementia. The nursing role in this DSCU includes both providing care and recommending treatment decisions. Intensive care nursing is offered so that the focus of care is one of "high touch" versus "high tech" (Hurley, Mahoney, & Volicer, 1995). Recommending treatment decisions is a component of advance proxy planning (Hurley, Bottino, & Volicer, 1994), which operationalizes the philosophy of the hospice approach to care (Volicer, Rheaume, Brown, Fabiszewski, & Brady, 1986). The levels mentioned in this chapter are explained in detail in chapter 9.

SPECIAL NEEDS OF PATIENTS WITH ALZHEIMER'S DISEASE AND THEIR FAMILIES

INEVITABILITY OF DEATH

The relentless progression of Alzheimer's disease and its consequences means that the patient will ultimately die from a complication related to the dementing process (Hurley, Volicer, & Mahoney, 1996). How individuals spend their final days and years depends on treatment decisions about providing palliative care options and the ability of clinical staff to provide comfort. The nursing staff must deal with the issue of limiting aggressive technological interventions.

I have to keep reminding myself that there is no hope for these patients. The very best we can do is to let them die comfortably and with dignity. It's not that simple, however. It's a real dilemma. It's an ethical problem, let's face it. As nurses, you know there are some possible treatments . . . and [the patients] *may* be okay. Or I guess the question is, how long do you want these patients to go on? They are declining functionally and mentally . . . it is a difficult situation for the caregiver.

The decision to avoid resuscitation attempts is a more clear-cut issue. The nursing staff members know that when cardiopulmonary resuscitation is attempted with a patient with late-stage dementia the likely outcome is death, sometimes survival in a much less functional state requiring acute care technology, and very rarely survival with the ability to return to the long-term care unit (Awoke, Mouton, & Parrott, 1992).

I can even see asking for a DNR [do not resuscitate] order upon admission; I don't think it's too soon for that. I think most people are capable of understanding that ultimately there is no hope for an Alzheimer patient and what CPR and DNR entail. The way I look upon the DNR order, is that if someone is fortunate enough to collapse from cardiac or respiratory failure, considering the prognosis of Alzheimer's disease, that may be the most comfortable way a patient could die.

Technology exists that can prolong life in some cases. Therefore, nurses need to consider withholding such technology in terms of not providing extraordinary measures to seek survival at all costs—and distinguishing that from taking someone's life.

Well, what I believe, and I don't know if it's correct according to the church, [is that] God would go along with keeping a person comfortable. We're not killing him. It's not euthanasia. . . . I think that there's a lot to be said for not trying to treat incurable illness and allowing natural death, if there is such a thing anymore. I don't feel uncomfortable, as far as my religion and profession are concerned, in allowing a patient to die. And I see it as almost a natural death, providing ultimate comfort—physically, spiritually, and emotionally.

ASSISTING THE FAMILY WITH THE TRANSITION TO LONG-TERM CARE

Caring for the patient means caring for the family as well. The nursing staff can support family members as they live through their emotional upheavals during a patient's dying process. Staff, as moral agents, are "caring" to both patient and family.

I think as troubled or demented as our patients are, they realize when you care for them. They know; they can tell by your voice, your smile, your touch. They can tell; they know.

I mean by caring for them, I don't mean that there is anyone here that we do not care for, but—it's to take their hand. It's to want to walk down the hall with them arm in arm; that means something to these people. We do a lot of hugging, with families as well as with the patients. There is a lot of touching. I tend to think that many families have been put through hell trying to keep their loved one at home. . . . And I always say to them, "How did you. . . ." Yes, I tell them what a wonderful job they did. "How did you ever do it for so long?"

Patients' responses can further complicate the family's emotional upheaval and challenge the nursing staff to protect the families' self-esteem. Objectively, the patient's declining abilities and close contact with the nursing staff mean that the patient will often respond better to staff than to family. Emotionally, this is very difficult for family members.

They [the family] want to think they still are very important. And many times we have to reinforce this because the patients don't know them. But we have to give them the pats on the back for what they have been through and what they have done. And I'm sure it's extremely difficult for them when patients will respond to us as staff members, because they see us everyday, and they often walk away from the wives. . . . It's adding another loss.

HELPING FAMILIES WITH THE INEVITABLE

Even though family members see the patient progressively decline, the notion of death can still be abstract. Without destroying hope or being so concrete that it could harm them, the nursing staff must try to prepare family members for the inevitable.

Mr. Ti's wife . . . I got to know her quite well. And she was adamant that she wanted everything done for Mr. Ti. Mr. Ti had tuberculosis and multiple medical problems. He had declined functionally a great deal; at one point he was sent to the acute unit for pneumonia. She was very upset at how they had to restrain him and just how the staff, not that the staff was bad to them, but how they reacted to an Alzheimer patient. When Mr. Ti returned, as I said, he continued to decline functionally. One day I sat down and spoke with [his wife]. We were planning on a family conference in a couple of weeks and I . . . brought up the fact about how . . . not all staff in the hospital know how to take care of an Alzheimer patient as well as we do, because we have had the experience. [Her husband] knows us, and knows our ways. He is secure on our unit. Then I . . . said, "You know, you wouldn't want him restrained again to have an intravenous, and for what? You can see his decline." We talked about it for a long time. And about tube feedings; we went right down the whole gamut. She agreed that she wouldn't want any of this. She wouldn't want him transferred. . . . She just wanted him comfortable. . . . And when he died, she seemed to be very happy with the way he died, as far as his comfort level. She also knew all of us, so she felt comfortable being with us and we could support her during his time of death.

Good communication is a prerequisite to the family's being able to receive the information and education they will need in order to be able to deal with the disease and its effects.

[Developing a professional relationship that allows for being able to bridge the emotional feelings and intellectual knowledge] is not going to happen with every family, because you can't get close enough to some families. But you can still educate them enough that they are more prepared.

PLANNING AND PROVIDING CARE

ASSESSMENT

The overall disease trajectory is one of decline, but each patient and family is unique. Vital information for guiding caregiving decisions must be collected and interpreted. The process of assessment includes both the patient and family as individuals and within the family context. Nursing actions are guided by knowing that the death of the patient is inevitable, whereas the survival of the family (at this DSCU, it is often an elderly wife) may be influenced by the patient's death, and thus is a major concern for nursing.

Patient Assessment

This patient population is very vulnerable and completely dependent on others for their most basic care. Nurses carry out medical interventions and provide comfort and protection 24 hours a day; thus, they know the patients very well.

At this point in their lives, we know them better than their families and they all know us better than they know their families. And we become their translators—we can tell if they have a urinary tract infection, or if they have a headache, or if they have a. . . We can tell the difference. If they cannot express their pain or anything like that, we have to pick up on it—through behavior changes.

Assessing Families

Nurses know family members by being on duty when they typically visit or call. When recommending treatment decisions, the nursing staff should consider what they believe to be in the best interest of the patient as well as family factors.

> Their [the family's] immediate health factor comes right into [the treatment decision]. You know if they are in pain right away. Their age might have something to do with it. How long the patient has been here and how we have seen the family struggle through the [consequences of late-stage Alzheimer's disease] come into it for me.

Recommending palliative care options means that the nursing staff must further assess the emotional state of the family as to whether they are prepared to make such a decision.

> I think they could be in a state of panic, confusion, bewilderment, whatever you want to say and not fully understand what comfort care means. Or they could feel that this [palliative care] was the right thing to do, but they're still not really comfortable with it. . . . There are differences . . . we can see that the patient may be ready for total palliative care—but the family may not be ready for it emotionally.

Families need to adjust to the DSCU, as do patients. One way to help family members adjust is to listen to and be responsive to their concerns by doing things not necessarily required by the patient but to please the family.

> She [the patient's wife] seems very pleased to have settled right in, and we've sort of enabled that too. We make sure the window is closed—you heard her concern about pneumonia. I mean, this is an older woman; she's lived with [the patient] for 52 years and so she thinks that a sweater over his shoulders is going to help, so we put the sweater over his shoulders. She is very pleased with how we have treated him and her both, up here. . . . She's trusting us, and I'm really surprised that it came this soon.

DEVELOPING INTERPERSONAL RELATIONSHIPS

A step in developing relationships is trying to understand what it is like for the family member who ultimately makes decisions for the patient. The notion of a special understanding of the feelings, thoughts, and motives of another is important to the development of nursing staff–family relationships (Olsen, 1991).

I just try to put myself in their situation and think about how devastating it would be. Of course, everybody has different personalities, but to come in and sit in that room for a family conference where there are maybe three nurses, a doctor, a priest whom they might not know, and a social worker whom they are probably most familiar with, but still haven't developed a relationship with yet. . . . So essentially the wife is sitting there and telling all of these strangers, "Sure, you don't have to do anything for my husband: You just keep him comfortable, that's fine; I don't want you to treat him." You have handed over your most cherished possession to a group of strangers and now they are saying, well, we don't want to [provide aggressive medical interventions] and they are giving you valid reasons. We need to tread softly.

TRUST

TRUTH TELLING AND FIDELITY

The ethical principles of truth telling and fidelity underlie the development of trust. Within the nurse-family professional relationship, nurses have the moral obligations of veracity, to tell the truth and not lie or deceive people (Veatch & Fry, 1987a), and fidelity, to remain faithful to one's commitments (Veatch & Fry, 1987b). These principles are carried out with kind honesty.

Number one is honesty. . . . Honesty with the family at all times, about everything. I think you do have to use a lot of tact, but I really think that nothing should be held back if they want to know. . . . I usually try to touch base with each of the [family members] that I see come in, depending on what's going on, how long I have known them. Sometimes it's just a hello, but I try to touch base with each one of them, and I think that's developing trust too. I can honestly say that I've never distorted the truth or, should I say, lied to a family [member] about his or her loved one. I do believe that in the course of a conversation, families develop trust when you go up to them and say, "He might seem a little sleepy today; that's because we had to start him on this new medication, but you should see a change in two or three days." I think they appreciate that and that if you have gone out of your way to talk to them about this, you are trusting them with that knowledge and you are looking at them as if they are intelligent and not inconsequential human beings that just come to visit every once in a while. I really have found that this is probably the best way. There are a few families that can't handle total honesty, or brutal honesty, is more what I call it, I guess. And then it's just called an avoidance. We don't avoid them, but we avoid talking about certain areas that we know they just couldn't handle at that time.

We will talk about almost anything that is happening, even if the patient is combative, but we don't talk about it as if it's a bad thing. [Being combative] is something, you know, we understand and unfortunately it goes with the disease—that usually it only lasts for a short period of time and we can handle it; we don't find a problem with it. When you develop rapport, the give and take, you are developing trust. Then when I do go to a family conference and I tell them we would rather not pass a nasogastric tube, they know I am being onest when I tell them my reasons—or hopefully they know that I am, because I haven't lied to them in the past, or tried to hide anything from them. This seems to work out well.

The nursing staff know they keep their promises. Families need to believe that staff will keep their promises, which is essential to trust.

How do you tell trust? . . . When I see wives backing off from visiting, this is one form of trust. Backing off on their frequent visits, I should say. . . . When I can see a change in their visiting patterns. Number one, they don't come in all teary-eyed, even though their husbands may have deteriorated or declined both mentally and physically. . . . I can see a strength in them, and they will come in for a few minutes and say, "Well, there is no sense in me staying here, he doesn't know who I am," where before they would be there for hours and be very teary and run up to you and say, "Is this wrong, is that wrong?" such as Mrs. W. does. I would say for the most part, it still takes a period of time, a period of adjustment, a period of developing trust. But there are verbal clues, and, as I said, the biggest thing is really backing off on their visitation because they don't feel they have to come up to make sure that [their husbands were] washed that day or fed that day.

There is a need to reach that point of trust.

We haven't reached that point of trust until families will be able to say and feel in their hearts "Sure, I believe that you will still feed him if I say no tube feeding." And "Sure, I believe you'll take care of him if I say don't treat him for infections." How do they know we are going to keep him comfortable just because we say so? It has to be an ongoing thing over a period of time before you can ask them to trust you enough that you ensure that their husband is comfortable and you will always try to feed him.

IMPACT OF TRUST

Communication improves as trusting relationships develop. Staff members do not know how much education has been provided to the family about Alzheimer's disease or how much denial may have been used as a coping mechanism, but they do know that there is a lack of understanding on the part of many families.

Family Teaching

Many staff–family interactions are used to teach about comfort and dementia, which can be used to promote the building of trust. Informed decisions mean that the family knows the impact of alternate courses of actions. The family needs to know that the nursing staff will actually do what they say they will do for the patient.

> I think it's a matter of learning to trust us. It's a big decision to make and it is difficult enough. I think they have to learn to trust us and then they also have to . . . say good-bye. . . . They have to realize that what they are doing is for the patient's benefit and for his comfort.

Mutuality in Decision Making

Helping the family make a decision does not mean parentalism. Nor does it mean abdicating professional responsibility by turning this responsibility over to the family, without a recommendation from a professional caregiver, because providing one may be too difficult for the staff. An example of mutuality versus dominance of decision making during one family conference occurred when, after making her wishes known, the wife looked to the professionals and said, "Do you agree?" The nursing staff interpretation was as follows.

> She needs that [reassurance], you know. She kept saying, "I want to know what you think." You know she kept throwing it back at us. And that's okay. We have our jobs to do. . . . I think when I talked to her yesterday and what I heard her say, and what Nurse N. said, is that she wanted us to make the decision with her. She was afraid to make it alone. Which I could understand. She didn't want to be solely responsible for this man dying, even in comfort, you know. . . . She wanted to know she did everything she could for him.

A second example illustrates how the nursing staff can preserve the patient's autonomy through the mechanism of substituted judgment.

> It seems it's easier for [wives] if they are not deciding this alone. One patient went very bad, very quickly, and the doctor wanted to talk to the wife about her changing him to complete palliative care. She's standing in front of the office saying, "Let me see; what do I really want, what do I

really want?" One of the nurses coming by said, "Excuse me, [maybe] I could just help you for a minute." This lady hadn't been with us for very long. [The nurse] said, "I just heard you saying, 'what do I want?' I would just like to say I understand what you are going through, but if you could only think of it this way: What would your husband want? You are acting on his behalf. You are his spokesperson. What do you think he would want? If you could just think of that." About two minutes later the lady said, "I know exactly what I want."

Staff Demonstration of Respect for Family Decision Making

Making the ethical principle of respect operational means that the nursing staff must respect another individual as someone who shares the same human destiny as oneself. Respect for families is demonstrated by staff members when they do not agree with a family's wishes, but they recognize the family's authority to make the decision for the patient and they abide by that decision. Since the patient can no longer exercise self-determination, respect for that person is maintained by family members who make treatment decisions.

> If [the patient is] a "no treat," then we won't treat with antibiotics; we will treat with morphine or comfort measures. We have to abide by the family's wishes. We may not always agree with them, but I think as professionals we should abide by them as if the patient had made the wish.

NURSING CARE WITHIN THE INTERDISCIPLINARY TEAM

Many goal-directed interventions can be carried out to prevent avoidable complications associated with Alzheimer's disease and to maximize the living potential of patients in the terminal phase. These goals can be viewed as a hierarchy and be related to ethical principles. Goals for all patients are safety, comfort, quality of life, and dignity.

Basic goals of safety and comfort are moral imperatives under the ethical principle of beneficence. Dignity is an essential and higher ordered goal and will be discussed with the principle of autonomy. (See chapter 13 for a further discussion on providing comfort to patients in the terminal stage of Alzheimer's disease and chapter 5 for methods to enhance quality of life.)

SAFETY

Safety fits within the ethical principles of doing good and avoiding harm. The DSCU nursing staff feared transferring patients to acute care units because those caregivers there are experts in striving for cure from the disease process but are typically limited in their knowledge of care required by patients with dementia. Limited specialized knowledge can result in acute care staff using restraints, which are seldom used in a dementia unit.

> [The patient] may not be safe. He might hang himself on whatever they would tie him down with. . . . I just think of his confusion if he is transferred. You know what I mean, it would get worse. . . . And the idea of sneakers on the patients, safety, I love our safety measures. It's really nice to know they aren't going to slip and fall on a wet floor because the housekeepers pay such good attention to the floors. . . . I just think it is important not to have him transferred.

COMFORT

Providing comfort is the hallmark of the hospice approach to care. Perhaps the efforts to legalize assisted suicide would not be an issue if patients with Alzheimer's disease and other terminal conditions could be assured that they would die a comfortable death (Sachs, Ahronheim, Rhymes, Volicer, & Lynn, 1995).

> What are we? We're a comfort unit. My priority is to provide care and comfort to Alzheimer patients and to be the primary nurse for the families of patients. . . . You know, comfort is really the only thing that we can ensure for these patients, to make sure that they are comfortable. We'd be negligent if we didn't come forth with it. I couldn't live with it, if I ran up against a doctor who would refuse to order something.

Staff members at the DSCU diagnose and treat discomfort. Infections in the terminal phase of Alzheimer's are often the immediate cause of death (Hurley, Volicer, & Volicer, 1996), and morphine and Tylenol are often used to treat the respiratory symptoms associated with a fever episode (Hurley, Volicer, Mahoney, & Volicer, 1993). Morphine has an additional effect of reducing labored breathing.

> Well, what we base it all on is comfort. The big thing is when someone is a level 5 [complete palliative care only], we usually do not work them up, so we don't know what's wrong with them. In this particular patient, previously when we worked up and treated his fever episodes and he developed a urinary track infection, this would be his behavior. He'd become more agitated and stop eating, so we knew this. When he became a level 5 and became agitated, he was evidently uncomfortable, and he would stop eating, I was told, "Well, let's just get a urine [sample]; if it's that, we can give him some Bactrim." And this is how he has been treated. So you will say, well, why don't we put him on some morphine? See, morphine

usually does relieve pain, but it also causes [patients] to be sleepy a lot
of times and if they still have the infection, then their eating decreases.
So we treat with comfort measures.

Comfort is an overarching patient goal and the focus for caregiving
actions, but regrettably, not all patients die "the good death."

I think maybe just by seeing various patients die and realizing that if
some of them had been made level 5s [complete palliative care], they
would not have suffered as much. I would honestly have to say that some
of our patients have . . . suffered while dying, to an extent anyway, not as
badly as they would have, had we not provided extra comfort measures.

The focus of care is providing comfort. Given the difficulty of being
sure that patients are free from discomfort, the nursing staff at the DSCU
have different concerns about using morphine.

Even when patients look comfortable, they aren't able to tell us in a lot of
ways, so you wonder if they aren't having internal pain or whatever. We
don't know what they are thinking, so you hope they are comfortable. By
their facial expressions, you think that they are, but . . . it's really tough.
The best method of learning is by experience, probably of seeing these
patients in varying degrees. It also helps us to provide more comfort
measures. Another big hang-up is that some nurses are very reluctant to
give out morphine. I don't feel uncomfortable giving morphine; I sort of
made my peace with myself that if a patient dies after being given morphine, he was dying anyway. I surely didn't kill him by giving him that
morphine. A lot of nurses feel very strongly, to the point that we have to
order [morphine] every 6 hours, or it won't be given if it's put down PRN
[whenever necessary], because they don't feel comfortable. I got angry at
first, but I understand it too, you know, if they more or less want me or
someone else to . . . take it out of their hands and say, "You have to give
it." Then that's fine too. But I really think the experience of working a long
time on the unit and dealing with dying patients has changed some of my
outlook and changed the levels that I might recommend. I think before,
when I first started working here, I'd say, it really was a lot to have a
patient as a level 5 [complete palliative care], even a bed patient, no matter what. It was suffering to see them like that. . . . There's no cure, there's
no hope, there's no sense to keep someone lingering because eventually
they become a contracted bed patient if you keep them going.

DIGNITY

Preserving dignity means that despite the incapacitation that occurs as
a result of Alzheimer's disease, the nursing staff must recognize the

worth and honor due this particular person. Staff members should treat patients as unique human beings that deserve respect, take actions to maintain patients' poise, bearing, and demeanor, and see beyond the superficial outward appearance to the intrinsic value of the individual. The DSCU is the patient's home, and caregivers are there to tend to the needs of each resident—from admission until death.

> You know, [patients] are just going to decline. But it's another thing to work with them on a daily basis and [know] they . . . are still human beings, they do have their own personalities no matter how different they are from what they were on the outside. These are the people we've grown to know and maybe the families don't know them at all anymore, because their personalities from before have essentially left them. I don't know if you could compare it to working with severely retarded children or something like that. . . . They should still be treated with respect, not as helpless, dying, debilitated persons.

CONCLUSIONS

Nurses as moral agents provide the care that patients, who are dying from the complications of a disease that has robbed them of their very personhood, are unable to provide for themselves. Gentle and kindly caregiving should be provided that incorporates ethical principles and clinical wisdom into care of the patient within their family constellation. Safety, comfort, quality of life, and dignity can be maintained regardless of the ravages to the body and mind caused by dementia.

REFERENCES

Awoke, S., Mouton, C., & Parrott, M. (1992). Outcomes of skilled cardiopulmonary resuscitation in a long-term care facility: Futile therapy? *Journal of the American Geriatrics Society, 40,* 593–595.

Fry, S. T. (1994). *Ethics in nursing practice.* Geneva: International Council of Nurses.

Henderson, V. (1977). *Basic principles of nursing care* (rev. ed.). Geneva: International Council of Nurses.

Hurley, A. C., Bottino, R., & Volicer, L. (1994, August). Nursing role in advance proxy planning for Alzheimer patients. *CARING Magazine,* (pp. 72–76).

Hurley, A. C., Mahoney, M. A., & Volicer, L. (1995). Comfort care in end-stage dementia: What to do after deciding to do no more. In E. Olson, E. R. Chichin, & L. Libow (Eds.), *Controversies in ethics in long-term care* (pp. 73–86). New York: Springer.

Hurley, A. C., Volicer, B. J., Mahoney, M. A., & Volicer, L. (1993). Palliative fever management in Alzheimer patients: Quality plus fiscal responsibility. *Advances in Nursing Science, 16*(1), 21–32.

Hurley, A. C., Volicer, B. J., & Volicer, L. (1996). Effect of fever management strategy on the progression of dementia of the Alzheimer type. *Alzheimer Disease and Associated Disorders, 10,* 5–10.

Hurley, A., Volicer, L., & Mahoney, E. (1996, March). Progression of Alzheimer's disease and symptom management. Supplement: Primary Care of Alzheimer's disease: A multidisciplinary challenge. *Federal Practitioner,* 16–22.

Hurley, A. C., Volicer, L., Rempusheski, V. F., & Fry, S. (1995). Reaching consensus: The process of recommending treatment decisions for Alzheimer patients. *Advances in Nursing Science, 18*(2), 33–43.

Nightingale, F. (1946). *Notes on nursing: What it is and what it is not.* Philadelphia: Lippincott.

Olsen, D. P. (1991). Empathy as an ethical and philosophical basis for nursing. *Advances in Nursing Science, 14*(1), 62–75.

Sachs, G. A., Ahronheim, J. C., Rhymes, J. A., Volicer, L., & Lynn, J. (1995). Good care of dying patients: The alternative to euthanasia. *Journal of the American Geriatrics Society, 43,* 553–562.

Veatch, R. M., & Fry, S. T. (1987a). Veracity. In *Case studies in nursing ethics* (pp. 117–135). Philadelphia: Lippincott.

Veatch, R. M., & Fry, S. T. (1987b). Fidelity. In *Case studies in nursing ethics* (pp. 137–154). Philadelphia: Lippincott.

Volicer, L., Rheaume, Y., Brown, J., Fabiszewski, K., & Brady, R. (1986). Hospice approach to the treatment of patients with advanced dementia of the Alzheimer type. *Journal of the American Medical Association, 256,* 2210–2213.

Advance Proxy Planning

Margaret Ann Mahoney, Ann C. Hurley, and Ladislav Volicer

C ollaborative health care decision-making models that include patients, family members, and multidisciplinary caregivers promise a comprehensive assessment of both ethical and clinical dimensions inherent in such decision (Mahoney, Hurley, Smith, & Volicer, 1992). By including more participants, the decision making becomes more complex and can create dilemmas based on competing values and beliefs and decisional delays due to conflicting needs and goals. When surrogates are needed to represent the wishes of patients who are incapable of participating in treatment decisions as occurs, with dementia of the Alzheimer type (DAT), the process becomes even more complex.

Policies and procedures that preclude unilateral decision making and are based on sound principles of ethical reasoning should be established. There may be incongruity between the treatment preferences of patients and decisions made by surrogates, based on perceptions of quality of life and satisfaction with care (McNabney, Beers, & Siebens, 1994). Surrogates have incorrectly guessed 41% of patients' answers to research questions, and the only predictor of accurate surrogate decision making was a specific discussion between the patient and surrogate about life support (Suhl, Simons, Reedy, & Garrick, 1994). Hospital policies seem to dictate practice patterns regarding life-sustaining interventions (Cugliari & Miller, 1994; Watts, Cassel, & Hickam, 1986), yet providers would like to see more patient participation in decision making (Solomon et al., 1993).

This chapter suggests that the process of advance proxy planning that was developed as a model of shared clinical decision making in the Dementia Special Care Units (DSCUs) at the Edith Nourse Rogers Memorial VA Hospital in Bedford, Massachusetts, be utilized to define "optimal care" and "quality of life" for each participant in the context of the individual experience of the disease process. Advance proxy planning involves professional caregivers who can communicate their knowledge about the progressive trajectory of DAT and offer the therapeutic expertise to provide clinical management of the symptoms of the illness, in a trusting relationship with family caregivers. The goal of advance proxy planning is to establish a therapeutic alliance between professional and family caregivers that continues through the subsequent phases of the disease. A hospice philosophy of care (Volicer, Fabiszewski, Rheaume, Brown, & Brady, 1986) is the foundation for this model of advance proxy planning. Caregiving goals are mutually defined to promote safety, comfort, quality of life, and preserve the patient's dignity.

DEVELOPING THE INFRASTRUCTURE

Well-constructed decisions must be formulated and evaluated. Clinical decision models need to support shared decision and incorporate legal mandates, ethical principles and professional standards of practices, and beliefs of family decision makers, as well as institutional policies.

FAMILY DECISION MAKING ABOUT HEALTH CARE

Health care institutions are required to inform patients of their right to participate in health care decision making, but often without institutional and professional policies that enhance shared decision making (Mezey, Evens, Golub, Murphy, & White, 1994). Many agencies have devised forms that are routinely administered when patients are admitted, and these are often interpreted as simply the right to refuse treatments. This has the potential to create an adversarial situation instead of promoting discussion and proactive decision making. During times of acute illness or medical crisis, patients and families may not be in the best position to make difficult choices. The stress of illness may block communication and affect the capacity to make sound decisions. Decisions made in haste may preclude discussion about the implications of choices, or the inherent risks and benefits of the proposed treatment. Health care decision making may be especially difficult for family members, who have been appointed as surrogates, and thus are required to support the patient's best interests ahead of their own. With advance proxy planning, there is ample opportunity for decisional review and for incorporating the beliefs of family members. These factors contribute to making a commitment to a well-formulated decision and decrease postdecision regret.

ETHICAL FRAMEWORK FOR COLLABORATIVE DECISION MAKING

Before entering into a dialogue with the families, the interdisciplinary treatment team must be in agreement about what constitutes optimal care for patients with advanced DAT. If clinicians do not discuss their own beliefs and values and do not have a shared conceptual agreement, then individual practice philosophies may prevent interdisciplinary collaboration. A process of values clarification allows providers to enter into moral discussions with a clear understanding of the terms being used, so that a foundation is established for the resolution of ethical dilemmas. When clinicians participate in health care decision making, "first, their actions, words, and presence help shape the patient's assessment of the best course of therapy. Second, their ability and willingness to carry out various decisions often define the range of options available to the patient" (President's Commission for the Study of Ethical Problems in Biomedical and Behavioral Research, 1983, p. 46).

Impediments to moral dialogue occur when people attach greater moral weight to acts than to omissions, based on their perceptions of causality. If a patient's death can be related to a professional's act, then that act could assume instrumental proportions in relation to the patient's demise. On the other hand, in the absence or omission of action on the part of the health care provider, the patient's terminal outcome would be attributed to his or her underlying disease process, independent of the health care professional. However, actions are not morally different from omissions. In either event, a different choice on the part of the health care professional may have affected the patient. The justification for acts and omissions is not found in attributions of causality, but is based on sound reasoning that is supportive of the patient's informed choice and is reflective of safe and prudent practice.

A closely related argument that may cloud ethical decision making is the distinction between withdrawing and withholding treatment. Not initiating therapy can seem more acceptable because it represents an omission instead of an action, yet this argument has been shown to lack ethical significance. If any ethical discussions involve this distinction, however, greater moral justification is needed to withhold therapy than to withdraw it. Based on the probabilistic nature of medical decision making (Elstein, Shulman, & Sprafka, 1978), the positive effects of an intervention are not completely certain before it has been initiated. After an intervention has been tried, if it is not beneficial, or creates burdensome side effects, then justification for its withdrawal has been clinically established. Decisions to withhold therapy, therefore, are more difficult to defend ethically, as the potential risks or benefits can only be surmised. Also, most decisions to withdraw treatment involve explicit decisions made by patients, families, and staff; whereas decisions to withhold therapy are commonly implicit and not usually discussed (President's Commission, 1983).

Health care providers, however, often have more trouble with withdrawing treatment once it has been initiated (Solomon et al., 1993). Moral proscriptions against patient abandonment and a reluctance to diminish the patient's hope and confidence for cure often have physicians resorting to "therapeutic privilege." This paternalistic practice is based on the ethical principle of beneficence, but it precludes open patient communication and has the detrimental effect of negating any truth telling by other health care providers.

The distinction between ordinary and extraordinary treatments is also not useful for ethical decision making. What is considered ordinary treatment in a large medical center, for instance, may very well be called extraordinary in a small community hospital. Advances in medical technology also change public perceptions of ordinary versus extraordinary treatments. The concepts of burden and usefulness of a treatment have advantages over other interpretations of ordinary and extraordinary, such as common versus unusual, or simple versus complex. Considering the usefulness or burdensomeness of a treatment allows examination of that treatment in relation to the patient, the condition, and the projected risks and benefits. Ethical decision making can more readily be applied to these elements, although it may be more difficult to make this distinction when considering less dramatic interventions, such as the use of artificial feeding.

There is the potential for disagreement about which outcomes can count as burdensome. Is financial cost relevant? Can family burden be taken into consideration? Is the sustained life burdensome, or just the treatment alone? The President's Commission for the Study of Ethical Problems in Biomedical and Behavioral Research (1983) found no medical treatments that a patient would be obliged to accept. However, a decision against aggressive medical intervention is not the same as deciding to forgo all care. When cure is not possible, aggressive nursing measures become paramount in maintaining the patient's dignity and comfort (Hurley, Mahoney, & Volicer, 1995). It is important for the members of the interdisciplinary team to achieve a shared understanding of these ethical distinctions, so that the process of advance proxy planning is not blocked by unclear communication, and ethically valid decisions can be made.

DEVELOPING INSTITUTIONAL POLICIES THAT SUPPORT ADVANCE PROXY PLANNING

Once the health care team has defined the shared values and beliefs of a moral community, then institutional policies must be in place that are supportive of that practice philosophy. Institutional policies must be tolerant of individual choice and reflect sensitivity and compassion to the patient's personal values. This harmony is not easily achieved in a hospital setting, where an estimated 80% of all deaths occur (Weiler, 1987). Since the mission of the hospital is treatment and cure, the process of dying may be prolonged by the application of highly technological treatments of questionable benefit to the underlying condition. Tensions often exist among health care professionals when palliative treatments are planned for the terminally ill in an acute care environment.

Health care institutions have a responsibility to ensure that there are appropriate procedures to enhance patients' competence, to provide for the designation of surrogates, to guarantee that patients are adequately informed, to overcome the influences of dominant institutional biases, to provide review of the decisions made, and to refer cases to the courts appropriately (President's Commission, 1983). Policies that define each of these considerations need to be in place to support advance proxy planning.

CONSENSUS BUILDING ABOUT OPTIMAL TREATMENT STRATEGIES

The formation of the therapeutic alliance on which advance proxy planning is based is accomplished by having consistent contact and good communication between members of the interdisciplinary team and the patient and his or her family. Because of the clearly articulated philosophy of a hospice approach to care (Volicer et al., 1986), the staff of the DSCUs have developed expertise in planning and providing care to patients with DAT that optimizes quality of life and maximizes comfort, which has been empirically verified. Patients in the DSCUs had lower observed discomfort than patients with DAT who were not cared for with a hospice approach (Hurley, Volicer, Mahoney & Volicer; 1993; Volicer et al., 1994).

Institutional policies and procedures that are supportive of the hospice approach to care have been operationalized at the DSCUs. The families are involved in making decisions about initiating aggressive medical interventions in advance of potential crises. The health care team meets to review the decisions that were made prior to admission, to share the results of their admission assessments, and to establish an interdisciplinary treatment plan (Mahoney et. al., 1992). A family conference is held about 8 weeks after admission to the DSCU to make the advance proxy plan (Hurley, Bottino, & Volicer, 1994). The advance proxy plan is based on inputs from the physician, nursing staff, and chaplain and include the patient's previous wishes as well as the family's interpretation of the patient's beliefs, goals, and values (see Figure 9.1).

The day before the family conference, the patient's physician meets with the nursing staff of the patient's unit to reach a consensus about the level of care the team believes is optimal for the patient so that this recommendation can be provided for family consideration (Hurley, Volicer, Rempusheski, & Fry, 1995). Providing a recommendation for the family to consider based on the nurses' interpretation of the patient's current status is less stressful than immediately presenting all options

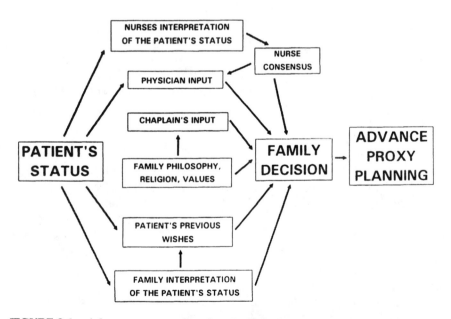

FIGURE 9.1   Advance proxy planning model.

From "Nursing Role in Advance Proxy Planning, by A. C. Hurley, R. Bottino, and L. Volicer, 1994, *Caring, 8,* p. 75. Copyright 1994, National Association for Home Care. Reproduced with permission.

to the surrogate. During the conference the patient's physician affirms the hospice philosophy, asks the family about the patient's previous wishes regarding medical interventions, discusses the patient's present condition within the context of the fact that DAT is currently incurable, presents the nursing staff recommendation and rationale, and begins the discussion.

All patients receive intensive nursing care so that the goal of maximum comfort is achieved (Hurley, Mahoney, & Volicer, 1995). In addition, five levels of care sequentially limit aggressive medical interventions (Volicer et al., 1986), with specific intensive care nursing interventions concomitant for each level.

1. Aggressive medical care includes aggressive diagnostic workups and therapy as indicated, resuscitation attempts (CPR) if necessary, treatment of coexisting medical conditions including transfer to an acute care unit if indicated, and tube feeding if normal food intake is not possible.
2. Complete medical care, as described above, but CPR is not attempted.
3. No CPR, nor is the patient transferred to an acute care setting for technological interventions. This excludes intravenous therapy. A patient would be transferred if an intervention is required to prevent discomfort, such as to repair a fractured hip.
4. No CPR, no transfer, and no aggressive workup or intravenous antibiotic treatment of intercurrent infections. Antipyretics and analgesics are given for fever and comfort (oral antibiotics may be prescribed for an apparent urinary tract infection manifested by dysuria).
5. No CPR, no transfer, no intravenous antibiotics, and no artificial feeding. This precludes the use of long-term feeding tubes, and patients are fed by natural means for as long as possible.

Decisions about levels of care are designed to operationalize the values and beliefs about the use of aggressive medical intervention for patients with an incurable illness that were expressed by the proxies during the family conferences. Within these levels of care, maintenance of the patient's safety, comfort, quality of life, and dignity is always the goal. Assessments of these indicators dictate decisions about optimal clinical management strategies. Initial selection of a level of care as an advance proxy plan is not an irrevocable decision and can be changed at any time. If the family has made the decision for complete palliative care, no more family conferences are routinely scheduled, for to do so would force the family to live once again through the difficult decision-making process. Furthermore, this might signal that the health care team has questioned their decision. Patients whose advance proxy plan is not complete palliative care are discussed as an annual family conference. Families may request a family conference at any time. The surrogate decision maker of all patients whose condition has worsened to the degree that they are placed on the seriously ill list are contacted by the physician, who describes the change in the clinical situation, states the current advance proxy plan, and asks for a confirmation that the family is still in agreement with the advance proxy plan. Thus making an advance proxy plan does not signal the end to further family and provider communication. During times of physiologic crisis, when the advance proxy plan is actually invoked, there is more communication.

Advance proxy planning involves more than decision making before a medical crisis occurs. Devising a cohesive philosophy of care among the members of the interdisciplinary team, establishing supportive institutional policies that apply across clinical settings, and developing consistent caregiving relationships improve teamwork and establish trust and rapport with the patients and families. Providers and families evaluate treatment outcomes, so that chronic illness can be managed within the parameters of sound clinical assessment, the patient's values, beliefs, and goals, and the appropriate utilization of health care resources. This is an established process of decision making that defines the optimal care that is provided for each patient.

ENHANCING DECISIONAL COMPETENCE

The patients in the DSCU in this discussion have advanced DAT and lack the cognitive capacity and judgment necessary for decision making. Therefore, family members who themselves have had role changes by assuming more responsibility for the family member with DAT (Brody, 1985; Cantor, 1983; Chenoworth & Spencer, 1986) now participate in decision making with members of the interdisciplinary health care team. Family members who speak on behalf of the patients must be able to participate in the decision-making process, which occurs after the family has transitioned from the role of primary caregiver and staff of the DSCU has assumed this role. When families decide to hospitalize the patient with DAT, their guilt, depression, and grieving must be addressed to reduce caregiver burdens as health care decisions are made (Mahoney, 1992). These symptoms of grieving seem to cycle around each loss

(Mahoney, 1992), as opposed to the linear trajectory that Kübler-Ross (1975) discovered with patients who are terminally ill.

SURROGATE DECISION MAKING MODELS

The advance directive informs the surrogate about the patient's wishes and goals. Two forms of advance directives exist: the living will and the durable power of attorney for health care decisions. Advance directives are usually written well before patients develop incapacitating diseases and may offer guidance in treatment preferences. But because they are written well in advance of the current illness, the language may be vague and nonspecific. Terms such as "terminal illness" and "extraordinary measures" must be interpreted by surrogates in the context of the current disease process, the patient's prognosis, and the specific interventions being considered.

When advance directives do not exist but the previous wishes of the patient are known, the substituted judgment standard is applied. The surrogate decision maker, possessing knowledge of the patient's preferences, acts as spokesperson. If the patient has not communicated any health care preferences to the family, then the best interest standard is used in which the surrogate makes a decision based on his or her judgment of what would be best for the patient.

LEGAL GUIDELINES FOR SURROGATE DECISION MAKERS

A family member is often the most appropriate person to be designated as a surrogate decision maker. Decisions made by surrogates are rarely subjected to judicial review. Only in unusual cases where there is a conflict or when the surrogate selects a highly unusual course of treatment do health care providers refuse to honor their decisions. The landmark Quinlan case was the first to issue an opinion on the rights of family members to refuse life-sustaining intervention on behalf of a patient. In 1976 the New Jersey Supreme Court granted the relief sought by Karen Ann Quinlan's father to allow the removal of ventilator support (*In re Quinlan,* 1976). Legal decisions have balanced the patient's right to privacy and self-determination while respecting the professional domain of medicine. Decisions about life-sustaining interventions require careful consideration, as they often affect more than one goal of the patient, that is, the prolongation of life and the relief of suffering. When these choices can be discussed with primary care providers, decisions can be made in advance that are stable over time and do not vary when the actual illness is experienced (Emanuel, Emanuel, Stoeckle, Hummel, & Barry, 1994).

CAREGIVING STRATEGIES FOR OPTIMAL MANAGEMENT OF PATIENTS WITH DEMENTIA

Family members often recognize the symptoms of DAT before the patient is aware of them. Therefore, family members play a critical role in dementia care. Health care providers work closely with patients and families during the initial diagnostic evaluation to exclude other organic or psychological causes for dementia. Once probable DAT is diagnosed, patients and families continue to need supportive providers who will manage the effects of this chronic illness, which may span from 2 to 20 years. Management of increasingly confused behaviors, with concomitant physical and psychological sequelae, is best accomplished by interdisciplinary teams who work closely with patients and families. Professional caregivers provide a continuum of care that includes home care, respite services, adult day health programs, and long-term care when patients need 24-hour skilled services. Health care decisions emerge from the therapeutic alliance that is formed between patients, families, and clinicians, so that advance proxy planning is a dynamic process of decision making for patients with DAT that is continuously evaluated and revised as the illness progresses.

EVALUATING THE PROCESS OF ADVANCE PROXY PLANNING

Several phases of investigations have examined the process and outcomes of advance proxy planning. In phase 1, a content analysis was conducted using a retrospective sample of 68 patient records that described the process and participants of family conferences during a 5-year period. The records contained documentation that quantitatively described the patient's condition and provided evidence of the patient's decisional incapacity. The baseline physical assessment data revealed that potential causes of reversible dementia had been assessed and ruled out. The medical records also gave no indication of any acute situation that would influence decision making or indicate that a medical emergency had precipitated a crisis. The decisions were truly made prior to the medical need for these life-sustaining interventions, which supported the notion of advance planning.

This patient population had very advanced DAT. Many were unable to communicate and relate to those around them. This rendered these patients unable to formulate or express a decision, so that it was necessary to have surrogate decision makers for this population. Wives were the most frequent proxy decision makers and were often accompanied by other family members and friends at the family conference. The health care providers who participated in the conferences were the medical director, the nurse practitioner, the nurse manager, the social worker, the chaplain, and the primary care nurse.

Level of care decisions were made during family conferences that were held within 8 weeks of a patient's admission to the DSCU. The nursing staff provided an initial recommendation for the family to consider at the family conference. The recommendation always included "do not resuscitate" status because of the poor outcomes of resuscitation in institutionalized demented individuals (Applebaum, King, & Finucane, 1990). Another recommendation made for almost all patients was that they should not be transferred to an acute care setting, unless required for comfort (e.g., treatment for a fracture). This recommendation was made because of the team's clinical experience that dementia patients' nutritional and functional states worsen in an acute care setting. The team also found that aggressive treatment in acute settings also compromised skin integrity, most likely because of the use of restraints to prevent patients from removing intravenous lines and catheters.

For patients who were bedfast and had limited ability to interact with their environment, the recommendation usually included palliative treatment of infections. This was based on the observation that antibiotic treatment is not effective in increasing survival in this patient population (Fabiszewski, Volicer, & Volicer, 1990). Neither does antibiotic treatment decrease patients' discomfort more than when only analgesics and antipyretics are used (Hurley et al., 1993). In addition, the diagnostic workup needed for the rational use of antibiotics inflicts a significant burden on the patient, who does not understand the need for blood drawing and cannot cough up a sputum sample, which then requires suctioning. Even when a complete workup is performed, the source of fever is not identified in 30% of episodes, decreasing further the benefit of this intervention (Fabiszewski et al., 1990). Furthermore, the treatment of infections with antibiotics does not slow the progression of DAT, and disease severity increased even more so in patients who received aggressive medical treatment (Hurley, Volicer, & Volicer, 1996).

Another recommendation made for all patients was avoidance of tube feeding. The team recommended that the patient should be fed as long as possible by natural means since this can be accomplished by adjustments of diet texture, use of dietary supplements, and skillful feeding techniques until the very terminal stage of the disease (Department of

Veterans Affairs, 1995). It is explained to the family members that tube feeding not only increases the patient's discomfort and often requires restraints to prevent the patient from removing the tube, but also prevents the patient from enjoying the taste of food and from interacting with staff members during feeding. Tube feeding often leads to significant complications, which include diarrhea and cramps, nausea, vomiting, abdominal distension, tubal obstruction and migration, infection, and leakage of stoma (Volicer, 1993). In addition, tube feeding not only does not prevent aspiration but actually increases the incidence of aspiration pneumonia (Pick et al., 1996).

At the family conference, the physician asked the family members about any previously expressed preferences about care. If no advance directive existed or previous wishes were expressed, then the best interest standard was applied in advance proxy planning. Some previous wishes had been formalized through living wills or expressed in discussions of organ donation. Other previous wishes were statements of beliefs, such as, "He never believed in keeping people alive with machines." Specific values or religious preferences were not expressly stated in the records reviewed in this sample. Religious expression was evident in a quote from one patient, a former nurse who often said about her incurable patients that she wished that "God would just take them." The family remembered this and viewed this frequently repeated sentiment as an indication of what the patient would want, given similar circumstances. Other patient preferences were expressed in terms of technology, stating that the patient "would not want to be kept alive by machines" or have "extraordinary measures" used.

In two instances, there were decisional conflicts. In one case, the family stated that they had discussed the use of respirators, and the patient would not want to be kept alive by one, but the family wanted aggressive medical treatment. In another instance, the family selected level 5 (complete palliative care), but the staff believed that the family did not understand the ramifications of their choice and the patient was initially treated as a level 3 (which was more congruent with the family's stated goals for optimal care) while the care team spent more time with the family to make sure that they were aware of the consequences of their decision. In each case, the family's decision was honored by the staff. This is essential if trust is to be established as the foundation of the therapeutic alliance.

THE DYNAMICS OF THE THERAPEUTIC ALLIANCE

In phase 2, proxy decision makers were interviewed before and after the family conferences to ascertain their understanding of the decision-making process and learn how they made decisions (Mahoney, 1992).

Family conferences were observed, audiotaped, and transcribed during the course of a year, using the method of participant observation and constant comparative analysis. All members of the interdisciplinary team supported this study, and 21 families consented to participate. The methods of grounded theory (Glaser & Strauss, 1967) were followed to describe an empirically valid model of the process of advance proxy planning. Analysis of these data led to the identification of four dynamics that characterized the formulation of the therapeutic alliance within the moral community that was comprised of members of the interdisciplinary team and the proxy decision makers. The family members participate in setting the goals for optimal care, and the staff organize their care plans to meet clinical objectives derived from these goals. This is the therapeutic alliance that is formed to constitute the moral agency of the patient within the formation of the moral community.

Prolonged engagement and observation of the interdisciplinary team provided the data to empirically validate the importance of interdisciplinary practice as the context for four dynamics that characterized the therapeutic alliance. Each dynamic contains the prefix *inter-*, which comes from the Latin word meaning "between, among, mutually, or reciprocally" (Costello, 1991, p. 701). The practice patterns of the interdisciplinary team operationalize these concepts, so that this theory is grounded in a moral community that is ethically justified, includes interdisciplinary team practices that are empirically documented, and has etymological roots that conceptually define the dynamics of the therapeutic alliance. In this grounded theory, the four dynamics that characterize the therapeutic alliance necessary for advance proxy planning in the moral community have been conceptualized as interest, interpretation, interagency, and intervention.

INTEREST

The word *interest* is derived from the Latin *inter + esse,* "to be," and means a feeling of having one's attention, concern, or curiosity particularly engaged by something; something that arouses such feelings, something in which one is interested; the power to excite such feelings; the quality of being interesting; concern or importance, a matter of primary interest; a business, cause, etc., in which a person has a share, concern, or responsibility; participation in a cause, or in advantage or responsibility; often, interests, a group exerting influence on, and often financially involved in an enterprise, industry, or sphere of activity; the state of being affected by something in respect to advantage or detriment; often, interests, benefit; advantage, as best interests (Costello, 1991, p. 702).

Interest requires an existential openness and a self-other awareness in order to be considered a member in the moral community with a legitimate concern for the patient, either through relation or professional role. Each member of the interdisciplinary team has personal and professional values and norms that influence the choices that were made in terms of roles and goals to be accomplished at the meetings. Moral elements, which include those personal and professional motivations, shaped by background and beliefs, education and training, ethical codes, legal mandates, social norms, and hospital policies, comprise this notion of interest:

> Real interests are neither the sum of our perceived interests nor perceived interests we happen to share with each other, nor perceived interests that happen to meet some independent (perhaps ideological) criteria for the good life. Rather, they simply are the interests that are responded to by the policies we arrive at via our participation in decision making. (Care, 1987, p. 74)

Through participation in the process of advance proxy planning, surrogates are also empowered to identify their own needs and goals. Each participant, both clinician and family member, has a personal interest in being at the meetings in order to fully participate, and this forms an interpersonal element. This interpersonal element, essential to the formation of the interdisciplinary team, is the capacity for self-other awareness (Buber, 1937), an ability to be existentially open to listen and respond to the communication at the meetings.

Without the dynamic of interest as it has been described, the formation of the therapeutic alliance may be blocked. Poor communication, mistrust, denial, or a lack of awareness of the patient's values and goals may lead to decisions that are clinically sound but may not constitute the person as a moral being. Decisions made in a crisis do not go beyond meeting the demands of the immediate situation. The personhood of the patient is not a factor in these clinical decisions. If that is the case, then disinterest, whether for personal or professional reasons, will interfere with the formation of the therapeutic alliance necessary to this process of advance proxy planning that should constitute the person as a moral being. The ethical standard for these decisions is the individual definition of self-determination, expressed as the interest of each participant in the decision-making process.

INTERPRETATION

Interpretation comes from the Latin *inter + praeire,* meaning "to go before, to lead" (Costello, 1991, p. 1059). A praetor was a magistrate in Roman times who administered civil justice. Currently, interpretation means "the act of interpreting; elucidation, explication; the meaning assigned to another's creative work, action, behavior, etc.; oral translation; the performing of a dramatic part, music, etc., so as to bring out the meaning or to demonstrate one's conception of it; the assignment of meaning to abstract symbols in a logical system" (Costello, 1991, p. 705). In this dynamic process of advance proxy planning, interpretation describes the communication of shared meaning. The event is understood in its context by all participants, so that the surrogates can make a truly informed decision.

Interpretation is defined as the process of assigning meaning to the shared events. The progression of the illness and the cognitive and emotional components identified in the literature on caregiver burden influence the process of interpretation. The knowledge and skill of the staff also are important to interpretation, so that an opportunity for real dialogue occurs. Having an appreciation of the effects of DAT on a family and understanding the personal history of the illness and the family caregiving patterns may better prepare the staff to provide support through the process of advance proxy planning. Interpretation is the basis for open communication. The ethical standard is derived from veracity, which requires truthful communication.

INTERAGENCY

Interagency is derived from the Latin *inter* + *agere*, "to drive, to do, act." An agent is defined as a "person or business authorized to act on another's behalf; a person or thing that has the power to act; a natural force or object producing or used for obtaining specific results; an active cause, an efficient cause; or a person who acts in an official capacity" (Costello, 1991, p. 26). *Interagency* is a term that has been coined to represent the process of shared decisions made on behalf of the patient by the surrogates, who participate as members of the therapeutic alliance in a principled moral community.

This dynamic ingredient is the actual decision making, in which the person is constituted as a moral being. The patient's values have been affirmed through expressing previous wishes; the decision is viewed in the context of the disease progression and supports the values of the patient, family, and staff. The responsibility for making the decision and for acting according to what has been mutually agreed is interagency. When these criteria are met, the surrogate decision makers feel comfortable with the decision and its moral justification, and there is little likelihood of experiencing postdecision regrets. Interagency is derived from the ethical principle of fidelity, which requires promise keeping.

INTERVENTION

Intervention comes from the Latin *inter* + *venire,* meaning to "come between disputing people, groups, etc., to intercede, mediate; to occur or be between two things; to occur incidentally, so as to modify or hinder; to occur between other events or periods; to interfere with force, or a threat of force; to become a party to a legal suit pending between other parties, especially in an attempt to protect one's personal interests" (Costello, 1991, p. 706). In this final step in the process of advance proxy planning, intervention describes the actions that are taken as a result of the decisions that have been made. Medical orders are written, care plans are developed, and families make realistic future goals. Intervention implies that all parties who participated in the decisions share the burdens, or benefits, of implementation. Congruence in decision making between values and beliefs of the participants can be evaluated in light of the actual care plans that are written to operationalize the decisions that were made. Mutual goal setting occurs, all participants feel a unity of purpose, and energies are aligned in a common cause, which is the optimal treatment strategy for the patient, as has been defined in the previous three dynamics. Intervention supports the ethical principles of beneficence and nonmaleficence.

SUMMARY OF DYNAMICS

Each of these dynamics is part of an interpersonal process that characterizes the therapeutic alliance within a moral community. In family conferences observed during this project, the decisions were not evaluated as being good or bad or based on norms external to the needs and concerns of each individual family. The goal of the family conference was to give the health care team directions within the context of the family's values and goals. The goal of the moral community was to make a decision that constitutes the patient as a moral being.

That is not to say that each family conference observed during this field research was ideal. There are many factors that can interfere with decision making. These include communication barriers that affect the level of participation that can be achieved, especially if defense mechanisms are activated. Conflicts can, and do, arise. Sometimes there were decisional delays, or the conferences were postponed until the family members were considered ready. The element of readiness is an important part of the planning process. Some families evidenced a high degree of ambivalence, and this is an important element to assess before plans are made for the family conference. Janis and Mann (1977) characterized this ambivalence as decisional conflict, which includes simultaneous, opposing tendencies within the individual to accept and reject a given course of action. The most prominent symptoms of such conflicts are hesitation, vacillation, feelings of uncertainty, and signs of acute emotional stress whenever the decision comes within the focus of attention. A major subjective characteristic of decisional conflicts is an unpleasant feeling of distress. (p. 46)

One consequence that is particularly relevant to advance proxy planning is the influence of past experiences. Janis and Mann (1977) found that their subjects relied on prior social training to help cope when they were in a situation they perceived as threatening. In this study (Mahoney, 1992), families related stories of other losses in their lives or other family tragedies. Where surrogate decision makers had previously encountered decision making about aggressive medical interventions or had relatives with DAT, these were often expressed in the context of the patient's previous wishes.

CONCLUSIONS

Advance proxy planning cannot be equated with only end-of-life decisions, but it is the backbone of the therapeutic alliance between professional and family caregivers. It is not an isolated event in time, such as the proxy form filled out on admission, or a static living will, or a necessary conference dictated by a medical crisis. Advance proxy planning is a process of decision making that mutually evolves in a moral community that is justified by the demands of the situation at hand, the policies of the institution, the philosophy of practice of the health care professionals, and the values and beliefs of the patients and families. Ethically valid decisions about life-sustaining interventions can be made by competent and informed persons based on an examination of the proportionate benefits and burdens in light of their individual circumstances and values. No single normative pattern exists that is not open to challenge if beneficence and self-determination are to be upheld for each individual patient.

Advance proxy planning, then, is a dynamic process of health care decision making that is based within the therapeutic alliance formed between the members of the interdisciplinary team and the proxy decision makers. This therapeutic alliance has been described by the concepts of interest, interpretation, interagency, and intervention. The orderly and ongoing nature of these decisions facilitates caregiving patterns and provides anticipatory guidance to providers and families before crises develop. When clinicians are proactive instead of reactive, the expertise of the providers and the personal goals of the family care-givers have a better chance of defining the best interests of patients who are unable to speak on their own behalf. Advance proxy planning is a shared decision-making model that is integral to providing compassionate care to patients and families who have dementia of the Alzheimer type.

REFERENCES

Applebaum, G. E., King, J. E., & Finucane, T. E. (1990). The outcome of CPR initiated in nursing homes. *Journal of the American Geriatrics Society, 38,* 197–200.

Brody, E. M. (1985). Parent care as a normative family stress. *Gerontologist, 25*(1), 19–29.

Buber, M. (1937). *I and thou* (R. G. Smith, Trans.). Edinburgh: T. & T. Clark. (Original work published 1923)

Cantor, M. H. (1983). Strain among caregivers: A study of experience in the United States. *Gerontologist, 23*(6), 597–604.

Care, N. S. (1987). *On sharing fate.* Philadelphia: Temple University Press.

Chenoworth, B., & Spencer, B. (1986). Dementia: The experience of family caregivers. *Gerontologist, 26*(3), 267–272.

Costello, R. B. (Ed.). (1991). *Webster's college dictionary.* New York: Random House.

Cugliari, A. M., & Miller, T. E. (1994). Moral and religious objections by hospitals to withholding and withdrawing life-sustaining treatment. *Journal of Community Health, 19*(2), 87–100.

Department of Veterans Affairs. (1995). *Alzheimer's disease: Natural feeding techniques.* [Videotape]. Chicago: Terra Nova Films.

Elstein, A., Shulman, L., & Sprafka, S. (1978). *Medical problem solving: An analysis of clinical reasoning.* Cambridge, MA: Harvard University Press.

Emanuel, L. L., Emanuel, E. J., Stoeckle, J. D., Hummel, L. R., & Barry, M. J. (1994). Advance directives: Stability of patients' treatment choices. *Archives of Internal Medicine, 154,* 90–96.

Fabiszewski, K. J., Volicer, B., & Volicer, L. (1009). Effect of antibiotic treatment on outcome of fevers in institutionalized Alzheimer patients. *Journal of the American Medical Association, 263,* 3168–3172.

Glaser, B. G., & Strauss, A. L. (1967). *The discovery of grounded theory: Strategies for qualitative research.* New York: Aldine.

Hurley, A. C., Bottino, R., & Volicer, L. (1994). Nursing role in advance proxy planning for Alzheimer patients. *Caring, 8,* 72–76.

Hurley, A. C., Mahoney, M. A., & Volicer, L. (1995). Comfort care in end-stage dementia: What to do after deciding to do no more. In L. Libow, E. Olson, & E. R. Chichin (Eds.), *Controversies in ethics in long-term care* (pp. 73–86). New York: Springer.

Hurley, A. C., Volicer, B. J., Mahoney, M. A., & Volicer, L. (1993). Palliative fever management in Alzheimer patients: Quality plus fiscal responsibility. *Advances in Nursing Science, 16*(1), 21–32.

Hurley, A. C., Volicer, L., Rempusheski, V. F., & Fry, S (1995). Reaching consensus: The process of recommending treatment decisions for Alzheimer patients. *Advances in Nursing Science, 18*(2), 33–43.

Hurley, A. C., Volicer, B. J., & Volicer, L. (1996). Effect of fever management strategy on the progression of dementia of the Alzheimer type. *Alzheimer Disease and Associated Disorders, 10,* 5–10.

Janis, I. L., & Mann, L. (1977). *Decision making.* New York: Macmillan.

Kübler-Ross, E. (1975). *Death: The final stage of growth.* New York: Simon & Schuster.

Mahoney, M. A. (1992). *Family decision making for patients with advanced Alzheimer's disease.* Unpublished doctoral dissertation, Boston College.

Mahoney, M. A., Hurley, A., Smith, S., & Volicer, L. (1992). Advance management preferences: The nurse's role in surrogate decision making about life sustaining interventions. In G. B. White (Ed.), *Ethical dilemmas in nursing practice* (pp. 45–58). Kansas City, MO: American Nurses Association.

McNabney, M. K., Beers, M. H., & Siebens, H. (1994). Surrogate decision-makers' satisfaction with the placement of feeding tubes in elderly patients. *Journal of the American Geriatrics Society, 42*(2), 161–168.

Mezey, M., Evans, L. K., Golub, Z. D., Murphy, E., & White, G. B. (1994). The Patient Self-Determination Act: Sources of concern for nurses. *Nursing Outlook, 42*(1), 30–38.

Pick, N., McDonald, A., Bennett, N., Litsche, M., Dietsche, L., Legerwood, R., Spurgas, R., & LaForce, F. M. (1996). Pulmonary aspiration in a long-term care setting: Clinical and laboratory observations and an analysis of risk factors. *Journal of the American Geriatrics Society, 44,* 763–768.

President's Commission for the Study of Ethical Problems in Biomedical and Behavioral Research. (1983). *Deciding to forgo life-sustaining treatment.* Washington, DC: U.S. Government Printing Office.

Solomon, M. Z., O'Donnell, L., Jennings, B., Guilfoy, V., Wolf, S. M., Nolan, K., Jackson, R., Koch-Weser, D., & Donnelley, S. (1993). Decisions near the end of life: Professional views on life-sustaining treatments. *American Journal of Public Health, 83*(1), 14–23.

Suhl, J., Simons, P., Reedy, T., & Garrick, T. (1994). Myth of substituted judgment: Surrogate decision making regarding life support is unreliable. *Archives of Internal Medicine, 154,* 209–217.

Volicer, L. (1993). Vignette on enteral feeding. *Journal of the American Geriatrics Society, 41,* 687–688.

Volicer, L., Collard, A., Hurley, A., Bishop, C., Kern, D., & Karon, S. (1994). Impact of special care unit for patients with advanced Alzheimer's disease on patients' discomfort and costs. *Journal of the American Geriatrics Society, 42,* 597–603.

Volicer, L., Fabiszewski, K. L., Rheaume, Y. L., Brown, J., & Brady, R. (1986). Hospice approach to the treatment of patients with advanced dementia of the Alzheimer's type. *Journal of the American Medical Association, 256,* 2210–2213.

Watts, D. T., Cassel, C. K., & Hickam, D. H. (1986). Nurses' and physicians' attitudes toward tube-feeding decisions in long-term care. *Journal of the American Geriatrics Society, 34*(8), 607–611.

Weiler, P .G. (1987). The public health impact of Alzheimer's disease. *American Journal of Public Health, 77*(9), 1157–1158.

Complexities of the Grieving Process in Spouses of Patients with Alzheimer's Disease

Yvette L. Rheaume and June Brown

I nvolvement of a person with AD and his or her family in a hospice program provides support in two important areas. The first is the provision of compassionate palliative care for the person who is dying from a fatal neurological disorder. The second is support of the family in the grieving process that continues during the entire course of the disease and the bereavement process after the patient's death. This second area involves support for the caregiver's own needs, which may have been neglected during the difficult and exhausting process of providing care for the patient.

Unlike traditional hospice programs, the major focus of emotional support in a dementia hospice program is directed toward easing the burden of grief in the spouse, since the patient who is cognitively impaired by Alzheimer's disease is unable to comprehend his or her approaching death (Volicer, Rheaume, Brown, Fabiszewski, & Brady, 1988). Hospice staff need to understand the disruptive effects in the spousal relationship that were caused by the progression of the disease and learn how to provide support to the families in the grieving process in AD.

This chapter will discuss anticipating the loss of the spouse, complex factors affecting grief adjustment, grieving, and grief therapy, and factors affecting adjustment. The case studies used to illustrate our points are fictitious but were derived from examples of grieving exhibited by the families we have cared for at the E. N. Rogers Memorial Veterans Hospital in Bedford, Massachusetts (Volicer, 1986).

ANTICIPATING LOSS OF AN AD SPOUSE

Inevitably in the progression of Alzheimer's disease, the spouse is deprived of both the opportunity to share and receive support from the Alzheimer patient and to share his or her grief. Witnessing a slow and lingering death may also generate unconscious fear of death in the spouse (Yalom & Vinogradov, 1988). An orderly grieving period is an unrealistic goal in the adjustment to the loss of a close relative with AD (Brown, Lyon, & Sullivan, 1988).

The experience of loss is inevitable. Anticipating the loss is an inescapable and painful process. The pain of emotional separation from the psychologically unavailable Alzheimer patient is ongoing, chronic, and seemingly unending. Few spouses are able to recover successfully from the resulting emotional distress without grief therapy.

To begin to understand the nature of grieving for the AD patient, it is necessary to assess the prolonged impact of Alzheimer's disease upon the spouse as the severity of illness alters virtually all normal life patterns. With the progression of the disease, the victim loses all functioning, including the sense of personal identity. Enmeshed in caregiving responsibilities, the spouse also experiences a loss of personal identity and suffers social isolation. As the disease worsens, the totality of care needed by the AD patient serves to separate the spouse from social interchanges that help define his or her sense of self. The sense of mastery and autonomy is lost as the spouse is absorbed by a total self-identification as a caregiver.

The experience of day-to-day caregiving responsibilities defers mourning. Consequently, spouse/caregivers are trapped in a kind of limbo where their need to grieve may go virtually unknown and untreated. This limbo often develops over a lengthy period of time wherein changes in the disease victim are subtle, and the impact upon family life is insidious and seldom fully understood. This is seen in the case of Mr. C.

> Mr. C. retired early from his job to care for his wife who was diagnosed with Alzheimer's disease. The patient, unable to comprehend what was happening to her, taunted her husband's awkwardness in "doing housework," her work. Later she physically fought his efforts to bathe and dress her. Mrs. C.'s illness created problems in sustaining old friendships. She had always been the catalyst for the couple's social life; without her, there was none. Her attempts to socialize created unpleasant and embar-

rassing interactions between Mrs. C. and their friends. Mr. C.'s attempts to prevent friends and family from noticing her symptoms created more emotional distance and misunderstanding. As the ongoing struggle to care for his wife seemed to preclude all else, his frustration and fatigue accompanied her decline. When his own health deteriorated and he became nearly incapacitated, Mr. C. was obliged to institutionalize his wife. Feeling alone and defeated, he was virtually immobilized by a sense of guilt and loss. Angry at the disease and the nonresponsiveness from his wife, he felt abandoned by life. He perceived himself as a failure in the "male role," and he was too old to resume competitive employment.

Because he was unable to continue in the demands of caring for his ill wife at home, Mr. C. perceived himself as a failure in the nurturing aspect of the "female role." Struggling to balance his thoughts, feelings, and actions, he became the "model" spouse who visited his wife often, devoting his life, at the age of 65, to one who did not know or notice him. Unable to accept that his wife's need for long-term care was not his fault, each visit confirmed his self-perceived guilt. Reassurances to the contrary seemed to him as patronizing.

Because many long-term care facilities suffer from a shortage of nursing help, staff may unwittingly encourage an overly attentive spouse, as in the case of Mr. C., to continue with overzealous bedside care. To do so may be detrimental to the caregiver's adjustment to the spouse's institutionalization. The excessive time, energy, and emotional involvement Mr. C. devoted to his institutionalized wife exemplify the myriad tragedies resulting from Alzheimer's disease that may go essentially untreated. As in the case described, grief reaction is suppressed or postponed in the expedience of coping with immediate care needs. Given the complexities in this case, the husband's grief remained suppressed until the necessary supportive and grief therapy helped him to regain his self-esteem and purpose in life.

All too often the bereaved block expressions of sadness in order not to inflict sorrow and pain upon others. They may choose to grieve in silence because often others do not give permission for their sadness. Prohibiting and inhibiting feelings of grief serve to intensify and prolong the mourning process. Liken and Collins (1993) have proposed three phases of predeath grief: avoidance, confrontation, and reestablishment. Figure 10.1 illustrates how to assess these phases of grief and suggests interventions.

PATHOLOGICAL GRIEVING

Pathological grieving is concomitant to the progression of AD. The patient with AD may live for years after the onset of illness, several years after losing those qualities that determine personality. Often the bereaved AD

Assessment   *Assess which phase of grief caregivers are in by:*

1. Asking open-ended questions (e.g., "What has it been like caring for your relative," or "How have things changed for you since your relative became ill?")
2. Observing for statements indicating avoidance (e.g., "I'm doing okay, I'll get by, " or "It's not really much different").
3. Observing for statements indicating confrontation of feelings (e.g., "I hate it; It's like caring for a complete stranger; I pray it will end soon," or "I'm lonely; I've lost the person I knew").

Avoidance Phase   *Allow caregivers to take the necessary time in the predeath avoidance phase by planning interventions that include:*

1. Being sympathetic to the overwhelming responsibility of being a caregiver and recognizing the caregiver's efforts.
2. Realizing that caregivers may need time before they are able to acknowledge the implications of a diagnosis of Alzheimer's disease.
3. Offering to provide information about Alzheimer's disease when caregivers feel ready.
4. Helping caregivers identify potential sources of emotional support for the future.
5. Being sensitive to caregivers' need to take "one day at a time" and not plan for the future yet.

Confrontation Phase   *Help caregivers cope with intense feelings during the predeath confrontation phase by planning interventions that include:*

1. Providing information about the grief process and commonly occurring emotional reactions that accompany grief.
2. Providing information about the physical symptoms that may accompany grief (e.g., shortness of breath, palpitations, and insomnia).
3. Acknowledging the difficult parts of caregiving, including the frustrations, disappointments, and sadness.
4. Encouraging caregivers to talk about what their relative was like before Alzheimer's disease.
5. Helping caregivers to identify how their life has been changed and what has been lost.
6. Encouraging caregivers to identify strategies to maintain pleasurable aspects of their life in the face of caregiving demands.
7. Discouraging the use of substances such as antianxiety agents or alcohol that mask or delay grief.
8. Informing caregivers about community resources that are available to assist them (e.g., Alzheimer's support groups).

Reestablishment Phase

1. Do not expect caregivers to reach this phase until after the relative dies.
2. Remind caregivers that even if their relative has seemed to have reached a "plateau," death can occur suddenly from an acute illness, such as pneumonia.

FIGURE 10.1   Interventions to facilitate predeath grief.

From "Grieving: Facilitating the Process for Dementia Caregivers," by M. A. Liken and C. E. Collins, 1993, *Journal of Psychosocial Nursing, 31,* pp. 71–76. Copyright 1993, Slack Inc. Reprinted with permission.

spouse is engaged in chronic mourning, with much of it in the presence of but isolated from the person mourned. Continuing to impede the spouse's adjustment to grief is the disease process that manifests itself in a fluctuating pattern of patient decline, with each loss of function having an acute quality. Cognitive and physical decline will usually reach a point when caregiving becomes a total disruption of normal life.

Many spouses carry bruises or worse from their efforts to provide daily care, or from the attempt to prevent the patient from wandering into unsafe environments or becoming lost. At the same time, hyperactivity, confusion, and suspicion may be pronounced in the AD patient, and fatigue is the constant companion of the spouse caregiver. At this point, institutionalization is often viewed as the only alternative. This, in turn, activates the caregiver's guilt, shame of failure, and betrayal, as well as separation anxieties. The decision to institutionalize a spouse is often resisted. Absolute despair and helplessness to continue the burden of care are the precipitants to institutionalization. What was resisted becomes a necessary objective. As institutionalization becomes the goal, adjustment to that decision may be seen as the final hurdle for the caregiver. In reality, the worst is not over, as is described in the following case.

> Mrs. S., whose business manager husband had full command of the family financial affairs, was totally unaware of his cognitive deficiencies when he began mismanaging both his customers' accounts and his own. Customers dwindled, as did his income, and then his savings. If he sometimes seemed preoccupied, the "press of business" provided a ready excuse and a concealment of a failing mind. It was also an easily accepted excuse by a spouse wanting to be supportive, yet unaware that the family economic base was crumbling. Suddenly, it seemed that there was no financial security, no future nestegg, insufficient income, and mountainous unexplained bills. Not for over a year would Mr. S.'s illness become so evident that diagnosis and medical treatment would be sought. In the meantime, Mr. S.'s seeming indifference fueled the flames of anger in his wife, who had to explain to bill collectors what she herself did not understand, find employment for herself, and view retirement years with cold, hard fear.
>
> Her rage grew as her husband's condition worsened. What she thought of as irresponsible money management, compounded by his emotional withdrawal and failure to assume his normal household responsibilities, left Mrs. S. feeling betrayed and deserted by her husband. She nagged him endlessly as she tried to force a solution for what had gone wrong in their lives. When her husband was diagnosed as having Alzheimer's disease, Mrs. S. instantly became a caregiver. She was still filled with rage, but she experienced guilt and shame for her previous anger toward his inexplicable behaviors. The now apparent fact that her husband had not

willfully blighted their lives served to increase her guilt. The numerous efforts made to educate her in how to manage his worsening behaviors were often lost in the personal battle to manage her own ambivalent and overwhelming emotions. Intellectually she knew how to respond and care for her husband's symptoms, but she was unable to transcend her own emotional chaos, and so abused him emotionally and, at times, physically. Family and friends who provided sympathy for her plight and support for her grief seemed to increase her guilt. She was unable to be in touch with her sorrow. Ultimately the decision was made to institutionalize Mr. S. This decision freed Mrs. S. from her massive burden of care but left her separated from any part of herself that she could respect or forgive, leaving her with the certainty that others must hate her as she had come to hate herself.

Firmly engaged in a pathological grief process grounded in rage, Mrs. S. was guided and redirected toward unlocking her grief. The process was complex and complicated by the interaction with her husband, who although severely demented was a continuing reminder of her intense emotions and unacceptable behaviors. Individual counseling led Mrs. S. to medical treatment for depression and hypertension. Family counseling served to enlighten other family members who had become locked in their own grief, isolating them from one another. Mrs. S. resisted group therapy, fearful that she would expose herself as the bad person she thought she was. In time she was able to accept group treatment and found release in the recognition that her actions and reactions to her husband were seen as normal by other members who had similar experiences. The group treatment gradually led Mrs. S. to forgive herself and to prepare for life without her husband.

Typically for most AD spouses, the relief of being freed from the burden of caregiving is quickly supplanted by loneliness and guilt. If the patient has a difficult adjustment to long-term care, the caregiver may suffer unwarranted guilt, concerned that he or she has precipitated an emotional overload to the spouse and the nursing staff. To compound this distress, as the personality of the AD patient recedes, the spouse clings to that which remains of the loved one once known, while an attempt is made to adjust to the ongoing changes. Each cognitive and physical decline is seen as a step toward death, a substantive reminder that the patient is dying, leaving the AD spouse more isolated.

COMPLEX FACTORS AFFECTING GRIEF ADJUSTMENT

Recovering from a significant emotional loss is a difficult task, requiring courage from the bereaved and considerable support and guidance from others. Grief reaction is universal (Bowlby, 1980) and generates intense mental suffering, deep sorrow, and painful regret (Peretz, 1970). The expression of such feelings is essential to work through the grief. Inhibition of these feelings is detrimental to health (Parkes, 1972; Weizman & Kamm, 1985).

Many studies indicate that AD family caregivers are at high risk for stress-related illnesses, total physical exhaustion, and situational depression (Fengler & Goodrich, 1965; O'Quinn & McGraw, 1985; Rabins, Mace, & Lucas, 1982). Some of the symptoms experienced by the fatigued caregivers may include sleep disturbance, feelings of physical exhaustion, and a sense of having lost control of their lives (Seltzer, Larkin, & Fabiszewski, 1988). Out of fear of losing control and falling apart, the bereaved may stop themselves from expressing any feelings. Frightened by the intensity of expressed feelings, still others keep an even tighter control of emotions. Maladaptive coping responses (Peretz, 1970) to grief include inhibited, delayed, or absent grief, chronic grief, depression, hypochondriasis, and exacerbation of preexisting somatic conditions, as well as the development of medical illnesses.

Physiological reactions to grief affect the physical and emotional well-being of the griever. The avoidance of mourning and the expression of grief feelings deny the existence of fear, sadness, and anger. In addition, the inhibition of grief feelings is harmful to the body. Acute grief has been identified as a syndrome with physiological symptomatology consisting of dyspnea, deep sighing, "lumps" or tight sensations in the throat, weakness, feelings of emptiness, exhaustion, decreased appetite, and insomnia.

Intense feelings of anxiety and tension may also be experienced. C. S. Lewis (1989) described grief as feelings of fear, a fluttering in the stomach, the need to yawn, or to keep swallowing. Physical sensation and tension are counterparts of emotion, and often somatic disturbances, headaches, backaches, colitis, spastic colon, asthma, rheumatoid arthritis, and sinus problems will develop (Weizman & Kamm, 1985). Masked grief reactions often manifest through physical and/or psychological symptoms of maladaptive behavior, as commonly seen in Alzheimer's spouses. The so-called neglected aspects of their own health and emotional well-being can symbolize grief suppression as well as jeopardize their very existence.

GRIEVING AND GRIEF THERAPY

Grief may be strong or weak, brief or prolonged, immediate or delayed; and particular aspects of grief may be distorted. There is a prolonged period during which the Alzheimer's patient may live in a state of being present physically but not mentally (Curl, 1992), which may lead to a distortion of reality for the spouse. Acknowledgment of grief may trigger intense feelings of guilt. Many spouses struggle with a sense that their feelings may somehow facilitate their partner's demise, and so those feelings and realities are denied.

The work of Elisabeth Kübler-Ross (1969) sharpened the focus on the process of dying and its corresponding psychological stages. Her concepts have been applied to the process of grief for dying patients and for the bereaved survivors. Approaching the death of a loved one precipitates a measure of grief and a sense of loss. Grieving is a process necessary to diminish the pain of loss. The complex and varied emotions experienced by a dying person are similar to grief reactions experienced by the mourning AD spouse.

In the earliest stages of Alzheimer's disease, before diagnosis, the spouse responds to the victim's symptoms with disbelief. The insidious process of disease onset and the difficulty of diagnosis foster the use of denial, described by Kübler-Ross (1969) as a mechanism of coping with overwhelming anxiety. What may appear as totally inexplicable symptoms in the Alzheimer patient serve to confuse, frighten, and activate recurring episodes of denial throughout the generally lengthy course of the illness as a mourning spouse generates a protective denial system to isolate himself or herself from information or persons who might confirm the irreversible condition.

The qualities of the relationship and the role that the dying person occupied in the family also determine reactions to grief. A particular grief reaction may be related to unresolved emotional issues in the relationship and the inability to achieve resolution. The lack of opportunity for an individual to prepare for the loss of a loved one generates intense and traumatic grief reactions. Intolerance of separation and the degree and importance placed on the security of attachment to a dying person will also influence grief reaction. A previously strong, dependent attachment to the AD spouse, along with intense anxiety at the briefest of separations, will determine a maladaptive grief response in the mourning spouse.

As the patient worsens, as symptoms of decline became more blatant, denial may not be possible. Anger will often supplant denial as an attempt to control feelings of despair. Anger may be, and often is, directed at doctors, nurses, and family members. Confronting the reality of impending death may involve considerable rage and resentment toward the Alzheimer patient. The spouse may be overwhelmed by guilt and confusion over these feelings and inadvertently create emotional distance from those who may be helpful. Throughout the course of the illness, these feelings recur in the spouse as the patient succumbs to each cognitive and physical decline.

Another response to grief, as described by Kübler-Ross (1969), is the attempt to "bargain" for an extension of life. This is a normal attempt to postpone death. This is also a period during which spousal ruminations often include reminiscences of the period of disease onset, with harsh self-recrimination (i.e., "I should have done . . . If only . . . "). The grieving spouse becomes trapped in futile efforts to rewrite history to effect a happy ending.

Similarly, confused by periods of seemingly clinical improvements in the victim, the spouse who is "bargaining" may become insistent upon treatment regimens that are aggressive and inappropriate for the patient, and may choose treatments that merely prolong suffering. Renewed efforts toward more intensive caregiving by the Alzheimer spouse may follow. Interwoven in the bargaining process is the growing sense of loss, of failure. Depression accompanies the myriad feelings in the relentless course of the illness. When the bargaining fails, withdrawn, brooding, and noncommunicative behavior in the grieving spouse is common. The sense of loss deepens as the spouse is confronted with other losses, including changing relationships with other family members, changing life styles, financial loss, and the ultimate loss through death.

Confronting and accepting the diagnosis of Alzheimer's disease and its terminal nature is a difficult task for spouses. As the personality of the patient recedes, the spouse clings more closely to what remains of the loved one, while an attempt is made to adjust to the ongoing changes. In the early stages, acceptance is usually limited to acknowledging those intellectual impairments resulting from profound disease within the brain. Throughout the course of the illness, the AD spouse struggles to accept a loved one, not as the person once known, but as a spouse becoming unfamiliar and strange. With the progression of the disease, each successive loss of cognitive and physical function seems to be an acute event. Each decline is seen as a step toward death, a substantive reminder that the AD spouse is dying. Anticipatory grieving, or mourning while a person is dying, may be helpful in leading to a greater acceptance of the ensuing death of the AD spouse and is a significant part of grief counseling.

In the terminal stages, the mourning AD spouse, weary and sad, may acknowledge that death is near and can begin to prepare for the inevitable loss. Yet, as all through the disease, sometimes the course alters as the patient recovers from a crisis or has a few good days, and the patient once again appears to improve or return to a higher level of functioning. Hope and denial thus replace acceptance, and the mourning

process begins once again. The impact of these fluctuations over a prolonged period serves to deplete the emotional energies needed for the
task of mourning.

A key element in understanding the experience of grief is the degree
of attachment in the spousal relationship (Dean, 1988). Loss may be virtually painless when there is little or no emotional attachment. Furthermore, the greater the social and/or personal distance from the AD
patient, the less painful the loss experience will be. However, there is
great impact from the cumulative effect of coping with numerous losses
in one's lifetime (Freeman, 1978). Attachment to the loved one has a complexity of form and degree that affects the course of grieving and grief
recovery. For the Alzheimer spouse, compounding the problem is the
realization that there will always exist a void, the emotionally incomplete
spousal relationship. Forever wishing the married life could have been
different, better, or more, the Alzheimer spouse experiences escalating
detachment, bitterness, and resentment.

The language of Alzheimer spouse is rich with phrases describing
themselves as being "married widows and widowers" (Levine, Gendron,
& Dastoor, 1984) or attending an endless wake or a continuous funeral.
Some describe visits to the late-stage patient as feeling like "viewing the
body." Spouses have described being with an AD patient drifting toward
a comatose state as "eerie" or "unearthly," experiencing what nursing
staff have described as a "macabre" period.

Unlike nursing staff who confirm the patient relationship through
physical contact as they provide care, the family can only sit at the bedside and wait for the impending death. The unconscious need to recap-
ture a sense of attachment and belonging continues throughout the
course of the illness. It may be experienced as a desperate need as death
seems closer. If, for example, the patient's hand should clasp the
spouse's hand or an errant smile appears, the spouse may feel that it is
an affirmation of their relationship. This is both comforting and fright-
ening to the spouse, seeming to sharpen the fear of loss.

Attachment becomes pathological when grieving for the AD victim
activates a maternal-like bonding (Brown, Lyon, & Sellers, 1988) within
the caregiver, as the afflicted spouse becomes increasingly dependent.
The obvious regression of the patient to the helplessness of infancy
intensifies and complicates the bonding and exaggerates the grieving
process as it expands to include mourning the loss of both the spouse
and the child the spouse has become. To acknowledge the existence of
pathological bonding is usually difficult for the AD spouse.

Another aspect that may intensify and prolong the grieving process is
the impulse to force feed the AD victim during the terminal phases of the

illness. In many cases, a spouse will attempt to feed the patient who is unwilling or, as in most cases, is unable to swallow. Even when the staff have requested spouses not to feed patients because of the risk of choking, spouses have been observed feeding dying patients much the way a parent coaxes a small child to eat. The significance of feeding, so basic to human need, may be a force too powerful to resist when it also embodies a sense of reattachment on a level that verifies to the mourning spouse the patient's acceptance of the spouse's presence and love.

Death may be expected, and though it is dreaded, it is also anticipated as a source of relief from the interminable dying process. Those spouses who have repeatedly experienced the patient's decline, the expectation of imminent death followed by the return to physical stability, often cope with the see-saw of emotions by denying trauma. The wish "that it were so" may cause them to say, "The worst is over." Many will say, "I've cried all my tears." Still others, friends, staff, and family members, may join with the denial because of their need to ameliorate further emotional pain for both the caregiver spouse and themselves. If sympathizers unknowingly collude with the AD spouse to shut off expressions of suffering that are too painful to hear, the spouse may accept the implied premise that there is a limit to what can be expressed, or felt, and their negative feelings create for them yet another sense of failure or shame, replacing the feelings of grief.

Exaggerated grief reactions, as described by Worden (1982, 1991), usually stem from an ambivalent relationship with the deceased. In the case of the mourning AD spouse, because of the prolongation of the illness with its insidious and destructive onset, excessive ambivalence between spouses usually exists. The nature of loss in AD causes exaggerated and vacillating emotional reactions in the spouse. At any time in the course of the illness, rage and guilt may emerge (Levine et al., 1984). When death does come, the bereaved are often encouraged not to mourn because the afflicted is at last freed from suffering. For some of the bereaved this is another reason for denying or holding back the expression of feelings. Thus the vital need to experience the sadness, to truly grieve the loss, is once more "forbidden" by internal and external forces. The grieving that frees them to remember and internalize the attachment as a source of strength for survival is lost in the cold void of loneliness.

Grief is often a misunderstood and neglected growth process (Faran, Keane-Hagerty, Salloway, Kupferer, & Wilken, 1991; Guilliland & James 1988). The AD spouse caught in the extreme of a protracted grieving situation discovers only too soon that family and friends are unprepared and emotionally unable to provide solace. Denied, though unintentionally, the opportunity to release emotions by talking and crying, incredible tensions and frustrations are perpetuated. In several clinical studies of families caring for relatives with Alzheimer's disease, it was found that families who did not participate in family support groups were at risk for clinical depression (Bergamn-Evans,1994; Cohen & Eisdorfer, 1988; Mittleman et al., 1995).

Grief work is a personal process that gives the mourners permission to express their pain, rather than allow it to be perpetuated. To work through grief, all feelings must be allowed expression. Within the organized structure of grief therapy, the bereaved are encouraged to release pent-up emotions and move toward phases of mourning that result in eventual grief resolution. Participation in grief therapy conveys a sense of commonality of feelings in the bereaved and reassures them that there is genuine support and commitment for the expression of grief. Thus, in the often painful and prolonged grieving process, personal growth is often possible, enabling the bereaved to attain the ability to abstract meaning from a previously totally destructive event, and to emerge with greater strength, self-trust, a sense of freedom than that experienced prior to the loss.

Failure to support the mourning spouse during the dying process and after may be a prologue to future emotional stress for the survivors. The rescue of the AD family may have to be attempted many times in the course of the disease that seems an endless rehearsal of death.

Alzheimer's disease therapy groups provide a welcoming, understanding milieu for suffering spouses. The practical information relative to caregiving is invaluable, as is the intense relief that may be engendered when joining with others with similar experiences and problems. However, if extensive group psychodynamic psychotherapy is not provided, the grieving process is seldom fully expressed (Wexler & Brown, 1993). Feelings of shame, because they are not "over it," may become the legacy for those who never learned their right to claim every aspect of the cruel process of grieving for the Alzheimer victim.

The hospice approach to care (Volicer et al., 1986) has been proposed as a way to institutionalize the grief work that is so necessary for spousal caregivers. The hospice staff needs to facilitate the adjustment of the patient, spouse, other family members, and friends to this approach to care.

FACTORS AFFECTING ADJUSTMENT TO HOSPICE CARE

At the E. N. Rogers Memorial Veterans Hospital in Bedford, Massachusetts, the Geriatric Research Education Clinical Center provides care with a hospice philosophy. Beginning with the first outpatient clinic visit, the family caregiver (usually the spouse) is helped by the staff consisting of the physician, nurse, and social worker to understand the progression of symptoms, treatment, and disease course, and to develop ongoing coping skills. The treatment philosophy under hospice care is explained, and advance proxy plans are discussed. A significant factor in providing support is staff recognition that the caregiver's continuing loss of control over events causes confusion, despair, and vacillating stages of grief. Therefore, medical information may need to be repeated frequently, caregiver efforts praised or gently corrected when needed, and feelings recognized and validated. Nurses and physicians provide ongoing medical support and education to patients and families, and social workers begin the lengthy task of grief therapy. Families are encouraged to participate in group or individual grief therapy to aid them in the onerous dual role of simultaneous caregiving and grieving.

Upon the patient's admission for long-term care, a more intensive grief is activated within the caregiver, who generally views the admission as an act of failure to cope. Nursing staff members, in addition to providing patient care, join with other staff disciplines, intermingling roles to reassure the caregiver that the admission was appropriate. The continuing education relevant to patient functioning provides a vital form of reality testing for the family members caught in the bewildering aspects of the patient's symptoms, which at times seem impossible to understand or accept.

A most significant aspect of family adjustment is the family conference, held within a few weeks of the patient's admission. The social worker and nursing staff prepare family members for the meeting in which they will be asked to make a decision for an advance proxy plan (Hurley, Bottino, & Volicer, 1994). The supportive atmosphere generated in the family conference encourages and allows the family to ask questions regarding any aspect of patient care, to better understand hospice care, and to select the level of aggressive or palliative treatment with which they are most comfortable. During this time, the family is provided with yet another level of support that encourages them to acknowledge the pain of their grief and their right to mourn. In the absence of the patient's participation in the decision making, the hospice staff serves as fill-ins to accept the family's feelings of pain and loss and to indicate they will stand with them through the mourning process.

Providing postdeath grief intervention is another function of the hospice approach, and spouses are encouraged to remain with their group to continue the benefits of psychodynamic group psychotherapy (Wexler & Brown, 1993). Other strategies are suggested by Liken and Collins (1993) and are illustrated in Figure 10.2.

Assessment   *Assess which phase caregivers are in by:*
1. Asking open-ended questions (e.g., "Tell me what it was like for you while your relative was ill," or "How have things changed for you since your relative's death?")
2. Observing for statements indicating avoidance (e.g., "It's over now, so I try not to think about it," or "They aren't really much different").
3. Observing for statements indicating confrontation of feelings (e.g., "It was terrible; I was relieved when my relative died," or "I've been really depressed; I miss my relative the way he was before Alzheimer's took him away from me").

Avoidance Phase   *Allow caregivers to take the necessary time in the postdeath avoidance phase by planning interventions that include:*
1. Reaching out to caregivers and letting them know you are available when they are ready to talk about their experience.
2. Maintaining contact with caregivers through periodic telephone calls.
3. Reminding caregivers about the grieving process and what is to be expected, including that it may take some time to realize what has happened to them.

Confrontation Phase   *Help caregivers cope with intense feelings during the postdeath confrontation phase by planning interventions that include:*
1. Asking open-ended questions (e.g., "Tell me about your reactions to your relative's death").
2. Reassuring caregivers that they will have "good days" and "bad days" and that this is normal during the grieving process.
3. Encouraging caregivers to talk with health care professionals as well as friends and relatives about feelings and experiences.
4. Helping caregivers find ways to replenish themselves and encouraging them to return to pleasurable activities as they are able.
5. Providing appropriate information about the grieving process.
6. Linking caregivers with community resources, such as bereavement support groups and groups for widows.

Reestablishment Phase: *Help caregivers reach the postdeath reestablishment phase by planning interventions that include:*
1. Encouraging caregivers to continue to tell their story.
2. Helping caregivers develop ways in which memories of their relative can be kept alive, e.g., organizing pictures, continuing to talk about their relative at family events, or making contributions in their relative's name.
3. Helping caregivers to anticipate difficult times (e.g., anniversaries, holidays, relative's birthday) and developing strategies to deal with these times.
4. Helping caregivers to identify unresolved aspects of the caregiving experience by use of open-ended questions (e.g., "When you think of the time you spent taking care of your relative, are there aspects of the experience that still trouble you?")
5. Encouraging caregivers to identify ways to gain perspective on their situation (e.g., writing thoughts in a journal and talking to others who have gone through a similar experience).
6. Being alert to the need for referral to psychological treatment for caregivers who are experiencing sustained depression or anxiety.

FIGURE 10.2   Interventions to facilitate postdeath grief.

From "Grieving: Facilitating the Process for Dementia Caregivers," by M. A. Liken and C. E. Collins, 1993, *Journal of Psychosocial Nursing, 31,* pp. 71–76. Copyright 1993, Slack Inc. Reprinted with permission.

In conclusion, families accepting hospice care are served by a philosophy of treatment that does not relegate death to the backstage, an intensive care unit environment, or other aggressive treatment areas removed from the hospice unit. Instead, death occurs where patients have lived in the long-term care setting. Death, therefore, is not hidden; its presence is unavoidable. Although this may be disturbing to families, it provides both patients and families the comfort of familiar faces and familiar surroundings in the final days and hours. It also reinforces the reality of AD as a terminal illness, making possible a fuller comprehension of loss and, therefore, a subsequent adjustment and recovery.

REFERENCES

Bergamn-Evans, B. F. (1994, March). Alzheimer's and related disorders: Loneliness, depression, and social support of spousal caregivers. *Journal of Gerontological Nursing,* 6–16.

Bowlby, J. (1980). *Attachment and loss: Attachment theory.* New York: Basic Books.

Brown, J., Lyon, P. C., & Sellers, T. D. (1988). Caring for the family caregivers. In L. Volicer, K. J. Fabiszewski, Y. L. Rheaume, & K. E. Lasch (Eds), *Clinical management of Alzheimer's disease,* Rockville, MD: Aspen Publishers. (pp. 29–41).

Cohen, D., & Eisdorfer, C. (1988). Depression in family members caring for a relative with Alzheimer's disease. *Journal of the American Geriatrics Society, 36*(10), 885–889.

Curl, A. (1992, November/December). When family caregivers grieve for the Alzheimer's patient. *Geriatric Nursing,* 305–307.

Dean, J. (1988). Grief and attachment. *Journal of Religion and Health, 27*(2), 157–153.

Farran, C. J., Keane-Hagerty, E., Salloway, S., Kupferer, S., & Wilken, C. S. (1991). Finding meaning: An alternate paradigm for Alzheimer's disease family caregivers. *Gerontologist, 31,* 483–489.

Fengler, A., & Goodrich, N. (1965). Wives of elderly disabled men. *Gerontologist, 19,* 175–183.

Freeman, L. (1978). Overcoming hurt and loss from childhood to old age. In *The sorrow and the fury.* Englewood, NJ: Prentice-Hall.

Gilliland, B., & James, R. (1988). *Crisis intervention strategies.* Pacific Grove, CA: Brooks/Cole.

Hurley, A. C., Bottino, R., & Volicer, L. (1994, August). Nursing role in advance proxy planning for Alzheimer patients. *Caring,* 72–76.

Kübler-Ross, E. (1969). *On death and dying.* London: Macmillan.

Levine, N., Gendron, C., & Dastoor, D. (1984). Existential issues in the management of the demented elderly patient. *American Journal of Psychotherapy, 37,* 215–223.

Lewis, C. S. (1989). *A grief observed: Special grief edition.* San Francisco: Harper.

Liken, M. A., & Collins, C. E. (1993). Grieving: Facilitating the process for dementia caregivers. *Journal of Psychosocial Nursing, 31*(1), 21–31.

Mittleman, M. S., Ferris, S. H., Shulman, E., Steinberg, G., Ambinder, A., Mackell, J. A., & Cohen, J. (1995). A comprehensive support program: Effect on depression in spouse-caregivers of AD patients. *Gerontologist, 35,* 792–802.

O'Quinn, J., McGraw, K. (1985). The burdened caregiver. In J. Hutton, & A. Kerny (Eds), *Senile dementia of the Alzheimer type.* New York: Alan R. Liss.

Parkes, C. (1972). *Bereavement.* New York: International Universities Press.

Peretz, D. (1970). Reactions to loss. In B. Schoenberg (Ed.), *Loss and grief: Psychological management in medical practice* (pp. 20–35). New York: Columbia University Press.

Rabins, P.V., Mace, N. L., & Lucas, M. J. (1982). The impact of dementia on the family. *Journal of the American Medical Association, 248,* 333–335.

Seltzer, B., Larkin, J., & Fabiszewski, K. (1988). Management of the outpatient with Alzheimer's disease. In L. Volicer, K. J. Fabiszewski, Y. L. Rheaume, & K. E. Lasch (Eds.), *Clinical management of Alzheimer's disease,* (pp. 13–28). Rockville, MD: Aspen Publishers.

Volicer, L. (1986). Need for hospice approach to treatment of patients with advanced Alzheimer's disease. *Journal of the American Geriatrics Society, 34,* 655–658.

Volicer, L., Rheaume, Y., & Brown, J. (1986). Hospice approach to the treatment of patients with advanced Alzheimer's disease. *Journal of the American Medical Association, 256,* 2210–2213.

Volicer, L., Rheaume, Y. L., Brown, J., Fabiszewski, K. J. & Brady, R. J. (1988). Ethical issues in the treatment of advanced Alzheimer dementia: hospice approach. In L. Volicer, K. J. Fabiszewski, Y. L. Rheaume, & K. E. Lasch (Eds.), *Clinical management of alzheimer's disease.* Rockville, MD: Aspen. (pp. 167–184)

Weizman, S., & Kamm, P. (1985). About mourning: Support and guidance for the bereaved. New York: Human Sciences Press.

Wexler, D., & Brown, J.(1993, May 28). *Group therapy for wives of Alzheimer's patients.* Paper presented at the annual meeting of the American Psychiatric Association, San Francisco.

Worden, J. (1982). Grief counseling and grief therapy. In *Attachment, Loss and the Tasks of Mourning.* New York: Springer.

Worden, J. W. (1991). Grief counseling and grief therapy; A handbook for the mental health practitioner (2nd ed.). New York: Springer Publishing Co.

Yalom, I. D., & Vinogradov, S. (1988). Bereavement groups: Techniques and themes. *International Journal of Group Psychotherapy, 38,* 419–457.

PART THREE

Implementation

Acceptance of Hospice Care for Dementia Patients by Health Care Professionals and Family Members

Daniel J. Luchins, Patricia Hanrahan, and Kim Litzenberg

L ike other patients with life-threatening diseases, dementia patients seldom have advance directives to guide their health care in the end stages of the disease (High, 1988; Sachs, Stockings, & Miles, 1989; Steiber, 1987; Volicer, Rheaume, Brown, Fabiszewski, & Brady, 1986). As discussed in chapter 9, family members must then make proxy decisions about end-stage care in conjunction with professionals. Palliative care is an important alternative to conventional care in end-stage dementia. The goals of palliative care focus on symptom relief and easing death rather than prolonging life. These goals apply to end-stage dementia patients. Their prognosis is poor and they have significant medical problems associated with the underlying condition, such as aspiration pneumonia. Although some end-stage dementia patients are in a vegetative state, others are at least intermittently aware of their environment. At this point the patients' quality of life appears to be quite poor, and they are often in need of palliative care in the form of symptom relief and pain control. Small-scale studies suggest that many families and professionals prefer palliative care for patients in the end stages of dementia (Danis et al., 1991; Volicer et al., 1986).

The delivery of palliative care through hospice programs offers important services to patients and family caregivers. Hospice programs include case management, help with medications and the patient's physical care, respite, and bereavement counseling. These services are included in the Medicare hospice benefit. A key part of hospice care is the 24-hour availability of hospice staff in case the patient's condition suddenly changes and he or she needs relief from pain or discomfort. Research on hospice care for cancer patients has found advantages over conventional care (Kane, Klien, Bernstein, Rothenberg, & Wales, 1985; Kane, Wales, Bernstein, Lebowitz, & Kaplin, 1984; Mor, Greer, & Kastenbaum, 1989). These advantages include better control of pain and symptoms, and greater satisfaction with care both among the patients and their families. Since Alzheimer's disease has been ranked as the fourth leading cause of death (Katzman, 1976), dementia patients and their families could also benefit from hospice care for assistance with late-stage illness.

WHAT IS APPROPRIATE HEALTH CARE
FOR END-STAGE DEMENTIA?

A central question in our research concerned the kind of health care that was considered appropriate for end-stage dementia (Luchins & Hanrahan, 1993). Is palliative care preferable for end-stage dementia patients? Is hospice care viewed as an appropriate alternative to conventional care? To get some guidance on these issues, three groups of people were surveyed:

1. Physicians who were involved in the care of elderly people;
2. Gerontologists from a variety of professions, such as, nursing, education, and social work;
3. Families of dementia patients.

The mailing list from the Gerontological Society of America (GSA) was the source for surveying all 819 members who were listed as physicians; of these, 514, or 63%, responded. From the remaining 6,000 GSA members, 1,000 gerontologists were randomly selected; of these, 676, or 68%, responded. The family caregivers were members of the Alzheimer's Association; of these, 218, or 44%, responded. At least one chapter from each region of the country was selected: in the Northeast, the New York City chapter; in the South, chapters from Miami and Memphis; in the Midwest, chapters from Rockford, Illinois, and Ann Arbor, Michigan; and in the West, chapters from San Francisco and Albuquerque.

Altogether 1,408 people, or 61%, of those we contacted responded to our survey. Nine tenths of the families who responded were caring for severely demented relatives and about half described their relative as being in the end stages of the disease. A large proportion of the physicians and gerontologists also provided care for dementia patients. Many respondents had experience in making terminal care decisions for end-stage dementia patients.

QUESTIONNAIRE

Before asking questions about appropriate health care, end-stage dementia was described in the following way. End-stage dementia occurs when the patient

- Needs complete assistance with eating and toileting
- Can no longer recognize the patient's loved ones
- Cannot do any of the things that used to make him or her happy
- Cannot talk anymore
- Is suffering from medical complications of dementia, such as falls or pneumonia

This description was drawn from stage 7 of the Global Deterioration Scale (Reisberg, Ferris, De Leon, & Crook, 1982).

Palliative Care

Professional and family caregivers were asked to assume that the patient's preferences for terminal care were unknown. The caregivers were then asked to choose from five levels of care ranging from the most aggressive at level 1, in which everything would be done to keep the patient alive, to palliative care only at level 5, in which medication would be used but only to keep the patient comfortable and not to cure acute infections (see Table 11.1). These levels of care have been used before to plan care in an institutional hospice program for demented patients described by Volicer et al. (1986), and also in a home hospice program developed by the Chicago Alzheimer's Association and Rush Alzheimer's Disease Center (Brechling, Heyworth, Kuhn, & Peranteau, 1989).

Hospice Care

Other questions concerned hospice care for dementia patients: Was hospice care viewed as an appropriate alternative to conventional care in end-stage dementia? Was home-based or institutional hospice care viewed as preferable? Were family and professional caregivers aware of hospice programs for dementia patients, as well as for cancer patients?

TABLE 11.1   Levels of Care

Level 1: Life-prolonging care would include:
  • Using antibiotics for acute infection, chronic medical problems, and pain
  • Using tube feeding, respirators, and resuscitation if the patient's heart stopped beating

Level 2: Care would include everything from level 1 *except* avoiding attempts to revive the person with electrical shock if his or her heart stopped beating.

Level 3: Care would be the same as level 2 *except* avoiding the use of a respirator if the person had difficulty breathing, as well as avoiding electrical shock to the heart.

Level 4: Care would include everything provided in level 3 *except* avoiding medication for acute illness that may end in death, such as pneumonia.

Level 5: As in level 4, everything would be done to keep the person comfortable, including medication for chronic illness and pain, *except* avoiding the use of feeding tubes if the person could not eat. Other elements of aggressive care that were excluded from other levels would also be excluded at this level, such as medication for infection, electrical shock to the heart, and respirators.

FINDINGS: ATTITUDES TOWARD PALLIATIVE CARE

The results of the survey were that the majority clearly favored palliative care (see Table 11.2). Two groups, physicians and family caregivers, were very close together in their views. The majority of family caregivers, 71%, viewed level 5, palliative care only, as the kind of care they would like their relative to receive in the end stages of dementia. Very few, only about 4%, preferred highly aggressive care at level 1. Physicians had similar views. The majority, 61%, preferred level 5, palliative care only. Just 2% thought the most aggressive care at level 1 was appropriate. Considerably more family caregivers preferred less aggressive care than gerontologists who were not physicians ($p < .05$). For example, 55% of gerontologists thought level 5, palliative care only, was appropriate compared to 71% of family members.

What Influenced Health Care Choices?

Among professionals and families, the most important factor was experience in planning for terminal care ($p < .05$). Professionals who had helped patients and their families to plan for terminal care were far more likely to favor palliative care. Among families, caregivers with prior expe-

TABLE 11.2 Distribution of Preferred Levels of Health Care for End-Stage Dementia Patients: Physicians, Gerontologists, and Family Members of Dementia Patients

Preferred levels of health care for end stage dementia	Physician (N = 513)	Gerontologist (N = 677)	Family member (N = 218)
Level 1: Do everything to prolong life	1.6% (8)	2.1% (14)	4.1% (9)
Level 2: Do everything but electric shock to restart the heart	2.5% (13)	6.9% (47)	3.7% (8)
Level 3: No respirator, no electric shock to restart the heart	17.9% (92)	18.3% (124)	15.1% (33)
Level 4: No respirator, no electric shock to restart the heart; also exclude medication for acute illness	16.6% (85)	17.6% (119)	5.8% (14)
Level 5: Also exclude tube feeding; focus on comfort and control of pain	61.4% (315)	55.1% (373)	70.6% (154)

riences with terminal care decisions were also more likely to choose less aggressive care.

ATTITUDES TOWARD HOSPICE CARE

The provision of hospice care for dementia patients received a great deal of support from most of the sample. Ninety percent of the professional and family caregivers viewed hospice care as an appropriate alternative for end-stage dementia. Although most of the group favored the hospice approach, they differed about where care should be provided.

Home Vs. Institutional Hospice

Professionals and family caregivers were asked whether they preferred hospice care for dementia patients at home or in an institution, such as a hospital or nursing home. About 70% of professionals preferred the home as the best setting for hospice care, while 56% of family caregivers thought institutional hospice care was a better alternative ($p < .00001$). Since families bear the major burden of home care, it is not surprising that they might favor institutional hospice. Family care for cancer patients in the National Hospice Study averaged 10 hours a day (Muurinen, 1986), with caregivers in the home-based hospice care group reporting greater burden than those whose relatives received hospital-based hospice care.

RELATED RESEARCH ON WHERE PATIENTS DIE

Although most families in our study preferred institutional hospice care, it is important to note that many families choose to care for their demented relatives at home. Recent research on this issue was conducted in cooperation with chapters of the Alzheimer's Association in Michigan (Collins & Ogle, 1994). More than 300 demented patients were followed over time, including 82 who subsequently died. These patients were most likely to die at home (41%) compared to in nursing homes (32%) or in hospitals (26%). In the 90 days before death, about a third remained at home and another third spent at least half of their time at home. Despite the extensive care needs of end-stage dementia patients, a fifth of the sample did not receive any help at home. Furthermore, among the patients who spent more than 45 of their last 90 days at home, only about half had a visiting nurse come out and only 27% had a physician home visit. These findings suggest the importance of making sure that families are aware of the help that they can receive through the Medicare hospice care benefit.

AWARENESS OF HOSPICE CARE FOR DEMENTIA PATIENTS

Turning back to our survey, since previous studies have found that the majority of hospice patients have cancer, we wanted to know whether the people in our survey were aware of hospice care programs for dementia patients. We found that most were not aware of available programs. Although 87% knew of hospice care programs for cancer patients, only 13% were aware of such programs for dementia patients ($p < .00001$). This finding led us, in our next study, to examine access to hospice care in end-stage dementia and the views of hospice staff on problems in the delivery of hospice services to these patients (Hanrahan & Luchins, 1995a).

ACCESS TO HOSPICE CARE PROGRAMS

Despite positive findings from evaluations of hospice care (Kane et al., 1984, 1985; Mor et al., 1989), relatively few dying patients receive hospice care services. A recent British study reported that only 7% of dying patients received hospice care (Seale, 1993). Policy analysts have long advocated expanding the hospice care approach to terminal illnesses other than cancer (Mor & Masterson-Allen, 1987; Seale, 1993). Previous studies have established that the majority of hospice patients have cancer (Mor & Masterson-Allen, 1987), but no studies have determined the proportion of hospice patients whose primary terminal illness was dementia. As we have just discussed, the majority of professional and family caregivers viewed hospice care as an appropriate alternative for end-stage dementia patients, yet most were unaware of such programs. This suggests an unmet need. In addition, the prevalence and costs of dementia indicate the importance of determining hospice utilization in the end stages of the disease (Bachman et al., 1993; Ernst & Hay, 1994; Rice et al., 1993; Weinberger et al., 1993).

How Many Patients with a Primary Diagnosis of Dementia are Enrolled in Hospice Programs?

To find out the extent to which hospices served dementia patients, we contacted 1,694 hospice programs that were known to the National Hospice Organization in 1990 (Hanrahan & Luchins, 1995a). Seventy percent of these hospices responded to our questionnaire (1,184 hospice programs). Our main question concerned the number of dementia patients in hospice programs who did not have some other terminal illness, such as cancer. In other words, their *primary* diagnosis was dementia. Another question concerned the number of patients whose dementia was secondary to another terminal illness, such as cancer or AIDS. Since we expected utilization of hospice care to be low for this group, hospice staff members were asked about their views on problems in serving dementia patients.

Results: Very Low Hospice Utilizaton

Although the responding hospices served 138,503 patients in 1990, less than 1% of those patients had a primary diagnosis of dementia and no other terminal illness (see Figure 11.1). Within this group, 80% were in the end stages of dementia. This appears to be a major gap in the service delivery system.

Primary & Secondary DX

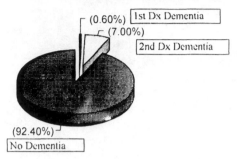

FIGURE 11.1   **Proportion of dementia patients in hospice programs.**

Dementia As a Secondary Diagnosis

Seven percent of hospice patients had dementia in addition to a terminal illness, such as cancer. Over half of the hospices (56%) served at least one patient with a secondary diagnosis of dementia.

Factors Related to the Enrollment of Dementia Patients

Although the enrollment of dementia patients in hospice programs was very low, three factors made the provision of hospice care for this population more likely. First, hospices that cared for patients with a secondary diagnosis of dementia were more likely to care for patients with primary dementia ($p < .001$). This suggests that the condition of dementia is not in itself a barrier to hospice care for end-stage dementia patients and that it is clinically feasible. Second, larger hospices were also more likely to care for dementia patients ($p < .01$). This finding argues against the need for specialized programs that are solely for dementia patients, since they appear to be readily served in general-purpose, large-scale programs. Third, for-profit hospices were more likely to enroll dementia patients. This suggests that the provision of hospice care in end-stage dementia is a fiscally sound option.

BARRIERS TO SERVICE DELIVERY

Since hospice care for dementia patients appears to be clinically and fiscally feasible, what accounts for such low use of hospice programs among dementia patients? In order to examine this issue, hospice staff members were asked about problems that had occurred in their efforts to serve dementia patients relative to other patients.

Difficulties Predicting Survival Time

According to hospice staff, the main obstacle was the difficulty in predicting the survival time of dementia patients. Eighty percent of the hospices viewed uncertainties about the survival time of dementia patients as a major problem in providing hospice care. Both traditional hospice guidelines and Medicare enrollment criteria require a prognosis of death within 6 months. This problem highlights the need to study factors that will predict death in end-stage dementia.

FEASIBLE CRITERIA FOR ENROLLING END-STAGE DEMENTIA PATIENTS IN HOSPICE PROGRAMS

Apart from the pioneering efforts of Volicer et al. (1993) in studying institutional hospice care, very little is known about factors influencing survival time in end-stage dementia. Research on empirically based standards for the enrollment of dementia patients in home hospice care programs is greatly needed.

In order to address the need for guidelines, we established and tested a set of enrollment criteria for the admission of end-stage dementia patients to hospice care (Hanrahan & Luchins, 1995b). These criteria were tested in a small pilot program developed in a collaboration between the University of Chicago and Meridian Hospice, Chicago, IL, followed by a replication in nine hospice programs (Hanrahan & Luchins, 1995). The criteria included advanced dementia and a history of medical complications (see Table 11.3).

RESULTS

Enrollment and Survival Time

Based on these criteria, 11 severely demented patients were enrolled compared to only 1 such patient in the year preceding the study. In the 2 years that the study continued, 8 of the 11 patients died. The enrollment criteria were successful in predicting a median survival time of 5 months, with an average of 7 months. The deceased patients had an average survival time of 3 months. Among the 3 surviving patients, the average length of stay was 16 months. Current Medicare reimbursement

TABLE 11.3   Hospice Enrollment Criteria for End-Stage Dementia Patients

I. Signs of very severe cognitive decline.
  A. May have the following (if known): Low mental status scores (MSQ or MMSE less than or equal to 1).
  B. All of the following impairments due to severe cognitive decline:
      Incontinence
      Needs assistance with eating
      Needs assistance with walking
      Needs assistance with bathing and grooming
      Very limited speech or cannot communicate meaningfully
      Unable to engage in purposeful activities

II. Serious complications. Patient should have a current or recent history of one or more of the following impairments:
      Difficulty swallowing food
      Aspiration pneumonia
      Dehydration
      Malnutrition
      Severe urinary tract infection
      Decubitus ulcers
      Septicemia
      Other serious complications

procedures allow for four billing periods: 90 days, 60 days, 30 days, and a fourth unlimited period. This means that even the long-stay hospice patients did not cause an undue burden to the hospice program.

CASE STUDIES: FAMILY CAREGIVERS' VIEWS ON HOSPICE CARE

Because hospice care for dementia is a relatively new concept, a qualitative study of five cases was used to describe family caregivers' attitudes and experience with Meridian Hospice. The purpose of the interviews was to find out why they chose hospice care for their relative, what they saw as helpful, and what problems occurred. Interviews were conducted with five African American family members whose demented relatives were enrolled in Meridian Hospice, who were available at the time of the study, and who were interested in participating. Subsequently, content analysis was used to identify common themes. This phase of our research benefited greatly from the assistance of Dr. Bernice Neugarten, who collaborated in structuring the research interview.

BACKGROUND AND REASONS FOR REFERRAL TO HOSPICE

Case #1

Mr. James was 87 years old. His wife, who was 86 years old, was diagnosed as having Alzheimer's disease. She was completely dependent in all activities of daily living, could no longer communicate, and had a history of falls and weight loss. Mr. James saw his choice as hospice care or nursing home placement, and chose the hospice program since keeping his wife at home was very important to him. He had previous experience with nursing homes, as he had placed his wife in a nursing home for a short time. However, he was completely dissatisfied with the care there, particularly the lack of individualized care. With the hospice program, he looked forward to being able to monitor the care provided to his wife at home. In addition, Mr. James requested assistance with medication bills, which had become overwhelming and which the Medicare hospice benefit would cover.

At the time of the referral, he performed all of the caregiving duties, leaving the house only to buy groceries. At those times he was extremely anxious since he had to leave his wife at home alone. Mr. James felt that he was referred to the hospice program because his physician recognized that his wife's care had become overwhelming for him, he was "desperate, physically and financially drained."

Case #2

Mrs. Thomas was 76 years old. Her husband had Alzheimer's disease. He was dependent in all activities of daily living and had a history of decubitus ulcers. Prior to their enrollment in the hospice program, Mrs. Thomas received help from a homemaker and a nurse from the Visiting Nurses Association. She had heard of the program before the referral but did not realize that hospice care could be provided at home until she talked with their doctor. The doctor explained that there was nothing more to be done to try to cure her husband's bedsores, and that medical care should now be focused on making him comfortable. Mrs. Thomas's primary purpose in enrolling her husband in the program was to obtain palliative care for him. She wanted him to be made as comfortable as possible, given that his bedsores would not go away. Although she was hesitant to accept the terminal prognosis, she related her use of hospice directly to the fact that her loved one was dying.

Case #3

Mr. Green was 90 years old. His wife, who also was 90, had been diagnosed with Alzheimer's disease. She could not converse beyond a greeting, was dependent in all activities of daily living, and had a history of falls due to mobility problems. Prior to their enrollment, Mr. Green received help with cooking and cleaning from a homemaker service. However, the referring physician reported that there was a great deal of tension between Mr. Green and the homemakers and that Mr. Green needed additional assistance with caregiving duties. Like Mr. James, Mr. Green felt that he was referred to the hospice program because his physician recognized that his wife's care had become overwhelming for him. In particular, Mr. Green said that putting his wife to bed was too much for him, as she could no longer walk. Thus he looked to the hospice program specifically for help with the physical care of his loved one.

Mr. Green also chose home hospice care over a nursing home, because keeping his wife at home was a priority for him. Some of his other relatives were in nursing homes, and he was not pleased with the care they received. He looked forward to being able to care for his wife himself and to monitoring the care provided by hospice staff.

Case #4

Mrs. Miller was 75 years old. Her mother, Mrs. Carson, had vascular dementia and was 102 years old. She could eat only soft foods with assistance, was dependent in all other activities of daily living, and had a history of falls and urinary infections. Her speech was minimal. Mrs. Miller lived in a separate apartment one floor below her mother and her two aunts, who were also demented. In order to care for her three demented relatives, she had a day nurse and a night nurse.

Mrs. Miller decided to use hospice care because the benefits were good. She and her doctor discussed the fact that her mother was terminally ill. However, her explanation of her decision to use hospice care was based on her feeling that she could use the hospice's help to arrange for medication and durable equipment. In addition, she thought she could benefit from regular checkups of her mother's health status at home by the hospice nurse.

Case #5

Mrs. Frank was 82 years old. Her husband, who was 83, had Alzheimer's disease. He also had a history of urinary tract infections and decubitus ulcers. At the time of the referral, Mrs. Frank had been caring for her husband by herself. She had heard about the hospice program; however, she did not have any direct experience with hospice care prior to their enrollment. She looked to the program to help her cope with the advanced stages of Alzheimer's disease.

CAREGIVERS' PERCEPTION OF HOSPICE CARE BENEFITS

Several kinds of hospice care services were seen as beneficial to both patients and family caregivers. Benefits that were mentioned included home visits by the hospice physician and nurses, palliative care, case-managed home health care, service provision in the home environment, and the high quality of staff care. Other services were especially important to the family caregivers themselves, notably respite, education, counseling, and bereavement services.

BENEFITS TO BOTH PATIENTS AND FAMILY CAREGIVERS

Home Visits

Visits by medical staff at home were especially important. Since the patients were usually unable to walk at this point, clinic visits were physically difficult for the caregiver, as well as time consuming and expensive. Before enrolling in the hospice program, for instance, Mr. Thomas's doctor would try to assess his needs and prescribe for him by phone, because Mrs. Thomas was not able to bring him to the clinic. Obviously, this was not a long-term solution, since it is difficult to treat a patient without seeing him. For these reasons, weekly physical checkups at home by the hospice nurse were viewed as very helpful by most of the caregivers. Home visits were also available from the hospice doctor.

Knowing that the medical staff was available around the clock was especially reassuring to the caregivers. For example, Mr. James called the hospice doctor when his wife fell out of bed and broke her arm. The doctor visited the home, examined Mrs. James, and arranged for her transfer to an emergency room. Because of home care, Mr. James was able to have his wife examined at home before taking more aggressive medical action. If this had been a circumstance in which aggressive treatment was inappropriate, it would have been avoided by using the hospice doctor.

Palliative Care

Caregivers whose relatives were currently suffering from complications appreciated the hospice staff's expertise in providing palliative care. An example is the assistance provided to Mr. Frank, which enabled him to die comfortably at home. When he first developed bedsores, Mrs.

Frank was concerned that she would not be able to care for him and placed him in a nursing home. While he was there, Mr. Frank gritted his teeth and stopped eating, became constipated, and was less alert. In Mrs. Frank's words, "He looked like he was passing out." In alarm at his condition, Mrs. Frank returned him home, where she received help from the hospice program. The hospice nurse gave him sponge baths and changed the pads on his bedsores. Once home he responded to spoon feeding by his wife and became more alert. In another example, Mrs. Miller reported that her mother was helped to feel more comfortable during her final days when the hospice nurse suctioned her lungs.

Case-Managed Home Health Care

Practical assistance with medication, medical equipment, and routine physical care were also seen as very helpful. The hospice staff ordered medication and equipment such as hospital beds and wheelchairs. Billing Medicare was also taken care of by the hospice. This relieved the caregivers of time-consuming tasks and provided them with financial assistance. Assistance from hospice home health aides was seen as very important. For example, Mr. James said the hospice relieved him of trying to provide care that he was unable to provide, namely, feeding and bathing his wife.

Home Environment

Home care allowed the families to monitor their loved ones' care very closely. They were also able to remain near each other until the end. For example, Mrs. Green would sometimes wake in the night and tug on her husband's bedspread. Although she couldn't speak coherently, Mr. Green felt that he could comfort her by talking to her when she awoke in the middle of the night.

Quality of Staff Care

Generally, the hospice staff was seen as very responsive to the needs of both the families and the patients. Mr. James, for instance, was especially pleased with the nurse's aide's ability to get his wife to eat without a struggle. The caregivers used such terms as "concerned," "understanding," "high quality," and "very helpful" to describe the staff.

BENEFITS TO FAMILY CAREGIVERS

Respite

While some caregivers did not need respite care, others found it extremely helpful. Because of respite care, Mr. James was able to leave his wife with the nurse's aide instead of alone while he shopped for groceries. Before her enrollment in the hospice program, he had been her sole source of care. Later, when he needed surgery, respite workers provided around-the-clock care for his wife for a month. Other caregivers needed less intensive respite. For example, a volunteer stayed with Mr. Thomas on Sunday, so that his wife could go to church.

Education

Those caregivers whose relatives had died at the time of the interview appreciated being taught by hospice staff about the signs and symptoms of approaching death.

COUNSELING

For some caregivers, the emotional support they received from the hospice staff was very helpful. Support from the hospice staff was reassuring to Mrs. Frank, who felt that she was not really alone because of the hospice program and could call any time, day or night. Mrs. Thomas reported that the hospice staff "hug you on the way in and on the way out and that's great for families coping with terminal people."

Bereavement Services

The caregivers whose relatives had died at the time of the interview greatly appreciated bereavement services. For instance, the bereavement coordinator helped Mrs. Miller to make funeral arrangements before her mother's death, consoled her, was there for the funeral and called later to see how she was doing. On the day Mrs. Miller's mother died, the hospice nurse took care of all of the arrangements. In Mrs. Miller's words, "I would not have known what to do without the hospice staff."

CAREGIVERS' PERCEPTION OF PROBLEMS

One problem reported by two caregivers was the lack of home health care by hospice staff on evenings and weekends. Mr. Green had to hire evening help separately from the hospice staff. Since help in the evening was his most important reason for turning to the hospice program, he was very disappointed. Mr. James also was unable to get the help he needed on weekends. Although he hired help through another agency, he felt that the quality of care was not nearly as good as that given by the hospice staff.

Assistance in planning a funeral was not seen as needed for two of the caregivers whose wives had not yet died. Although the hospice staff respected their choice to forgo working with the bereavement counselor, the caregivers found the hospice staff's questions regarding planning for their wives' deaths to be intrusive and felt that these matters were personal family issues.

IMPLICATIONS OF THE CASE STUDIES

The reasons for referral to hospice care reflected the extensive and technical care needs of patients in the end stages of dementia and, essentially, documented the relevance of hospice services to families who were struggling to care for severely demented patients. These needs included assistance with palliative care and the demanding physical care requirements of patients who were incontinent and needed assistance to eat and to move. Care for patients with end-stage dementia was especially overwhelming to those caregivers who had no other help.

Once hospice care was provided, there appeared to be a good fit between the kinds of services offered and the needs of both patients and family caregivers. In general, the caregivers interviewed were very satisfied with the care provided by the hospice staff. In addition, it is apparent from the caregivers' reports that the patients themselves benefited from the skilled and individualized palliative care provided at home.

The major problem area reported in the interviews was that the timing of hospice services did not always fit the need. Providing care for a terminally ill person (with any diagnosis) persists throughout the weekend and evening. Therefore, to be maximally beneficial, or in some cases to be helpful at all, hospice programs should make arrangements for service to be provided during the hours most needed by the particular caregiver. It is, of course, important to note that some hospices are able to provide weekend and evening care, so these problems are not typical of all hospice programs.

While the caregivers varied in their need for specific services, such as respite and bereavement counseling, most felt that help from hospice staff allowed them to better manage the final stages of their loved ones' illness. In fact, it is a tribute to the hospice staff that they have been able to individualize their treatment plans so that the different needs of almost all of the caregivers and patients were met. For example, Mr. James was not interested in discussing or planning for his wife's death. Although he was offered help from hospice staff with the practical and emotional implications of his wife's dying process, he did not feel pressured by the staff to discuss these issues. In summary, the hospice program seemed to meet many needs of both patients and family caregivers and to be well accepted by them. The lack of universal need for some hospice services did not take away from the overall benefit of hospice care.

REPLICATION STUDY

Because staff from 80% of the hospice programs viewed the issue of predicting survival time as a major problem in serving dementia patients, further research was conducted on this issue (Hanrahan & Luchins, 1995c, 1995d). In our next study, we attempted to repeat findings that our enrollment criteria could identify appropriate patients for hospice care—in other words, patients who were likely to have an average survival time of 6 months or less (Luchins, Hanrahan, & Murphy, 1996). The purpose of the replication was to expand the study to institutional hospice settings, as well as replicate our findings with home hospice patients. This study, which is in progress, includes nine hospice programs in the Midwest that provide care both at home and in nursing homes. Data on 47 patients in two cohorts has been collected over 4 years. Enrollment in this phase of the study stopped 6 months prior to the end of the study period in order to allow for a six-month follow-up period.

CRITERIA

Our enrollment criteria continued to focus on patients who were impaired in all or most activities of daily living and could no longer engage in purposeful activities. Patients also had either current complications or a history of recent complications that are typical of late-stage dementia (e.g., difficulty swallowing food). For most patients, the severity of the dementia corresponded to stage 7 of the Global Deterioration Scale (Reisberg et al., 1982).

MEASURES

We found that the hospice programs needed some help in identifying appropriate patients. Hospice staff members were thus asked to rate patients in activities of daily living, to do a mental status test with any patients who were able to participate (Kahn et al., 1960; Folstein, Anthony, Parhad, Duffy, & Greenberg, 1985), and to determine the patients' stage on an adaptation of the Global Deterioration Scale (Reisberg et al., 1982) called Functional Assessment Staging, or FAST (Reisberg, 1988). Because patients were required to have recent complications, hospice staff also completed a medical complications checklist (MCC), which consisted of a list of common complications of end-stage dementia and documentation of when the problem occurred (current vs. within the past year). Complications included swallowing problems, aspiration pneumonia, malnutrition, dehydration, decubitus ulcers, urinary tract infections, septicemia, seizures, fractures or broken bones, and deep vein thrombosis. The checklist was based on common complications in advanced dementia according to physicians who responded to our previous survey (Luchins & Hanrahan, 1993). Hospice staff members were also asked to characterize the palliative care plan with regard to whether or not medications could be used for acute illness.

We also collected measures of appetite, nourishment, and mobility that were used by Schonwetter et al. (1990) in a study of survival time among cancer patients. Performance ratings of *appetite* ranged from 1 = normal to 5 = refuses fluid; *nourishment* was scored 1 = heavy to 5 = extreme cachexia; and *mobility* was rated 1 = normal to 5 = unable to turn in bed.

Survival time consisted of the number of days between enrollment in the hospice program and the patient's death, or if the patient was not deceased, the number of days from enrollment until November 31, 1992, for the first cohort and until March 31, 1995, for the second cohort.

PRELIMINARY FINDINGS

Survival Time

Preliminary findings have been analyzed for the 36 patients in the first two years of the replication, combined with the 11 patients in our 2-year pilot study with Meridian Hospice, for a total of 47 patients. The hospice enrollment criteria predicted a median survival time of 4 months and a mean survival time of 6.9 months; 38% survived more than 6 months. The 37 deceased patients had a mean survival time of 4.5 months, while the 10 patients (21%) who were still alive averaged a survival time of 15.7 months.

Correlates of Survival Time

FAST scores and mobility ratings were significantly related to survival time. However, 41% could not be scored on the FAST, as their disease progression was not ordinal. Among patients who could be scored on the FAST and who had reached stage 7C (mobility impaired, one intelligible word a day or less), mean survival time was 3.2 months; 92% were deceased and only 17% survived longer than 6 months (N = 12). These patients appear to be good candidates for the hospice program, given the current eligibility criteria. In contrast, those who could be scored and had not reached this stage had a mean survival time of 18 months. Because the enrollment criteria suggested that patients have impairment in most or all ADLs, relatively few patients were in this group (N = 5). All of these patients were still surviving and all had survived for more than 6 months. These patients do not appear to fit current requirements for hospice enrollment. Those whose disease progression was not ordinal averaged a survival time of 8.6 months (N = 12); 92% were deceased, but 7 (58%) survived for more than 6 months. Mean survival times among these three groups differed significantly ($p < .001$, analysis of variance [ANOVA], F = 11.52). All pairwise comparisons were also significant (Tukey-B Test, $p < .05$).

Influence of the Palliative Care Plan

When both FAST status and the care plans were examined, each had an effect on survival time (see Table 11.4). Patients whose care plans called for the use of medication for acute illness had longer survival times than those without this provision, $p < .01$. For the nonordinal group, even though all were enrolled in the hospice program, there was a threefold difference in mean survival between those who received medications for acute illness (14.9 months) and those who did not receive medication (5.2 months). This finding is similar to the life-prolonging effect of treating fever observed by Volicer et al. (1993), in those with less severe disability. This effect of treatment suggests that nonordinal end-stage dementia patients, with impaired mobility and better preserved language, might be suitable for hospice care if their palliative care plans were conservative, and not appropriate if more life-prolonging care was anticipated.

Service Characteristics: Staff Time Per Patient

Nurses clearly provided the vast majority of service time to dementia patients in hospice care, with certified nurses's assistants providing the bulk of care at an average of 18 hours a month per patient and licensed practical nurses providing 5 hours. Senior companions averaged 7 hours of monthly care per patient in addition to 5 hours from other volunteers.

TABLE 11.4   Survival Time: Effect of Palliative Care Plan
and Patient Status on the FAST

FAST status*	N = 25	Medications used for acute illness survival time	Medications not used** survival time
Less than stage 7C	4	24.2 months (SD = .2) N = 2	17.5 months (SD = 2.8) N = 2
At or past stage 7C	11	4 months (SD = 3.9) N = 6	2.6 months (SD = 4.3) N = 5
Not ordinal	10	14.9 months (SD = 6.2) N = 5	5.2 months (SD = 3) N = 5

ANOVA, $F = 19.95$, $p<.001$
*FAST status, main effect, $F = 24.6$, $p<.001$.
**Use of medications, main effect, $F = 9.8$, $p<.01$.

Bereavement counselors offered 2 hours of monthly care per patient. The medical director, social worker, administrator, and secretary all provided an hour or less of care per month. The per diem rate for the Medicare hospice benefit was $104.03/day in 1995. The utilization of staff time would appear to be well within the limits of Medicare reimbursement. Additionally, patients in nursing homes continued to receive Medicaid. In Illinois, Medicaid reimbursement for hospice patients was limited to 95% of the usual rate.

RELATED RESEARCH ON SURVIVAL TIME

Other research by Volicer et al. (1993) suggests that patients with severe dementia who have a fever are likely to die within 6 months. In examining death certificates, Kukull et al. (1994) found that pneumonia is also a common cause of death in end-stage dementia.

CONCLUSIONS

In summary, family and professional caregivers have very positive attitudes toward palliative care for patients in the end stages of dementia and view hospice care as an appropriate alternative. However, hospice care is rarely available for these patients. The primary barrier to hospice enrollment is the difficulty in predicting survival in end-stage dementia. Recent research suggests that severely demented patients may be ready for hospice enrollment if they

1. Need assistance in all of their activities of daily living
2. Have current or recent medical complications, especially if accompanied by fever
3. Have low scores on performance ratings of mobility
4. Have FAST scores of stage 7C or greater (among those who can be scored)
5. Have impaired mobility, among those who cannot be scored on the FAST, and a conservative palliative care plan

Alternatively, one should at least consider adapting the hospice model to new populations by dropping a 6-month survival time as an enrollment criterion. A terminal condition, together with a need for skilled nursing, has been suggested as an enrollment criterion for AIDS patients and might be equally appropriate for end-stage dementia patients.

Once in hospice, the clinical care needs of dementia patients were readily accommodated by hospice staff. Most of the care was provided by the nursing staff, particularly certified nursing assistants. The services provided by the hospice programs appeared to be well within the reimbursement level of the Medicare hospice benefit. The needs of family caregivers, as well as patients, appeared to be well met by the hospice program.

ACKNOWLEDGMENTS

This research was made possible by generous support from the University of Chicago Hospitals' Home Care Research Grants, the Alzheimer's Association/Mr. and Mrs. Neil Bluhm Pilot Research Grant, and research grants from the Alzheimer's Disease Research Committee of the Illinois Department of Public Health. The authors also appreciated the thoughtful reviews of the questionnaire used to assess appropriate care for end-stage dementia patients by faculty associated with the University of Chicago's Center on Aging, Health, and Society, particularly Christine Cassel, M.D., and Greg Sachs, M.D. We are also grateful for reviews of the survey instrument for determining access to hospice care by Edward F. Lawlor, Ph.D., director of the University of Chicago's Center on Health

Administration Studies, and Kendon J. Conrad, Ph.D., associate professor, School of Public Health, University of Illinois. We appreciate John J. Mahoney and Galen Miller, Ph.D., of the National Hospice Organization and Thomas Kirk of the Patient and Family Services Department of the Alzheimer's Association for their thoughtful reviews of our questionnaires. Our pilot study with Meridian Hospice was made possible by the untiring efforts of the staff in extending hospice care to dementia patients. The contributions of then Executive Director Marie Van Gemert and Peggy Jones, B.S.N., were essential to the study. Bernice L. Neugarten, Ph.D., of the University of Chicago's Center on Aging, Health, and Society, played a substantial role in structuring the case studies from Meridian Hospice. For their assistance with our replication study, we are also very grateful to the following hospice programs: Henry Ford Hospice, LaGrange Memorial Hospice, Hospice of the North Shore, Horizon Hospice, Evangelical Health Service Hospice, West Towns VNS Hospice, VNA Hospice of Chicago, and the Hospice of Northeastern Illinois.

REFERENCES

Bachman, D. L., Wolf, P. A., Linn, R. T., Knoefel, J. L., Cobb, J. L., Belanger, A. J., White, L. R., & D'Agostino, R. B. (1993). Incidence of dementia and probable Alzheimer's disease in a general population: The Framingham Study. *Neurology, 43,* 515–519.

Brechling, B. G., Heyworth, J., Kuhn, D., & Peranteau, M. F. (1987). Extending hospice care to end-stage dementia patients and families. *American Journal of Alzheimer's Care Related Disorders Research,* pp. 21–29.

Collins, C., & Ogle, K. (1994). Patterns of predeath service use by dementia patients with a family caregiver. *Journal of the American Geriatrics Society, 42,* 719–722.

Danis M., Southerland L. I., Garrett J. M., et al. (1991). A prospective study of advance directives for life-sustaining care. *New England Journal of Medicine, 324*(13), 882–888.

Ernst, R. L., & Hay, J. W. (1994). The U.S. economic and social costs of Alzheimer's disease revisited. *American Journal of Public Health, 84,* 1261–1264.

Folstein, M., Anthony, J. C., Parhad, I., Duffy, B., & Gruenberg, E. (1985). The meaning of cognitive impairment in the elderly. *Journal of the American Geriatrics Society, 33,* 228–235.

Hanrahan, P., & Luchins, D. J. (1995a). Access to hospice care for end-stage dementia patients: A national survey of hospice programs. *Journal of the American Geriatrics Society, 43,* 56–59.

Hanrahan, P., & Luchins, D. J. (1995b). Feasible criteria for enrolling end-stage dementia patients in home hospice care. *Hospice Journal, 10*(3), 47–54.

Hanrahan, P., & Luchins, D. J. (1995c). *Survival time among demented hospice patients.* Miami: American Psychiatric Association.

Hanrahan, P., & Luchins, D. J. (1995d). Reply to Dr. Maletta. *Journal of the American Geriatrics Society, 43*(10), 1175–1176.

High, D. M. (1988). All in the family: Extended autonomy and expectations in surrogate health care decision-making. *Gerontologist, 28,* 46–51.

Kahn, R. L., Goldfarb, A. I., Pollack, M., & Peck, A. (1960). Brief objective measures for the determination of mental status in the aged. *American Journal of Psychiatry, 117,* 326–328.

Kane R. L., Klien S. J., Bernstein L., Rothenberg R., & Wales J. (1985). Hospice role in alleviating the emotional stress of terminal patients and their families. *Medical Care, 23*(3), 189–197.

Kane, R. L, Wales, J., Bernstein, L., Lebowitz, A., & Kaplan, S. (1984, April). A randomized, controlled trial of hospice care. *Lancet,* 890–894.

Katzman, R. (1976) The prevalence and malignancy of Alzheimer's disease. *Archives of Neurology, 33,* 217–218.

Kukull, W. A., Brenner, D. E., Speck, C. E., Nochlin, D., Bowen, J., McCormick, W., Teri, L., Pfauschmidt, M. L., & Larson, E. B. (1994). Causes of death associated with Alzheimer disease: variation by level of cognitive impairment before death. *Journal of the American Geriatrics Society, 42*(7), 723–726.

Luchins, D. J., & Hanrahan, P. (1993). What is the appropriate level of health care for end stage dementia patients? *Journal of the American Geriatrics Society, 41,* 25–30.

Luchins, D. J., Hanrahan, P., & Murphy, K. (in press). Criteria for enrolling dementia patients in hospice. Under review.

Mor, V., Greer, D. S., & Kastenbaum, R. (Eds.). (1989). *The hospice experiment* (2nd ed.). Baltimore: Johns Hopkins University Press.

Mor, V., & Masterson-Allen, S. (1987). *Hospice care systems: Structure, process, costs and outcome.* New York: Springer.

Muurinen, J. (1986). The economics of informal care: Labor market effects of the national hospice study. *Medical Care, 24*(11), 1007–1017.

Reisberg, B. (1988). Functional Assessment Staging (FAST). *Psychopharm Bull, 24,* 653–659.

Reisberg, B., Ferris, S. H., De Leon, M. J., & Crook, T. (1982). The Global Deterioration Scale for assessment of primary degenerative dementia. *American Journal of Psychiatry, 139*(9), 1136–1139.

Rice, D. P., Fox, P. J., & Max, W., et al. (1993). The economic burden of Alzheimer's disease care. *Health Affairs, 12*(2), 164–76.

Sachs, G., Stocking, C., & Miles, S. (1989). Empowerment of the elderly: Increasing advance directives? *Gerontologist, 29,* 190A.

Schonwetter, R. S., Teasdale, T. A., Storey, P., et al. (1990). Estimation of survival time in terminal cancer patients: An impedance to admission. *Hospice Journal, 6,* 65–80.

Seale, C. (1993). Demographic change and the care of the dying, 1969–1987. In D. Dickenson, & M. Johnson (Eds.), *Death, dying and bereavement* (pp. 45–54). London: Sage Publications.

Steiber, S. R. (1987). Right to die: Public balks at deciding for others. *Hospitals,* *61*(5), 72.

Volicer, B. J., Hurley, A., Fabiszewski, K. J., et al: (1993). Predicting short-term survival for patients with advanced Alzheimer's disease. *Journal of the American Geriatrics Society, 41,* 535–540.

Volicer, L., Rheaume, Y., Brown, J., Fabiszewski, K., & Brady, R. (1996). Hospice approach to the treatment of patients with advanced dementia of the Alzheimer type. *Journal of the American Medical Assocation, 256*(16), 2210–2213.

Weinberger, M., Gold, D. T., Divine, G. W., et al. (1993). Expenditures in caring for patients with dementia who live at home. *American Journal of Public Health, 83*(3), 338–341.

Barriers to Providing Hospice Care for People with Dementia

Joyce Simard and Ladislav Volicer

People with dementia of the Alzheimer type (DAT) and other progressive dementias have not typically been identified as appropriate patients for hospice services, even though in late stages these diseases should be considered terminal illnesses because there is no available treatment and because they lead to premature death (Katzman et al., 1994). Why, then, has this significant population, over 4 million Americans, been excluded from receiving hospice services? Barriers from a variety of sources have made it difficult for this population to access the services that will help patients die the "good death" and families of patients to receive support and counseling.

Many people with dementia live in nursing facilities, a significant number in Dementia Special Care Units (DSCUs). Since the 1980s DSCUs have emerged as a care option for residents with DAT. There are currently over 3,000 DSCUs offering a variety of services to residents and their families (U.S. Congress, Office of Technology Assessment, 1992). DSCUs have been designed to provide a secure environment for residents in the middle stage of the disease, when wandering into other residents' rooms and the risk of elopement becomes problematic for staff and other residents (Volicer & Simard, 1996).

Some DSCUs keep residents until death, with an "aging in place" philosophy (Volicer & Staff of the Dementia Study Unit, 1992). However, the usual policy is to transfer the resident to an Advanced Care Unit (ACU) or to another area of the nursing facility when the resident is no longer ambulatory (Leon, 1994). Rather than an emphasis on activities and keeping residents actively engaged in their daily routine, the ACU places more emphasis on nursing care because the residents are completely dependent in all activities of daily living. Whether persons with DAT are in a DSCU, ACU, or another part of the nursing facility, they will eventually move into the last stage of the disease. At this point, residents, their families, and staff could benefit from the services offered by a community hospice program. Sadly, the Medicare Hospice Benefit is accessed for very few persons with late-stage DAT despite the fact that they are eligible to receive it (Hanrahan & Luchins, 1995).

Some hospice programs report that 1% or fewer of their patients have Alzheimer's disease (Luchins & Hanrahan, 1993). Most place DAT in the "other" category and do not even bother to track this type of patient. The reasons for the low utilization of the hospice benefit are varied. Barriers develop from all involved—physicians, families, nursing facilities, and hospice programs. To break down these barriers, we must understand each entity's point of view and show how it is a "win-win" situation for all involved to partner with each other. Only then will residents and their families who have lived with the disease for so many years be able to take advantage of the benefits that so many other terminally ill patients and families experience—a comfortable death, surrounded by compassionate caregivers.

SELECTION OF APPROPRIATE HOSPICE PATIENTS

In the early 1960s, hospice providers began offering services to patients with cancer. With the advent of AIDS, the population that hospice programs served began to change. This increased the awareness that patients with other types of diseases could and should receive hospice services. However, patients with DAT were rarely found in the hospice programs. They are a "hidden" population. Patients with DAT either live in a nursing home, where hospices rarely provided care, or are at home with family, seldom leaving the house. Physicians did not think of patients with DAT as appropriate for a hospice referral, and families who care for their loved ones at home typically avail themselves of few community services and simply do not know that the Medicare Hospice Benefit can be used for DAT.

Recently, the National Alzheimer's Association has begun to provide education for families, advising them of their right to elect the Medicare Hospice Benefit for their loved one. The National Hospice Organization (NHO) formed a task force and wrote a guide to assist hospice providers in determination of eligibility for the patient with nontraditional diagnoses (Stuart et al., 1995). With a rise in the number of hospice programs, developing and sustaining a census that supports the hospice is an important element of each hospice's business plan. Since there will be over 4 million Americans with DAT, and elders who are the highest risk age group are also the fastest growing segment of the population, hospice providers have become increasingly interested in caring for patients with DAT.

PREDICTION OF 6-MONTH SURVIVAL

One of the main barriers to the involvement of Alzheimer patients in a hospice program is the need for prognosis of 6 months or less of life, which is a requirement for accessing the Medicare Hospice Benefit. The course of a progressive dementia is highly unpredictable, with periods of stabilization occurring even in advanced DAT. Because death is caused by the complications of dementia and not by the dementia process itself, it is very difficult to predict when the patient will have less than 6 months to live.

Several factors that affect the long-term survival of dementia patients have been identified. These include age, gender and duration of illness (Burns, Lewis, Jacoby, & Levy, 1991), rate of dementia progression (Brodaty, McGilchrist, Harris, & Peters, 1993), degree of cognitive and functional impairment (Burns et al., 1991; Evans et al., 1991; Heyman et al., 1987; Hier, Warach, Gorelick, & Thomas, 1989; Knopman, Kitto, Deinard, & Heiring, 1988), behavioral problems (Knopman et al., 1988; Walsh, Welch, & Larson, 1990), presence of hypertension (Hier et al., 1989) and other physical illness (Burns et al., 1991), depression (Burns et al., 1991), cachexia (Evans et al., 1991), and wandering and falling (Walsh et al., 1990). However, only two studies investigated short-term survival, approaching the 6-month hospice certification requirement. The first study reported that 1-year survival can be predicted by performance on a cognitive test battery, with a deficit in expressive language indicating an especially poor prognosis (Kaszniak et al., 1978). The second study analyzed factors associated with 2-year survival and found that predictor variables were age, gender, and functional and behavioral impairments (Van Dijk, Dippel, & Habbema, 1994) and comorbidity (Van Dijk, Van de Sande, Dippel, & Habbena, 1992).

More recently, several lists of criteria for the involvement of patients with dementia in hospice programs were published (see Table 12.1). However, none of these criteria are based on objectively analyzed data demonstrating

TABLE 12.1   Clinical Criteria for Inclusion in a Hospice Program

Criteria	Sources					
	1	2	3	4	5	6
Inability to dress independently	x					
Inability to bathe properly	x				x	
Inability to walk	x	x	x	x	x	
Bedbound			x	x		
Increasing weakness		x				x
Poor appetite						x
Eating difficulties		x				
Needs to be fed					x	
Difficulty swallowing	x			x	x	
Consistent weight loss	x	x				x
Lean body mass <70% of IBW						
Increasing cognitive deficits						x
Decreased verbalization			x			
Able to say half dozen words	x			x		
Able to say only 1-2 words			x	x	x	
Mini-Mental Examination score <4				x		
Mini-Mental Examination score ≤1					x	
Increased dependence in ADLs		x				
Fecal and urinary incontinence	x			x	x	
Needs total assistance with ADLs						
More lethargic or withdrawn		x				x
Ability to smile lost				x		
Functional Assessment Stage >7B			x			
Cannot do what made them happy					x	
Unable to recognize loved ones					x	
Verbalizing fear of dying		x				
Verbalizing acceptance of death		x				
Family needs emotional support		x				
Avoidance of hospitalization		x				x
No tube feeding			x			x
No antibiotics			x			x
Recurrent infections						x
Other serious medical problems	x			x		

1. *Medical Guidelines for Determing Prognosis in Selected NonCancer Diseases,* by B. Stuart, L. Herbst, D. Kinbrunner, M. Preodor, S. Connor, T. Ryndes, C. Cody, & K. Brandt, 1995, Arlington, VA: National Hospice Organization.
2. Okun, S. N. (1995). Responding to change. *Hospice Care PRN 4* (1), 2–3.

TABLE 12.1   *(continued)*

3. Kinzbrunner, B. M. (1993, May). Non-malignant terminal diseases: criteria for hospice admission. *Academy of Hospice Physicians Newsletter,* pp. 3–6.
4. Old Colony Hospice, Stoughton, MA. (ND). *Hospice referrals for end stage neurological disease.* Stoughton, MA: Author.
5. Hanrahan, P., & Luchins, D. J. (1995). Feasible criteria for enrolling end-stage dementia patients in home hospice care. *Hospice Journal, 10,* 47–54.
6. Trinity Hospice of Greater Boston. (ND). *Non-oncolgic diseases/criteria for admission.* Brookline, MA: Author.

that they are actually predictive of 6-month survival. Furthermore, the criteria do not have operational definitions and it is not specified exactly which, how many, or what combinations predict 6-month mortality. In summary, these criteria are a list of characteristics of late-stage dementia, which may or may not be related to 6-month survival.

Quantitative criteria for the inclusion of dementia patients in a hospice were proposed by Community Hospice Inc. (1994). All patients considered for this hospice program are evaluated by three scales: Karnofsky, modified activities of daily living (ADLs), and a summary of descriptive scales. The end stage of Alzheimer's disease is defined as the patient being bedbound or chairbound, unable to effectively communicate with words, having markedly decreased appetite and/or intake, and having a Karnofsky score of 5 or less, an ADL score of 12 or less, and a descriptive scale score of 19 or less.

These definitions and scales do not accurately characterize patients with end-stage DAT. The cutoff points for Karnofsky and ADL scores may be too high because the Karnofsky score of 4 (disabled; requires special care and assistance) would apply to patients with even moderate dementia and the ADL score of 12 would accept patients who are still able to bathe, dress, toilet, and transfer with assistance instead of being completely dependent. The descriptive scales instrument does not apply well to dementia patients because it includes cachexia, pain, and dyspnea, which are rarely observed even in advanced dementia.

The prediction of survival in advanced dementia is complicated because most scales that measure dementia severity lack the sensitivity to detect further progression of dementia. Many scales have a "floor effect" in which the score can go no lower, even when the patients deteriorate further. However, the progression of dementia into the very late stages can be detected by using the Bedford Alzheimer Nursing Scale–Severity (BANS-S), which was developed specifically for patients with advanced dementia (Volicer, Hurley, Lathi, & Kowall, 1994). BANS-S combines ratings of interaction ability (speech, eye contact), functional deficits (dressing, eating, ambulation), and occurrence of pathological symptoms (sleep–wake cycle disturbance, muscle rigidity/contractures). The 7-item BANS-S has a range of 7 (no impairment) to 28 (complete impairment) (see Table 12.2). The scale has good reliability and reproducibility and construct validity. The BANS-S score obtained within 3 months of death correlates with the extent of DAT pathology in the hippocampus (Volicer et al., 1994).

Even with the BANS-S, however, it was not possible to predict 6-month survival in stable patients with advanced dementia. Because most deaths of dementia patients are caused by infections (see chapter 2), we have postulated that the prediction of 6-month survival may be possible when the patient developed a fever episode. We have found that older age and higher severity of DAT at the time of the fever episode, palliative care, and hospital admission for long-term care within 6 months of the onset of fever were positively associated with the likelihood of mortality within 6 months of the onset of fever (B. J. Volicer, Hurley, Fabiszewski, Montgomery, & Volicer, 1993). This predictive model was converted to nomograms to facilitate the calculation of probability of dying within 6 months for patients with advanced DAT. The nomograms permit direct determination of the probability by connecting age and disease severity of an individual patient (L. Volicer, Volicer, & Hurley, 1993). To allow for differences in management strategy and time from admission to long-term care to fever development, four different nomograms were constructed (see Figure 12.1).

Applying this model to a different patient population, it was found that the percent who died ranged from 16% among those for whom the model predicted a probability of survival less than .25 to 53% among those for whom the model predicted a probability of survival of .75 or greater (B. J. Volicer et al., 1993). Thus the model was better at defining patients who will not die within 6 months than at selecting those who will definitely die during that time period. The other limitation of this model is

TABLE 12.2 BANS Severity Scale

---

1. DRESSING: Independent—Completely Dependent
2. SLEEP-WAKE CYCLE: Regular—Disrupted
3. SPEECH: Intact—Mute
4. EATING: Independent—Completely dependent
5. WALKING: Independent—Unable even with help
6. MUSCLES: Flexible and full joint motion—Contracted
7. EYE CONTACT: Always maintained—Never maintained

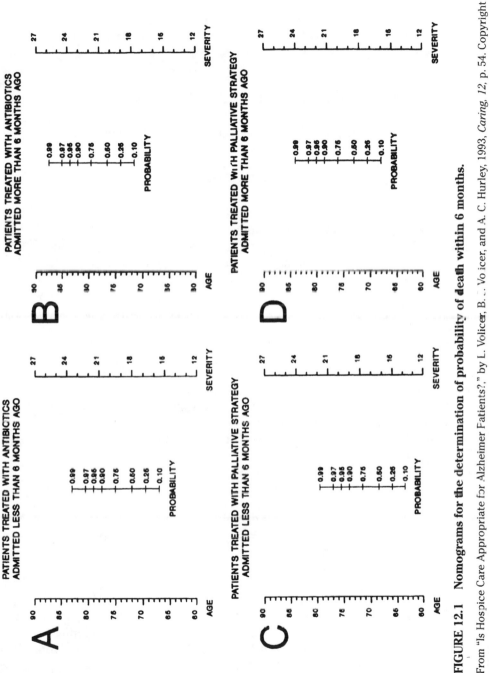

FIGURE 12.1 Nomograms for the determination of probability of death within 6 months.

From "Is Hospice Care Appropriate for Alzheimer Patients?," by L. Volicer, B. J. Volicer, and A. C. Hurley, 1993, *Caring, 12*, p. 54. Copyright 1994 by the National Association for Home Care. Reproduced with permission.

237

that it was developed using a patient population at a Veterans Administration Medical Center that was mostly male and younger than the general nursing home population. Further work is required to improve the prediction of 6-month survival in patients with advanced dementia.

CHALLENGES FOR THE HOSPICE PROGRAMS

Once the patient is identified for hospice services, several challenges occur for the hospice. The first is getting the physician to make a prognosis of 6 months or less of life, given the uncertainty of this prediction. This is a significant problem, because Medicare has initiated focused reviews of patients living longer than the 210 days of the benefit with an emphasis on monitoring nontraditional patients. Hospice programs are uneasy to enroll patients who are not clearly in the terminal stage of DAT because the program can retroactively be denied reimbursement for these patients. Some hospice programs offer a palliative or supportive care program to patients who are terminal yet not "actively dying." A hospice program provides consultative services and volunteers. The hospice absorbs the costs and does not bill Medicare until the patient is clearly dying. At this point, the patient elects the Medicare Hospice Benefit. All hospice services are then provided and Medicare is billed.

A hospice may decide to begin working with the patient when it appears he or she has 6 months or less to live and the decline in the patient's health status continues. The family then elects the hospice benefit for the patient, as the patient with end-stage DAT cannot make this decision. This permits the hospice to begin working with the family and patient and to develop a relationship with them. If the patient improves, the hospice can take him or her off the benefit and continue providing some services under the palliative care program. The patient can be picked up under the next benefit period when his or her condition worsens. Hospice programs have historically provided care to those who do not qualify for hospice benefits. Because of the difficulty of making the survival prognosis of 6 months or less, patients with DAT are good candidates for palliative or supportive care programs.

Once the patient is enrolled in the hospice program, the hospice staff has the challenge of developing a plan of care with a patient who is unable to participate in end-of-life decisions. Staff members should make all efforts to develop the plan of care with the nursing facility's interdisciplinary team, the patient, and the family. A patient in the end stage of DAT is usually unable to communicate, and the family often does not begin to think about the number of decisions that will need to be made in the terminal stage until their loved one is unable to make these decisions. The hospice must rely on the attending physician, family members, and facility staff to decide how the last months and weeks will be lived. Now that patients are being diagnosed earlier, it is hoped that decisions regarding end-of-life treatments will be made when the patient can still participate in the discussions. Until then, the hospice provides support for the family and, if the patient is in a nursing facility, includes staff in the development of the hospice plan of care.

Another challenge for a hospice is the DAT patient who is dying from another disease and is in the earlier stages of dementia, when behaviors typical of DAT require special approaches and communication skills (Volicer, Hurley, & Mahoney, 1995). Most hospice staff members have not received training on how to serve this population. Fortunately, the local chapter of the Alzheimer's Association can offer books, videos, and hands-on training classes. The DSCUs may also offer hospice staff opportunities to be included in training classes. Learning to care for a patient with a different reality takes time and commitment from the hospice staff. Only then will staff members be able to care for a patient with early-stage dementia in a way that decreases risk for the staff and is less stressful for the patient.

ROLE OF PHYSICIANS

Educating family physicians is an important step in "finding" patients. Doctors are the traditional health "gatekeepers" and can be of enormous help in referring patients to a hospice program. DAT patients and their spouses are of a generation that generally view doctors as authoritative and knowledgeable. These families will usually follow a physician's advice. When asked if they know about hospice programs, most physicians will respond that they know what hospice care involves for cancer patients. Physicians either do not know that a hospice program covers nontraditional diseases or they cannot fathom what a hospice would do to improve the life of an end-stage DAT patient, especially one in a nursing facility. They almost totally overlook what a hospice program can do for the caregiver and the facility staff.

Therefore, informing physicians and facility staff of the "right" of a DAT patient to access the Medicare Hospice Benefit is a positive step to reaching this patient. It may be the only time in the entire disease process that Medicare, a program the patient has supported with taxes over the years, will help. Physicians must learn how the hospice benefit pays for medications and supplies and offers nursing support, along with clergy and social work services, for the family that will continue for a year after the patient's death (Health Care Financing Administration, 1992).

Physicians may fear the hospice will take over, that they will lose control of their patients' care. When they realize that they must approve the hospice plan of care, that no treatment is changed without their approval, and that all their visits are covered by Medicare, physicians are more willing to refer patients to a hospice.

ROLE OF FAMILIES

Family members, especially the spouse of the DAT patient, have for the most part provided care without help. Seventy percent of families never use community services. They are understandably reluctant to allow anyone into their lives when they have carried on for so long alone. Living with someone who has DAT is a lonely experience, especially for the well spouse. Friends are embarrassed by the behavior of their friend. They do not know how to handle the unusual behaviors, so they gradually stop inviting the couple to "get togethers". The well spouse becomes totally focused on getting through the day, with little thought about what he or she needs. When and if the spouse recognizes the signs of impending death, he or she may not even know how to reach out for help.

Many patients with DAT live with the disease for 15 or 20 years, although the average life span is 8 years (Volicer et al., 1987). Eight years is a long time to get used to being isolated. The Medicare program that most seniors feel will take care of them as they age does not. Most patients with DAT are not even covered by Medicare if they are admitted to a nursing facility. The majority of residents admitted to a DSCU are admitted from home and do not have the 3 hospital days that would qualify them for Medicare coverage. Even if they have been hospitalized with a broken hip, which is not uncommon for a DAT patient, rehabilitation potential is so low that they do not qualify for the number of covered days an oriented patient receives.

Even when physicians approve and refer the patient, the family members themselves may decide not to access the hospice benefit. It may be difficult for them to have the nursing facility staff take over the care, since hospice care providers are a tangible sign that death is near. Family members may not be ready to face the impending death. Caregivers have lived with the disease for so long, they do not believe that their loved one is really going to die.

INVOLVEMENT OF NURSING HOME FACILITIES

The nursing facility needs to understand how a hospice program can enhance the services being offered. Many times the family of a DAT patient becomes almost impoverished as a result of the disease. The hospice benefit reaches out to offer practical help at no cost to the patient. The nursing facility staff must not only know how to advocate for the resident to access the hospice benefit, but must be able to develop a partnership with the hospice so that there is a unified delivery of care.

Nursing facilities for many years have fought the image that they were places patients went to die. Recently, because of the emphasis on containing costs, the managed care industry has been developing partnerships with nursing facilities. Nursing facilities are less costly than rehabilitation hospitals and are developing specialized units or business units that concentrate on rehabilitation. They provide separate entrances for younger managed care patients so that the patients will not have to see or interact with chronically ill elderly residents. Nursing home facilities may not be eager to become involved with residents who have no chance of rehabilitation and those who are dying—unless they see a business advantage to providing hospice services.

In the early development of the hospice movement, Medicare underwrote grants to determine the cost effectiveness of hospice care (Manard & Perrone, 1994). Hospice in fact was managed care before managed care had a name. Studies show that the majority of expense for the Medicare recipient is spent in the last 3 months of life (Lewin-VHI Inc., 1995). Managed care companies are including hospice coverage in their menu of services, and the nursing home equipped to offer skilled care may also be able to provide the inpatient benefit. Reimbursement for this benefit may be about $300 per day. Managed care companies are also looking for nursing facilities that can provide a full range of services, from subacute medical care and rehabilitation to hospice care. A nursing facility may contract with a local hospice to provide the care or may opt to provide the services using their own staff. It makes good business sense for nursing facilities to offer hospice services.

Another concern nursing facilities have with hospice program is that it might have a negative impact on their total Medicare days. Medicare reimbursement is significantly higher than Medicaid, and the reimbursement for Medicaid is in jeopardy. Many states are now talking about cutting reimbursement to nursing facilities. The Medicaid program that provides funding for a significant number of residents is seen as being fiscally out of control. States strapped for funds in a tight economy are trying to find ways to control costs, and cutting back on Medicaid services is high on the hit list. Most nursing facilities lose money on Medicaid residents. However, most facilities accept them for admission to keep their beds full and to stay out of trouble with discrimination issues. Residents who are admitted from acute care facilities, where they have been patients for at least 3 days, usually qualify for Medicare Part A skilled benefits. If however, they chose to elect the Medicare Hospice Benefit, they cannot receive Medicare skilled care. In November 1995, hospital discharge planners were mandated to begin informing patients of their right to access the Medicare Hospice Benefit (Health Care Financing Administration, 1996). This has the potential to seriously erode Medicare reimbursement for nursing facilities.

Hospice programs aware of this dilemma may agree to provide some free hospice services with the agreement that when residents have exhausted their Medicare days, the hospice would receive the referral. Services may include pain management consultation and some social service or hospice visits. Providing free services is less problematic for a hospice that has a number of reimbursable patients in a nursing facility. The hospice staff members do not have to make special visits, but they must see residents when they are seeing other patients. Referrals to a hospice are generated by nursing facility staff members who have an understanding of how the hospice not only can help the residents and their family but can support the staff.

Educating the nursing facility staff is relatively easy. Local hospices are eager to provide educational inservices as part of their community outreach programs. Equally important is the nursing facility's agreement to educate the hospice team. In order for the hospice to be sensitive to issues the nursing facility faces with regulations and reimbursement policies, they must begin a relationship by asking to understand. One of the seven habits of "highly effective people" outlined by Covey (1989) is "Seek to understand." When a climate of acceptance is apparent, the nursing facility is less defensive about providing care to "their" residents.

The nursing staff may feel that they are already providing hospice care, as they have been caring for dying residents for as long as nursing facilities have been in business. Additionally, many nurses are uncomfortable with the high dosages of pain medication that hospice programs authorize and are unwilling to "allow" a resident to decide to cease taking food or liquids. Another significant concern is financial. With the prospect of financial fines as a result of poor survey outcomes, nurses may fear that surveyors will cite them on weight loss or overuse of medication. In other instances, staff members feel that a hospice will try to take over resident care yet continue to leave them responsible for the 24-hour care.

DSCU staff members seem to have an especially difficult time letting go of their residents. They often feel a part of a resident's extended family or, in cases when the family is not involved with a resident, they fill the role of the family. Average patient stay on a DSCU is 3 years, and staff turnover is typically low (McCracken & Gilster, 1992). Involving a hospice in patient care is to admit that that is dying. That may be difficult for nurses who have been intimately involved with a patient for years.

When hospice administrators take the time to develop a respectful relationship with a nursing facility, involve facility staff in the development of the hospice plan of care, and offer practical assistance, nursing facility staff can be their strongest ally. The hospice staff representatives must offer to be present at surveys to answer any questions surveyors may ask, as hospice care in nursing facilities is still relatively new and surveyors must also be educated. As long as the hospice plan of care and the facility's plan of care are unified and the appropriate documentation is in order, there should be no concerns. As a matter of fact, a hospice supports quality of life and residents' rights to make decisions on how they wish to live their lives—two important features of care monitored by surveyors.

It is helpful to have a "hospice" section in the medical record, with a copy of the hospice plan of care, the signed election statement, and progress notes for hospice documentation. If hospice nurses document in the hospice section, they should also document in the nurses' notes and make a reference to their hospice note. Communication is the key to coordinated care. The hospice staff must relay any concerns to the nursing staff so that they can follow up when hospice staff member leaves. The facility must also understand that a resident must not be hospitalized without the approval of the hospice staff. One goal of hospice care is to support patients so that they can die at home. In this case, "home" is the nursing facility. A brightly colored sticker on the front of the chart identifying the resident as a hospice patient and giving the phone number to call with any change of condition is a helpful method of avoiding any unnecessary hospitalization. When the hospice provides staff education programs, administrators must make a special effort to meet with the facility's night staff, as they are frequently present when a crisis arises.

Another useful step in developing a strong partnership between the hospice and a nursing facility is for the hospice to meet with the facility's medical director. Enlisting the support of the director will help gain referrals from attending physicians. The medical director needs to understand how the hospice care is implemented in the nursing facility and know that additional bereavement services are available to a patient's family and the facility's staff up to a year after the resident's death.

Following families after the deaths of their loved ones is a unique component of a hospice program. Social workers in nursing facilities do not have time to provide follow-up care, and families who have provided care at home have many adjustment problems. In particular, families who have lived with DAT for so many years may need help in making a new life for themselves. This seems to be especially true for spouses. In many cases, well spouses have been cut off from friends and have been isolated in their caregiving role. They do not even know how to live alone again. Hospice bereavement counselors can support the grief process and help find meaning to life when there are no more caregiving responsibilities.

Providing hospice services to the patient with DAT who lives at home or in a nursing facility is a challenge for many involved individuals and institutions. The barriers that may surface as the cultures of the hospice and that of the nursing facility meet, are not insurmountable. Involvement in a hospice program is called the hospice benefit and it is just that: a benefit for the patients, their families, and the facility's staff. As hospices begin to embark on a new journey with a very special population, they will come to know millions of people who desperately need them.

REFERENCES

Brodaty, H., McGilchrist, C., Harris, L., & Peters, K. E. (1993). Time until institutionalization and death in patients with dementia: Role of caregiver training and risk factors. *Archives of Neurology, 50,* 643–650.

Burns, A., Lewis, G., Jacoby, R., & Levy, R. (1991). Factors affecting survival in Alzheimer's disease. *Psychological Medicine, 21,* 363–370.

Community Hospice Inc. (1994). *Community Hospice: Admission criteria.* Phoenix: Author.

Covey, S. R. (1989). *The seven habits of highly effective people.* New York: Simon & Schuster.

Evans, D. A., Smith, L. A., Scherr, P. A., Albert, M. S., Funkenstein, H. H. & Hebert, L. E. (1991). Risk of death from Alzheimer's disease in a community population of older persons. *American Journal of Epidemiology, 134,* 403–412.

Hanrahan, P., & Luchins, D. J. (1995). Access to hospice programs in end-stage dementia: A national survey of hospice programs. *Journal of the American Geriatrics Society, 43,* 56–59.

Health Care Financing Administration. (1992). Code of federal *regulations: Part 418. Hospice care* (pp. 567–579). Washington, DC: National Archives and Records Administration.

Health Care Financing Administration. (1996). *Medical technical amendment on notification of availability of hospice benefit* (p. 42). Washington, DC: Author.

Heyman, A., Wilkinson, W. E., Hurwitz, B. J., Helms, M. J., Haynes, C. S., Utley, C. M., & Gwyther, L. P. (1987). Early-onset Alzheimer's disease: Clinical predictors of institutionalization and death. *Neurology, 37,* 980–984.

Hier, D. B., Warach, J. D., Gorelick, P. B., & Thomas, J. (1989). Predictors of survival in clinically diagnosed Alzheimer's disease and multi-infarct dementia. *Archives of Neurology, 46,* 1213–1216.

Kaszniak, A. W., Fox, J., Gandell, D. L., Garron, D. C., Huckman, M. S., & Ramsey, R. G. (1978). Predictors of mortality in presenile and senile dementia. *Annals of Neurology, 3,* 246–252.

Katzman, R., Hill, L. R., Yu, E. S. H., Wang, Z.-Y., Booth, A., Salmon, D. P., Liu, W. T., Qu, G. Y., & Zhang, M. (1994). The malignancy of dementia: Predictors of mortality in clinically diagnosed dementia in a population survey of Shanghai, China. *Archives of Neurology, 51,* 1220–1225.

Knopman, D., Kitto, J., Deinard, S., & Heiring, J. (1988). Longitudinal study of death and institutionalization in patients with primary degenerative dementia. *Journal of the American Geriatrics Society, 36,* 108–112.

Leon, J. (1994). The 1990/1991 national survey of special care units in nursing homes. *Alzheimer Disease and Associated Disorders, 8*(Suppl. 1), S72–S86.

Lewin-VHI Inc. (1995). *An analysis of the cost savings of the Medicare hospice benefit.* Washington, DC: National Hospice Organization.

Luchins, D. J., & Hanrahan, P. (1993). What is appropriate health care for end-stage dementia? *Journal of the American Geriatrics Society, 41,* 25–30.

Manard, B., & Perrone, C. (1994). *Hospice care: An introduction and review of the evidence.* Washington, DC: National Hospice Organization.

McCracken, A. L., & Gilster, S. D. (1992). Desires and perceptions of staff concerning work performance in a dedicated Alzheimer's facility. *American Journal of Alzheimer's Care, 7,* 16–22.

Stuart, B., Herbst, L., Kinbrunner, B., Preodor, M., Connor, S., Ryndes, T., Cody, C., & Brandt, K. (1995). *Medical guidelines for determining prognosis in selected non-cancer diseases.* Arlington, VA: National Hospice Organization.

U.S. Congress, Office of Technology Assessment (1992). *Special care units for people with Alzheimer's and other dementias: Consumer education, research, regulatory, and reimbursement issues* (OTA-H-543). Washington, DC: U.S. Government Printing Office.

Van Dijk, P. T. M., Dippel, D. W. J., & Habbema, J. D. F. (1994). A behavioral rating scale as a predictor for survival of demented nursing home patients. *Archives of Gerontological Geriatrics, 18,* 101–113.

Van Dijk, P. T. M., Van de Sande, H. J., Dippel, D. W .J., & Habbema, J. D. F. (1992). The nature of excess mortality in nursing home patients with dementia. *Journal of Gerontology, 47,* M28–M34.

Volicer, B. J., Hurley, A., Fabiszewski, K. J., Montgomery, P., & Volicer, L. (1993). Predicting short-term survival for patients with advanced Alzheimer's disease. *Journal of the American Geriatrics Society, 41,* 535–540.

Volicer, L., Hurley, A. C., Lathi, D. C., & Kowall, N. W. (1994). Measurement of severity in advanced Alzheimer's disease. *Journal of Gerontology, 49,* M223–M226.

Volicer, L., Hurley, A. C., & Mahoney, E. (1995). Management of behavioral symptoms of dementia. *Nursing Home Medicine, 3*, 300–306.

Volicer, L., Seltzer, B., Rheaume, Y., Fabiszewski, K., Herz, L., Shapiro, R., & Innis, P. (1987). Progression of Alzheimer-type dementia in institutionalized patients: A cross-sectional study. *Journal of Applied Gerontology, 6*, 83–94.

Volicer, L., & Simard, J. (1996). Establishing a dementia special-care unit. *Nursing Home Economics, 3*(1), 12–19.

Volicer, L., & Staff of the Dementia Study Unit. (1992). "Ideal" DSCU not so ideal. *Gerontologist, 32*, 129.

Volicer, L., Volicer, B. J., & Hurley, A. C. (1993). (November). Is hospice care appropriate for Alzheimer patients? *Caring Magazine, 12*, 50–55.

Walsh, J. S., Welch, H. G., & Larson, E. B. (1990). Survival of outpatients with Alzheimer-type dementia. *Annals of Internal Medicine, 113*, 429–434.

Providing Palliative Care for the Terminal Alzheimer Patient

Sally J. Smith

The philosophy of care at the Dementia Special Care Unit of the Edith Nourse Rogers Memorial Veterans Hospital (ENRMVH), Bedford, MA, is based on the hospice or palliative care approach (Volicer, Rheaume, Brown, Fabiszewski, & Brady, 1986). This humane method of care strives to provide the patient with maximum comfort by increasing nursing, recreational, and other pleasurable interventions while minimizing aggressive medical interventions that may cause discomfort. The degree to which medical interventions are minimized is based on the decisions reached at a family meeting in which the philosophy of care of the program is described to the health care proxy or family members of the Alzheimer patient. These decisions, which assign patients to one of five levels of care (Volicer et al., 1986), are made shortly after admission to long-term care when the patient is generally well and death is not imminent (Volicer & Fabiszewski, 1988). In a 1993 survey, Luchins and Hanrahan found that the majority of gerontology professionals and family members of dementia patients would choose the least aggressive level of care for end-stage dementia patients. (See chapter 12 for a discussion of the inclusion of persons with Alzheimer's disease in hospice care.) This chapter discusses how decisions that guide the provision of nonaggressive care are put into practice when the patient becomes terminally ill.

Both the patient's family and caregivers need reassurance that the dementia patient can be kept comfortable without resorting to advanced technological interventions. Both must be confident that this shift from aggressive medical interventions to palliative care does not mean that the patient will receive less care. In fact, each patient receives intensive nursing measures to provide comfort during the inevitable dying process. The paradigm of high touch has replaced high-tech care and is believed to be paramount in the interdisciplinary care of dementia patients at ENRMVH.

To understand how to provide comfort to the person with end-stage Alzheimer's disease, it is necessary to understand the process that the patient undergoes during his or her last days of life. There is little in the literature that describes the dying process of the Alzheimer patient. Most of the hospice literature focuses on the patient dying of cancer. The dying process has been described as a transitional course for both patient and family in which the patient "fades away" (Reimer, Davies, & Martens, 1991). Most authors agree that the dying process is an individualized experience, shaped by the person's history, which includes the type of illness that is causing the death and prior patterns of behavior. As with life, no two deaths are the same, even given the same diagnosis. However, a pattern did emerge when the dying process was examined, as recorded in the nursing notes in patient's medical records at ENRMVH. After the death of 24 end-stage Alzheimer patients at ENRMVH, a medical review revealed the onset and duration of symptoms that preceded death. These observations are reported in this chapter along with other related research.

In their study of terminally ill elders, McCracken and Gerdsen (1991) concluded that the terminal phase of life begins when the dying individual starts to turn from the outside world and withdraws into the internal self, thus conserving energy. The dying process observed by McCracken and Gerdsen lasted for a mean duration of 21 days. In the retrospective chart review of end-stage Alzheimer patients at ENRMVH, there was a time span of 5 to 38 days in which the nurse's notes indicated that the patient was in a dying process. This time span was measured from the first nursing documentation of one of the signs of the dying process, usually food refusal, to the time of the patient's death.

DECREASED APPETITE

During the dying process, the body goes through a physical shutting down procedure with characteristic signs and symptoms. In all of the terminal patients at ENRMVH, the first sign of this shutting down was a decreased appetite or food refusal. Many experienced hospice professionals believe that this disinterest in food and fluids in the last days of life is part of an adaptive process that allows a terminally ill individual to die with less suffering (Andrews, Bell, Smith, Tischler, & Veglia, 1993; Billings, 1985; Brown & Chekryn, 1989; Enck, 1994; Musgrave 1990; Zerwekh, 1983). However, the emotional and social importance that society places on providing food and fluids to those who cannot obtain it for themselves is almost overwhelming. Love and concern for others are commonly expressed with food. It is hard to imagine a gathering of loved ones without the provision of food. When individuals or groups wish to assist those less fortunate, they often send food. We only need to recall holidays such as Thanksgiving, Christmas and Hanukkah to understand how well ingrained the belief is that to love or nurture is to provide food. Therefore, all persons involved in the care of the dying patient must be educated about the benefits and burdens of artificial hydration and nutrition in the dying process.

Brown and Chekryn (1989), both experienced palliative care nurses, published a table outlining the possible risks and benefits of artificial hydration for the dying patient. The probable benefits of withholding artificial hydration are a decrease in vomiting, dyspnea, choking, peripheral edema, and the length of time of the dying process. Terminal dehydration may cause an electrolyte imbalance, which produces what the authors refer to as a "natural anesthesia." In contrast, intravenous hydration may preclude care in a familiar surrounding such as home or a palliative care unit. The benefits of artificial hydration—decreased dry mouth and thinner respiratory secretions—may not be balanced by removing the patient from familiar surroundings and staff. Brown and Chekryn (1989) concluded that withdrawal from food and fluids was part of the body's preparation for death and was beneficial to the patient. Other research supports and emphasizes the concept that allowing the dying patient to determine the amount and type of intake is a comfort measure (Ahronheim 1996; Andrews et al., 1993; Enck, 1994; McCann, Hall, & Groth-Juncker, 1994).

The anorexia of the dying patient goes beyond a lack of interest in food and fluids to include actual physical difficulties with eating and swallowing. Patients studied at ENRMVH became disinterested in food 5 to 38 days before death. From 4 to 17 days before death, 80% choked on food or liquids, and all were completely unable to swallow 1 to 4 days before death. Because this program does not advocate artificial nutrition or hydration, natural means of providing whatever nutrition that the patient may desire and be able to take were explored. Small amounts of highly nutritious, well-tolerated liquids were offered frequently. In this stage of the dementia, staff and family should be made aware that there is a fine line between coaxing and coercion. Cool, not icy, thick liquids are often tolerated best. Partially melted ice cream, smooth fruit yogurt, cool Ensure, or Sustecal are often accepted and enjoyed in small amounts until the patient is no longer able to swallow. At that time, the patient may be kept comfortable by offering a single ice chip at a time to melt under the tongue or in the cheek.

LETHARGY

Lethargy was another early sign of shutting down and the beginning of the dying process. It occurred 5 to 17 days before death in two thirds of the ENRMVH patients. The remaining one third of the patients were already bedbound and minimally responsive prior to entering the dying process. Comfort was promoted for the lethargic patient by allowing him or her to remain at bedrest, thus conserving all remaining energy. All activity of daily living tasks were taken over by the caregivers, including positioning and feeding. As with decreasing intake, family members may become dismayed when the patient no longer is strong enough to tolerate getting out of bed daily. It is helpful to inform them that any energy that the patient has left may be available for communication with others if it is conserved with bedrest.

CARDIOVASCULAR CHANGES

In dying dementia patients, the heart rate may become rapid, and early into the dying process it may even double, but with hypoxia, the heart rate and blood pressure often decrease and irregular rhythms may occur. If infection is present, the heart rate may remain high. As peripheral circulation decreases, the body may become diaphoretic. The surface of the skin feels cool even when the patient is mildly febrile. Depressed metabolism reduces the amount of heat liberated from the body, but internal temperatures may remain normal or high. Skin over the bony prominences may first become mottled or cyanotic, which is often followed by the skin of the whole body. The nail beds and oral mucosa often become deeply cyanotic shortly before death occurs. In the population studied at ENRMVH, fever, probably due to dehydration or infection, occurred in 100% of the patients, 1 to 15 days before death. Pallor, cyanosis, and/or mottling occurred 1 to 4 days before death in two thirds of the patients studied. These cardiovascular signs of impending death do not appear troublesome to the patients. Hypotension and cardiac arrhythmias are not symptomatic when the patient is at bedrest. Cool, cyanotic, or mottled extremities can be wrapped in soft, warmed blankets for comfort. Fever may or may not be uncomfortable for the individual patient, and the level of discomfort must be carefully assessed because breaking a fever may produce discomfort with additional diaphoresis, necessitating a bed linen change. External methods of reducing a fever, such as ice packs on the pulse points or ice blankets, are never comfortable and should not be used. If necessary, acetaminophen taken orally or rectally reduces fever effectively and promotes comfort.

The decrease in cardiac output affects the kidneys significantly, causing a decrease in urinary output. Eighty percent of the population studied had a severely decreased urinary output 1 to 4 days before death. Careful attention to skin care, with special focus on keeping each patient clean and dry, kept the patients comfortable. No catheters were used and there were no cases of urinary retention. Because urinary output is severely diminished, some dependent edema may occur, but none was noted in the records reviewed.

RESPIRATORY CHANGES

The respiratory system shuts down in a manner closely linked to the cardiovascular system. Inadequate cardiac output may lead to pulmonary congestion. Pulmonary secretions may also be present if the patient has pneumonia, a very common proximal cause of death in late-stage dementia patients. Signs of the respiratory system shutting down may include breath sounds that are diminished, irregular, rapid, or audible even without a stethoscope. As the respiratory system shuts down, carbon dioxide levels increase, but the brain becomes less sensitive to this elevation and periods of irregular respiration and/or apnea occur with increasing frequency. In the records reviewed, an increased respiratory rate was documented in 80% of the patients 1 to 19 days before death. Fifty percent were congested enough to require suctioning at least once or twice in the last 1 to 15 days of life. Labored breathing and/or dyspnea was reported in less than 20% of these patients. Most articles that discuss the dying process with and without artificial hydration describe this diminished need for suctioning as a great benefit resulting from terminal dehydration (Brown & Chekryn, 1989; Enck, 1994; Levy & Catalano, 1985; Musgrave, 1990; Zerwekh, 1983). Oxygen at a low-flow rate (2 to 3 liters a minute is usually adequate), delivered in the least disruptive manner available (usually a nasal cannula), and morphine in low doses can suppress the sensation of air hunger and provide comfort. Short-acting benzodiazepines in low doses orally or sublingually can decrease the anxiety associated with dyspnea. If excessive secretions are present, positioning the patient on his or her side promotes drainage of the secretions orally (Long, 1996). Gentle chest percussion can loosen thick mucous secretions and help the patient raise and expectorate them. Suctioning should be avoided unless absolutely necessary because it causes great patient distress and the irritation of a suction catheter produces increased mucous production. If necessary, gentle oral or oropharyngeal suctioning with a tonsil tip or Yankour device can be helpful. Atropine in small doses or a scopolamine patch can be used to decrease excessive secretions.

MUSCULOSKELETAL SYSTEM CHANGES

A decreased supply of nutrients produces changes in the musculoskeletal system. Extreme weakness is common in all muscle groups. Muscles of the tongue and palate weaken and sag as the patient becomes too weak to clear the large airways. Secretions in these large airways move and vibrate with every respiration, causing a sound commonly referred to as a "death rattle." This respiratory noise is very distressing to the family and some staff members, but patients do not seem troubled by it. This weakness is best handled with bedrest. Side positioning or some mild postural drainage may be helpful in relieving the rattling respirations. Scopolamine or atropine will decrease the secretions and relax the smooth muscles of the tracheobronchial tree, decreasing this distressing noise. Restlessness, picking, or repetitive motions may be present due to a decrease of oxygen in the brain and a change in metabolism. This restlessness was found in 50% of the patients studied 4 to 6 days before death. If restlessness is extreme and the patient is strong enough, short periods of time in a reclining chair may promote comfort.

GASTROINTESTINAL SYSTEM CHANGES

The shutting down of the gastrointestinal tract leads to decreased or absent bowel sounds. The rectal sphincter relaxes and fecal incontinence may occur. If the patient has had little or no oral nourishment prior to this shutting down, the gastrointestinal tract is relatively empty and few digestive juices are present. There is minimal gastric distention and/or distress. However, if the patient has been hydrated, vomiting or distention may occur. In the study sample, only about 20% of the patients had any nausea or vomiting reported within 5 to 6 days before death. Antiemetics, such as prochlorperazine (Compazine) or trimethobenzamide hydrochloride (Tigan), delivered via rectal suppository, are very effective if given regularly to avoid repetitive nausea and vomiting. The phenothiazines (e.g., chlorpromazine hydrochloride) and antihistamines (e.g., diphenhydramine hydrochloride) are effective if the nausea has a vestibular component or occurs with hiccoughs (Levy & Catalano, 1985). Scopolamine or atropine can be effective with intractable retching. There was no intractable retching found in the studied patients. Nasogastric tubes, which could be used to relieve stomach distention, are very uncomfortable and should be avoided if at all possible.

Dry mucous membranes, especially of the mouth, may occur with terminal dehydration. This is the most common discomfort reported by dehydrated terminal cancer patients (Brown & Chekryn, 1989; Musgrave, 1990; Zerwekh, 1983). Dry mouth is readily alleviated with careful attention to mouth care. Ice chips and sips of whichever liquid the patient tolerates on a frequent basis help to keep the mouth moist. If thick mucous is present on the oral mucosa, a 50% or less concentration solution of hydrogen peroxide can be used on a gauze pad or face cloth to wipe away debris. Moistir spray (Kingswood Laboratories, Indianapolis, IN), an artificial saliva, sprayed onto the dry tissues is very soothing and simple to use. The lips can be kept moist with a thin layer of petroleum jelly. Dryness of the mucous membranes was found in 50% of the records reviewed during the 2 to 9 days before death. Another 17% of patients were reported to have dry skin turgor, but none had skin breakdown.

Constipation is present in almost all terminally ill patients due to the slowing down of bowel motility, the use of narcotics, and dietary changes. Bulk laxatives, such as psyllium, are useless and can be harmful in this population because they depend on an adequate intake of liquid. Stool softeners are not effective. If necessary, a local stimulant such as a glycerin or bisacodyl (Dulcolax) suppository may be necessary for evacuation of the large bowel. If necessary, and if the patient is able to safely swallow, a mild large bowel stimulant such as lactulose (Enulose) can be effective in preventing impaction. Diarrhea is seldom a problem in the terminal dementia patient. If loose stools are present, they are usually secondary to a fecal impaction with liquid stool moving around it. The best treatment for impaction and overflow loose stool is manual disimpaction and prevention of further impactions with a stimulant suppository every 2 to 3 days.

MENTAL STATUS CHANGES

The nervous system is dulled by the buildup of carbon dioxide and other waste products. The senses may be dulled and pupillary responses may be slowed. Sleeping may be increased, and eventually the patient becomes unresponsive. In the ENRMVH study, changes in patients' mental status resulted in increased confusion and disorientation. Two thirds of the patients became unresponsive 1 to 2 days before death. Because of the advanced dementia of the study population, changes in cognitive status were not found. Seizures may occur shortly before death, but there were none in the population studied. Phenytoin (Dilantin) by mouth or lorazepam (Ativan) sublingually or intramuscularly may be necessary if the seizures are recurrent or intractable. No medication is necessary for a single, isolated seizure.

McCracken and Gerdsen (1991) reported seven emotional/spiritual/mental signs of approaching death: withdrawal, vision-like experiences, restlessness, decreased socialization, unusual communication, giving permission, and saying good-bye. The progressive cognitive decline of patients with Alzheimer's disease makes the identification of those signs in this population very difficult. Withdrawal occurs as the dying patient detaches and lets go of relationships and surroundings. Socialization is reduced, causing distress in many family members. Loved ones should be encouraged to sit quietly with the dying person or converse in soft, soothing tones, without imploring the patient to communicate. The anxiety of the family can be communicated to the patient, causing the patient to have distress, which may be difficult to alleviate. Visions or hallucinations may occur, and the patient may appear to be talking to his or her parents or other loved ones who are deceased. In her presentation to the 1995 National Alzheimer's Association Conference in Chicago, Joanne Rader (1995) reported a patient, who was usually anxious and noncommunicative, stating clearly that "the angels are coming" shortly before her death. These visions are generally happy or comforting and not disturbing like many of the hallucinations experienced by dementia patients. Family and staff must understand and support a patient who is having such visions.

Many patients seem to need the permission of their loved ones to die comfortably. Again, it is difficult to believe that this is possible in the advanced dementia patient with severe cognitive deficits. However, recently, one patient in the ENRMVH with advanced Alzheimer's disease had been fading very slowly. His wife, who was also in poor health and lived too far away to visit regularly, sent him frequent cards and letters, which were read to him by the staff. The last letter he received informed him that she was too ill to ever visit again and that she understood the frailty of his health. She closed by stating that it was all right to stop struggling to survive and that she hoped to be with him soon "in heaven." This patient died quickly and peacefully shortly thereafter. It is our conclusion that optimal patient comfort occurs when families and staff accept unusual communications from the patient and feel able to say good-bye with honesty and love.

As described above, most of the characteristics of the dying process are neither painful nor unbearably burdensome for the patient. In the population studied, only 50% percent of the patients had any period of moaning or appearing uncomfortable. They were all effectively made comfortable with small doses of narcotics, usually morphine, on a regular or as-needed basis. Experienced staff can effectively a assess patient's comfort even in advanced dementia by understanding verbal and nonverbal cues from the demented patient (Hurley, Volicer, Hanrahan, Houde, & Volicer, 1992; Marzinski, 1991). Understanding the natural dying process of late-stage dementia patients helps the staff to respond to the needs of these individuals in this transition from life to death.

REFERENCES

Ahronhelm, J. (1996). Nutrition and hydration in the terminal patient. *Clinics in Geriatric Medicine, 12*(2), 379–391.

Andrews, M., Bell, E., Smith, S., Tischler, J., & Veglia, J. (1993). Dehydration in terminally ill patients. Is it appropriate palliative care? *Postgraduate Medicine,* 93(1).

Billing, J. (1985). Comfort measures for the terminally ill. Is dehydration painful? *Journal of the American Geriatrics Society, 33*(11), 808–810.

Brown, P., & Chekryn, J. (1989, May). The dying patient and dehydration. *Canadian Nurse,* pp. 14–16.

Enck, R. (1994). *The medical care of terminally ill patients.* Baltimore: Johns Hopkins University Press.

Hurley, A., Volicer, B., Hanrahan, P., Houde, S., & Volicer, L. (1992). Assessment of discomfort in advanced Alzheimer patients. *Research in Nursing and Health,* 15, 369–377.

Levy, M., & Catalano, R. (1985). Control of common physical symptoms other than pain in patients with terminal disease. *Seminars in Oncology, 12*(4), 411–430.

Long, M. C. (1996). Death and dying and recognizing approaching death. *Clinics in Geriatric Medicine, 12*(2), 359–368.

Luchins, D., & Hanrahan, P. (1993). What is appropriate health care for end-stage dementia? *Journal of the American Geriatrics Society, 41,* 25–30.

Marzinski, L. (1991). The tragedy of dementia: Clinically assessing pain in the confused, nonverbal elderly. *Journal of Gerontological Nursing, 17*(6), 25–28.

McCann, R., Hall, W., & Groth-Juncker, A. (1994). Comfort care for terminally ill patients: The appropriate use of nutrition and hydration. *Journal of the American Medical Association, 272*(17), 1263–1266.

McCracken, A., & Gerdsen, L. (1991). Sharing the legacy: Hospice care principles for terminally ill elders. *Journal of Gerontological Nursing, 17*(12), 4–8.

Musgrave, C. (1990). Terminal dehydration: To give or not to give intravenous fluids? *Cancer Nursing, 13*(1), 62–66.

Rader, J. (1995). *Reinventing the American nursing home.* Presented at the Fourth National Alzheimer's Disease Education Conference, Chicago, IL.

Reimer, J., Davies, B., & Martens, N. (1991). Palliative care: The nurse's role in helping families through the transition of "fading away." *Cancer Nursing, 14*(6), 321–327.

Volicer, L., & Fabiszewski, K. (1988, January/February). The use of medical technology in advanced Alzheimer's dementia. *American Journal of Alzheimer's Care and Related Disorders and Research,* pp. 11–17.

Volicer, L., Rheaume, Y., Brown, J., Fabiszewski, K., & Brady, R. (1986). Hospice approach to the treatment of patients with advanced dementia of the Alzheimer type. *Journal of the American Medical Association, 256,* 2210–2213.

Zerwekh, J. (1983, January). The dehydration question. *Nursing 83,* pp. 47–51.

The Experience of Jacob Perlow Hospice: Hospice Care of Patients with Alzheimer's Disease

Paul R. Brenner

BACKGROUND ON THE MODERN HOSPICE MOVEMENT

ORIGINS

The origins of the modern hospice movement are found in the vision and work of Dame Cicely Saunders, M.D., in England (Beresford, 1993). Reacting to the inadequate and inappropriate treatment she observed dying patients receiving in hospitals, she set about to create an alternative. At first this was understood to be an institutional alternative to the hospital, that is, an actual place where the dying would receive care designed to meet their needs and to which their loved ones could come and visit at any time, and stay if desired, without the typical hospital restrictions and decor.

Dr. Saunders, who is also a social worker and registered nurse, established some of the most distinctive characteristics of hospice care. The first of these is interdisciplinary, rather than multidisciplinary, care. Dr. Saunders pioneered the creation of teams that integrated the skills and perspectives of physicians, nurses, social workers, chaplains, volunteers, and other care providers for the creation of a unified plan of care. Interdisciplinary care is not hierarchical but collaborative and interdependent.

The second characteristic is the necessity of serving the family along with the patient, and to extend care for the family into the bereavement period. The patient and family are served together as a unit of care in a hospice program.

The third charcteristic is that chronic pain management requires an entirely different kind of response than acute pain management. The goal is to intervene in the pain cycle, to stop the pain, and then to prevent its return so that patients do not have to live on the dehumanizing merry-go-round of alternating episodes of pain and relief.

When the hospice model at St. Christopher's, London, crossed the Atlantic and was first planted on American soil in New Haven, Connecticut, the setting shifted from caring for patients in a hospital-like alternative care facility to the idea of keeping patients in their own homes, supporting their families, and helping families care for their own. In the United States, hospice care has primarily been part of a home care program, using inpatient care as a backup for needs that cannot be managed at home.

DATABASE OF HOSPICE

In 1974 when the New Haven Hospice began operations, there was no access to reimbursement for hospice services. The New Haven Hospice secured a founding grant for 3 years that limited it to serving patients with cancer. Therefore, cancer care shaped very fundamentally the way hospice services developed and were structured, along with the assumptions that were made about end-of-life care, treatment, and costs. The database of patients served by the early hospices of the 1970s was almost exclusively elderly, middle class, and White. The individuals who were working in communities to establish hospice programs were mostly middle class, White, middle-aged, and female. There was a congruence of values and assumptions between hospice caregivers and those receiving the care. This emphasized:

- Truth telling: Educated consumers were not just making choices about the kind of care they wanted and did not want; they also were asking for a level of truth telling that was not a characteristic of medical management of the time. Not wanting to be "protected" and turned into victims, the patients wanted to be empowered for participation in their care and the decisions that affected them.
- Choice: Educated consumers with a 1960s-shaped consciousness were choosing the kind of dying they wanted: not one with the heroics and suffering of futile care in an impersonal acute care setting, but one that was comfort-oriented, in their own homes, and with

loved ones participating. There was a clear concept of what constituted a "good death" and what did not.
- Nuclear families: The presence of a family member in the home,
  especially during the day, was necessary as the hospice program
  provided only intermittent skilled and supportive noncustodial care.
  Such caregiving in the home was mostly done by women: wives,
  daughters, daughters-in-law, and sisters. Without those caregivers
  the hospice was limited in what it had to offer and could accomplish. Many hospices even required the presence of an active family caregiver as part of their admission criteria. Without a caregiver,
  there could be no admission to a hospice.
- Volunteerism: Hospices found a warm response in the hearts of
  many people throughout communities in the United States. Many
  had been influenced by the books and lectures of Elisabeth Kübler-
  Ross (1969), and they stepped forward to get involved and make it
  possible for the hospice movement to grow and thrive. Including
  nonprofessionals in direct service was a call to action to which there
  was enormous response. Volunteers frequently made the difference
  between what hospices could accomplish in relationship to what
  could be paid for through limited reimbursements or donations.

THE HOSPICE MEDICARE BENEFIT

It was the 1970s' patient database and hospice experience that provided
the basis in the early 1980s for the addition of hospice care as a reim-
bursed service, first in Medicare[1] and later in Medicaid. This benefit not
only provided an avenue for financial stability for the services hospices
provided, but also created the first consistent national standard to define
hospice care. This included the responsibility to

- manage the entire terminal stage of an illness, identified as the last
  6 months of life expectancy;

---

[1]Effective November 1, 1983, hospice care became a benefit provided through
Medicare, Section 1861(u), of the Social Security Act. Conditions of participation
are set forth in 42 CFR Part 418.42. CFR 418.100 is an additional condition applicable only to hospices that provide short-term inpatient care and respite directly
rather than through contractual arrangements. Section 1866(a)(1)(Q) of the act
as added by 4206(a)(1)(C) of the Omnibus Budget Reconciliation Act of 1990, P.L.
No. 101-508, requires hospices to file an agreement with the Secretary of Health
and Human Services to comply with the requirements found in Section 1866 of
the act regarding advanced directives.

- provide core professional services, including physician, nursing, psychosocial, and spiritual counseling, support services, and volunteer services, as well as access to all other needed services, including pharmacy, Durable Medical Equipment, and medical supplies, special therapies, and transportation;
- provide a continuum of home care and inpatient care with an annualized utilization of no more than 20% of all services as inpatient and no less than 80% of all services as home care;
- provide 1 year of bereavement care for family members following the death.

When Congress established a medical hospice benefit in 1982, many new providers entered into the hospice market and there was a rapid proliferation of programs. According to the National Hospice Organization, as of 1995 there were over 1,800 hospices in the United States certified to provide the Medicare and Medicaid benefits.[2]

DIVERGENCES

At the same time this rapid development and expansion in hospice program occurred, AIDS appeared with a unique trajectory very different from cancer, in a patient census that was young and stigmatized, with no medical cure, and with few treatments. The assumptions that were the basis of Medicare–Medicaid benefits did not match the realities of the needs of individuals with AIDS.

Also at this time, Children's Hospice International,[3] an advocacy and educational organization, was chronicling the needs of children and adolescents with irreversible illnesses. With this patient population, too, the limits imposed by Medicare–Medicaid benefits inhibited an appropriate hospice response to end-stage care, especially as children tend to be treated very aggressively to the end.

Finally, other weaknesses in the ways hospice benefits were structured became evident as barriers of access to hospice care. Those who did not readily fit the hospice benefits criteria included:

- persons who live alone;
- persons with long term-chronic illnesses;

---

[2]Information provided by National Hospice Organization. 1901 North Moore St., Suite 901, Arlington, VA 22209.

[3]Children's Hospice International, 2202 Mt. Vernon Avenue, Suite 3C, Alexandria, VA 22301.

- persons who do not have a primary care physician;
- persons who live alienated from the dominant medical and social systems;
- persons and prisoners with special conditions, such as handicapping conditions, mental illnesses or addictions;
- persons for whom English is not the primary language;
- persons of non-European cultures;
- refugees, immigrants, and migrants;
- persons with different cultural assumptions and understandings of family, health, disease, choice, truth telling, treatment, grief, dying, death, and decision making.

Against this background, few hospices or others in the medical field believed at the time that persons with Alzheimer's disease and related disorders were appropriate for hospice care.

THE ENDING OF LIFE

Hospice care was established in the belief that the ending of a human life is a significant personal, family, and social event, and how that ending occurs and the meanings that are attached to it can be influenced profoundly through hospice care.

With perhaps no other population is that fundamental assumption more challenged than by the person with advanced Alzheimer's disease. After all, persons with Alzheimer's are not able to be an active participant in their own care. Because of their condition, they cannot make decision for themselves, nor can they articulate any meaning and value statements.

There is something within our dominant culture that does not seem to know how to ascribe humanity, dignity, worth, and value to these persons who seem at such a distance. Often times institutional care becomes something like "keeping" them until they die, not knowing what to do with them until that happens. There may even be a tendency in some settings for professional caregivers to treat them like animals with the long shadow of the old asylum mentality still at work.

ANATOMY OF A PROJECT

BACKGROUND OF JACOB PERLOW HOSPICE

It is within this matrix that Jacob Perlow Hospice undertook a special project to test these assumptions, to develop a program of services targeting this population, and to offer a model to guide other hospices in admitting patients with advanced Alzheimer's disease. Jacob Perlow Hospice is incorporated as a special program of Beth Israel Medical Center in New York City. After many years of maintaining a supportive care program, Beth Israel made the decision to establish a comprehensive hospice program, which became operational in 1988. A dedicated 8-bed inpatient unit was created and located in the Petri Campus of the Medical Center, to provide acute symptom management for problems that could not be met through home care. The hospice currently has an average daily census, both home and inpatient care, of about 100 patient-family units. The service area of the hospice includes Manhattan, Brooklyn, Queens, and the Bronx.

CHALLENGE OF ALZHEIMER'S DISEASE

In the spring of 1990 a proposal to establish a pilot project to offer hospice services to patients with end-stage Alzheimer's disease was presented to Jane Weber, the director of Jacob Perlow Hospice, by Dr. Susan Goldfein, a volunteer with the New York City Chapter of the Alzheimer's Disease and Related Disorders Association (ADRDA)[4]. Susan's mother, who had a dual diagnosis of cancer and Alzheimer's disease, had been one of the first patients served by the hospice. Susan had been the family caregiver. The value she had found through the support and assistance of the hospice team formed her vision for an expanded role for a hospice for Alzheimer's patients. The proposal included a list of possible markers that, when combined, identified the progression of dementia in patients to the end stage. These markers, which guided the hospice admission criteria, were developed for this proposal by Dr. Barry Reisberg.[5]

During the 1980s little attention was paid to Alzheimer's patients within the hospice movement. The prevailing conventional wisdom was that hospices had little or nothing at all to offer patients without cognition. Cognition was central to the hospice's ability to have patients collaborate in their care and prepare themselves emotionally, spiritually, and relationally for their deaths. It was also unclear what role there was for pain management and symptom control, because assessing pain could not be done with the patient's participation. Some questioned whether Alzheimer's patients had any experience of pain at all.

---

[4]Alzheimer's Disease and Related Disorders Association, New York City chapter, 420 Lexington Avenue, New York, NY 10170.

[5]Dr. Reisberg worked directly with Jacob Perlow Hospice in creating the criteria that were used as part of this project.

Fortunately, this conventional wisdom was not heeded. Weber understood the issue as one of access to care and was willing to take the hospice staff on a learning experience under the assumption that the hospice did have a role to play, even though that might be different from its role with persons with cancer, AIDS, advanced heart disease, or anyone with cognition.

The demographics of Alzheimer's disease in the New York City area are compelling, with over 75,000 living cases. The disease occurs in 6% of the general population over 65 years of age, and 20% of those 75 and over. The disease can take anywhere from 3 to 25 years to progress to the advanced stage, and confirmation of diagnosis requires autopsy. By the year 2050 it is estimated that over 14 million persons in the United States over age 65 will have Alzheimer's. On the average, somewhere between 60% and 70% of residents in nursing homes have some form of dementia.

Central to the historic mission of the hospice movement is to support families in their care of a loved one at home. Certainly, families who have a member with Alzheimer's are stressed by years of caregiving and could benefit greatly from support, especially as they face the ending of life and want their loved one not to be institutionalized, if that is not necessary.

Caring for someone during the final months of life is especially exhausting. When there is so much physical care that needs to be done to maintain skin integrity, prevent bedsores, maintain hygiene, and so on, assistance is often needed. Physical care to enhance comfort ties directly to the historic mission of the hospice movement.

INVOLVEMENT OF THE ROBERT WOOD JOHNSON FOUNDATION

With assistance from Jean Marks, the associate executive director of the New York City chapter of ADRDA, the proposal was submitted in 1992 to the Robert Wood Johnson Local Initiatives Funding Partners Program, and subsequently approved. In 1993 the project was initiated.

Three primary goals were established:

1. Increase access of persons with Alzheimer's disease and related disorders to hospice care through education and outreach.
2. Provide a full complement of hospice home care and inpatient care services appropriate to meet the needs of patients and families.
3. Create a model that demonstrates the role of hospice care for Alzheimer patients and their families.

An interdisciplinary team was formed to manage the project. Its members included:

Jane Weber, Project Director
Richard Geltman, M.D., Medical Director
Brenda Mamber, ACSW, Supervisor of Social Work Services
Cheryl Avellanet, R.N., Director of Clinical Services
Meri Spector, R.N., Clinical Nurse Specialist
Robert Schley, CSW, Clinical Social Worker
Rima Starr, Music Therapist
Madeline Milgroom, Research Analyst

The funders of the project included the Robert Wood Johnson Foundation, the Forchheimer Foundation, the Dextra Baldwin McConagle Foundation, and the Butler Foundation.

PROJECT HISTORY

An intense project of this nature was a first for Jacob Perlow Hospice. The Hospice operated as a clinical program of services, and a research project was a major undertaking. Nurses, social workers, chaplains, and other caregivers were accustomed to documenting services, but not the kinds of information that were needed for the project. It may seem naive to acknowledge this now, but in 1993 it was not clear that not everyone in the clinical staff was interested in the project for its "research" value, and at times that proved challenging to the project.

A second major development was that the leadership of the project changed three times due to changes in the leadership of the hospice itself. Nevertheless, the project team remained stable throughout the 3 years.

GOAL ONE:
EDUCATION AND OUTREACH TO INCREASE ACCESS

The first task of the hospice project team was to create a brochure to describe the hospice's program for Alzheimer's care. This brochure was widely distributed to reach potential sources of referral and as many persons as possible who are directly affected by the disease. Due to the isolation of some patients and their families, however, the brochure has been limited in its effectiveness.

Next, a short videotape presentation was created. The tape features a music therapy session with a patient and two family members. This presentation demonstrated the value of the role of the hospice in the care of end-stage dementia patients. Not only did the patient in this videotaped scenario become involved and engaged, but the family members were able to experience some meaningful interaction with their loved one again.

Hospice team members have offered many presentations about the program, including:

- Annual Mayoral Conference on Alzheimer's Disease, sponsored by the New York City Department on Aging;
- Columbia University School of Public Health;
- Eldercare;
- Self-Help Community Services;
- New York City Chapter of the ADRDA and Alzheimer Support Groups;
- Rocky Mountain Alzheimer's Association;
- New York State Hospice Association;
- National Hospice Organization.

Access to care has significantly increased across the project history, as can be seen in Table 14.1.

GOAL TWO:
PATIENT–FAMILY CARE

Although not all data from the project are yet available for detailed analysis, a profile of patients with Alzheimer's has emerged (see Table 14.2). In addition to the basis demographic information about the patient, there is also information about how many days of care were involved and the location of the death. This profile is interesting in comparison to the characteristics of the total census of the hospic, as given in Table 14.4. As can be seen from Table 14.4, the typical Alzheimer patient the hospice has served is a White female over age 75 who has Medicare coverage and who will die at home.

TABLE 14.1   Patients Enrolled in Project

Year	Patients admitted
1993	29
1994	32
1995	33

TABLE 14.2 Demographic Summary

Total patients served	Number	Percentage
Race		
White	82	87.26
Nonwhite	12	12.74
Status with Caregiver		
Patient lived with		
caregiver	59	62.32
Other Living		
Arrangement	35	37.68
Religion		
RC	24	26.05
Jewish	40	43.16
Protestant	12	12.77
Other	18	17.67
Gender		
Male	25	26.60
Female	69	73.29
Age		
50–64 years	3	4.71
65–74 years	10	11.36
75+ years	81	84.46
Payer Source		
Medicare	88	93.40
Medicaid	4	4.55
Other	2	2.27

According to the New York City chapter of the ADRDA, the reason for such low non-White numbers may be that Alzheimer's is underreported and/or underdiagnosed among communities of color. There may also not be the kinds of formal support in those communities for families who have a member with Alzheimer's disease. A third possibility is that the genetic base of the disease may not be as prominent within those communities. For reasons not yet determined, however, there are significantly fewer persons of color who were served by the Alzheimer's Hospice Project.

NURSING HOME OUTREACH

New York State blocked access to nursing homes by hospice programs until recently, so relationships were just now being established as the project was developing. However, the hospice's Alzheimer's Program was central to the establishment of a contract with Cobble Hill Nursing Home

TABLE 14.3 Service Summary Information

Site of death	Number	Percentage
Home	50	71.58
Inpatient Unit	16	22.86
Nursing Home	5	16.67
(year 3 only)		
Days of care		
Total days all patients	16,493	
Total Inpatient days	493	
Average daily		
Alzheimer's census	15	
Total nursing home		
days	78	
Length of stay prior		
to demise of patient		
00–07 days	12	16.26
08–30	16	22.60
31–60	9	12.59
61–90	3	5.15
91–120	6	9.07
121–200	10	13.51
201+	15	21.59
Total days on program,		
deceased patients		
Total care days,		
all patients	12,149	
Average length of		
stay per patient	154.5	
Median length of stay	72.8	

in Brooklyn, which has an extensive continuum of care for residents with Alzheimer's disease. Since services were implemented only in 1995, the hospice program at Cobble Hill has not yet reached its potential, so its impact on the project was limited.

ADMISSION ISSUES

It was one of the goals of the program to work within the 6-month prognosis requirement of the Medicare–Medicaid hospice benefits. Prognos-

TABLE 14.4   Patient Demographics

Category	Total hospice patients (%)		Alzheimers patients only (%)	
Race	White	70%	White	89%
	Non-White	30%	Non-White	11%
Third party payer	Medicare	67%	Medicare	96%
Gender	Female	58%	Female	80%
Age	50–64	17%	50–64	2%
	65–74	23%	65–74	9%
	75+	50%	75+	89%
Site of death	Inpatient unit	45%	Inpatient unit	23%
	Home	55%	Home	76%

ticators were based on functional assessment guidelines to determine a life expectancy of less than 6 months. These included:

- Limited vocabulary,
- Loss of interest in smiling,
- Inability to walk without assistance,
- Inability to sit up,
- Difficulty in eating,
- Recent weight loss,
- Urinary and bowel incontinence,
- Urinary tract infections,
- Pneumonia.

Of these prognosticators, the final four are the most significant. During the course of the project these prognosticators were refined through usage. The present practice of Jacob Perlow Hospice utilizes the new guidelines issued by the National Hospice Organization (1996) and deems admissions appropriate when the patient is noncommunicative, has had recurrent infections, is experiencing weight loss, and is eating very little.

THE ROLE OF CAREGIVERS IN PROGNOSTICATION

The hospice began its work with Alzheimer's patients with the assumption that medical criteria could be developed that would guide admissions within the 6-month prognosis requirement of Medicare–Medicaid. However, it became clear that medical criteria alone were not adequate and would not provide a secure prognostication of life expectancy. The variable that must be considered in relation to the medical criteria is the role of the family caregiver. Patients who have caregivers whose life purpose has become the care of their loved one will tend to live longer.

For example, the caregiver of one patient in the program is the patient's daughter. The caregiver, who was not married, had moved in with her mother to take care of her. The daughter continues to take care of her mother at home, spending hours carefully feeding her and giving her skin care. The patient has lived far beyond the time expected of other patients with the same medical conditions. Patients whose caregivers have begun to let go and who have a life independent of patient caregiving will live a more appropriate time receiving hospice services.

OTHER ISSUES RELATED TO ADMISSION AND TREATMENT

The first issue regarding admission and treatment has to do with *informed consent* and *patient participation* in care. Because of a limited cognitive state of a person with end-stage Alzheimer's, the patient is usually not capable of making his or her own decisions. Therefore, it is important to have a family member or significant other with durable power of attorney make health care decisions. This is the person the hospice team works with as decisions need to be made, such as whether pneumonia will be aggressively treated or not.

Second, family members have struggles and issues, beginning with their own exhaustion, which continue through the long steady decline of their loved one. They have experienced one unending funeral, and at the end, have what seems to be the shell of the person they have known and loved. Because there is a genetic factor with Alzheimer's disease, there may also be concerns about others in the family developing the disease. After the death, there is often a reluctance to verify the diagnosis through an autopsy.

The clinical staff of Jacob Perlow Hospice has seen two discernible tendencies in families. On the one hand, there are family members who are very fused into their caregiver roles, are reluctant to allow others to become involved in direct care, and are hesitant to take time for respite and rest away from the patient. On the other hand there are those who have begun to let go and make the emotional separation. Some may resist getting too involved directly. Both groups need different kinds of psychosocial and spiritual support.

Third, hospice staff members, both paid and volunteer, are accustomed to getting verbal feedback from patients, which helps to validate their work and to give meaning and purpose to their constant presence with dying and death. For patients with Alzheimer's disease, however, there is no satisfaction to be derived through meaningful verbal engagement. Education, support, and skilled supervision are needed to assist staff members in finding satisfaction in their work with these patients.

PATIENT AND FAMILY CARE

The primary symptoms for patients with Alzheimer's disease tend to focus on three major problem areas:

1. Swallowing and feeding,
2. Pain control,
3. Bowel and urinary management.

Symptoms exhibited by family caregivers tend to include

1. Anxiety,
2. Exhaustion,
3. Sense of failure and blaming.

First, there is an important *educational role* for the nurse with the family caregiver. While affirming the value and benefit of the care that has been given in the past, it is helpful to clarify that the progression of symptoms is related to the progress of the illness, not the failure of caregiving efforts. Helping family members to focus on problem-solving actions in response to specific situations empowers them and validates their role to the very end.

Second, the *assessment process* is complicated by the patient's cognitive limits. Therefore the observation skills of the nurse become more critical, along with the experience of the family caregivers.

Third, the *treatment regime* to respond to problems exists within current hospice patterns of practice. The difference is that the day-to-day care is totally dependent on family members and/or home health aides.

A nurse can help caregivers to establish a routine of proper positioning in bed and can offer instruction on the use of pillows or cushions to support contracted limbs, the use of egg-crate or alternating-pressure air mattresses, the frequent changing of softened bedclothes, and the use of music and touch. This inclusion can empower families to assist in pain management and affirm the value of their role and their caregiving.

Careful instructions for feeding and suggestions to promote swallowing can be given to family members, including the kinds of foods to prepare, and to avoid, how to feed, how to use a portable suction, and which agents to use to reduce thick oral secretions. The issue of tube feeding frequently surfaces through the expression of fear that by not "force feeding" the patient, the patient will starve to death. The guilt that is stirred is very painful. For religious caregivers, the assistance of the hospice chaplain may be helpful in resolving this issue.

PAIN MANAGEMENT

With advanced Alzheimer's disease, physical pain is often the result of

- Constipation or diarrhea,
- Lodged food particles,
- Contractures,
- Bed sores,
- Urosepsis.

The most effective means to achieve relief, according to the experience of the project's team, is low-dose morphine sulfate in the form of Roxanol (20 mg/ml) in doses of 5 to 10 mg sublingually, q14h PRN. The effects of morphine can be observed in diminished agitation, improved swallowing, less choking, and overall relaxation. During the final 48 hours of life rectal morphine can be given (20mg q4h a.t.c.) as well as Tylenol suppositories q4h PRN for T>100 to help ensure maximum comfort.

Part of the educational and supportive work of the nurse with family members is to instruct caregivers to medicate the patient before undertaking any activity that is going to alter the patient's position, such as bathing, feeding, dressing, and transferring from bed. When swallowing is reduced, bowel management is challenging. The use of Dulcolax® suppositories q.o.d. has worked. For patients who can swallow, liquid Senekot® or Senekot granules mixed with food is effective. Harris flush is effective as a way to relieve abdominal gas distress. Fennel tea is a mild, pleasing carminative drink.

If an indwelling Foley catheter is needed, Foley care is given 3 times a day. The prophylactic use of a bladder-acidifying agent, such as mandelamine or vitamin C, is effective. These measures greatly reduce the incidence of urosepsis.

Finally, in accord with a study, by Fabiszewski, Volicer, and Volicer (1990), the team does not recommend the use of intravenous antibiotics for the treatment of infections.

ATTENDANT CARE

Home health aides are the most frequently used service by Alzheimer patients in home care. The utilization recorded in the course of this project is an average of 131 visits per patient, or approximately 524 hours of care. It is this support that makes the difference in the ability of families to keep a patient at home rather than seek an institutional placement. The expenses of this support, when spread across a patient's entire length of stay, can help make it manageable.

VOLUNTEERS

It has been our experience that few volunteers work comfortably directly with Alzheimer patients. Most are involved in providing respite care and support for family members. One volunteer, however, who plays music for patients, derives great personal satisfaction and fulfillment from doing this work.

MUSIC THERAPY

Music therapy has been used effectively with a number of patients in the program. Because music response has been sited in one of the most primitive areas of the brain, there may be a response to music when there is little response to anything else. The music therapist in the hospice carefully researches with family members songs and tunes that were especially beloved by the patient, usually at an earlier time of life. Music is often connected to specific happier times of life. It is often a great comfort to family members to see the patient respond and experience some kind of connection. It is a glimpse of the person they always knew and loved, and that is comforting when rational communication is almost nonexistent.

BEREAVEMENT

Family members in the program who have made the greatest use of hospice bereavement services have been the daughters of patients who did not have families of their own. Unlike their siblings who had built-in support through spouses and children, these daughters had, to some degree, become enmeshed in the care of the parent who was dying. One of the issues that has emerged involved helping family members learn how to restructure their lives after the patient dies. However, the constellation of grief tends to fall within the ranges seen with family members of non-Alzheimer patients. Nothing unique or distinct as a bereavement issue has been noticed by the hospice team or staff.

GOAL THREE:
DEMONSTRATION/MODEL

The final goal of the project is to demonstrate the role of hospice care and to articulate this as a viable application of hospice philosophy and practice. One aspect of this goal is to do adequate research on the patients served. At the beginning of the second year of the project, the research staff position was filled, the recommended software was purchased, and complete data collection was begun. Before the study could begin, however, it was necessary for the hospice to receive approval from the Beth Israel Medical Center's Committee on Scientific Activities (COSA).

Because the research depends on consistent data collection on patients, it has been necessary to work with the home care nursing staff. A videotape was made about data collection for use as a refresher for staff nurses and an orientation for new staff members. After some experimentation it was found that the most efficient way to perform the tests needed for data collection involved admitting the patients into the hospice unit for the initial blood work and scans. Families also found this method preferable to performing these tests on an outpatient basis. The goal was to have data on at least 50 to 60 patients by the end of the project so there would be an adequate sample.

An issue that has emerged through patient care has been pain management, one of the fundamental aspects of hospice care. The fact that there are no tools to identify and measure pain in noncognitive, nonverbal, demented patients has been a challenge to the team. One of the major commitments of the third year of the project has been to develop a means to assess pain.

HOSPICE INTEREST IN ALZHEIMER'S CARE

Since the beginning of this project in 1993, more and more hospices have begun to aid patients with advanced Alzheimer's disease. According to the National Hospice Organization, in 1995 Alzheimer's represented 2% of the total care of all patients.

PROJECT DOCUMENTATION

The final summary works of the project still need to be completed. One summary will be scientific and research oriented, whereas the other will be more descriptive and clinical. These findings will present the final learnings of the project. It is the intention of the project to have these studies published and to make formal presentations as well.

COSTS

Is "doing the right thing" by serving Alzheimer patients and their families also financially viable in the presently uncertain reimbursement environment? Through the funding of the project, additional support was available to assist with expenses, particularly for the music therapist and home health aide services. However, the assumption that was made at the beginning of the project was that on completion of the grant the program would be able to sustain itself through current levels of reimbursement (almost exclusively Medicare) and special funds the hospice has established to support uncompensated services. That assumption at present seems optimistic.

Whether the hospice will be able to continue the additional home health aide support at the levels it has been providing is a serious question at this time. Although some families are able to hire private duty aides, most are not. It may be that without supplemental funding, fewer patients may be able to be supported at home and will need nursing home placement.

GOVERNMENT POLICY SHIFT

In 1995 both the Health Care Finance Administration (HCFA) and the Office of Inspector General have undertaken a review of hospice practice involving the admission of noncancer-diagnosis patients, and patients with a length of stay beyond 210 days of care. Because the average length of stay of patients with Alzheimer disease is much longer than that of the average cancer patient, this review has the effect of questioning the role of hospice care with Alzheimer patients. Already, focused medical review of two Alzheimer patients served by Jacob Perlow Hospice has had one patient declared ineligible for continued reimbursement through Medicare.

It is not clear how this kind of action will affect other hospice providers, which may be discouraged from taking a proactive approach to the care of patients with Alzheimer's disease. This action certainly is not encouraging hospice programs to extend access of care to more difficult and complex patients and families. Such activity also seems to indicate a fundamental misunderstanding of the dying process itself, its predictability, and the role of nonmedical psychosocial considerations in determining the needs of patients and families at the end of life.

CONCLUSIONS

Dame Cicely Saunders is reported to have said, "You matter to the end of your life." Patients with end-stage Alzheimer's disease and related disorders, due to their cognitive limitations, challenge some values by which society measures worth. However, in its treatment of patients as individuals, in its commitment to ensure that patients' pain is assessed with great care and patience and is addressed effectively and adequately, in its dedication to respect patients, honor their lives, and accord them value, Jacob Perlow Hospice is demonstrating that its basic principles and mission have a critical role to play in the care of these patients and their families.

REFERENCES

Beresford, L. (1993). *The hospice handbook* (pp. xix–xxv). Boston: Little, Brown.
Fabiszewski, K.J. Volicer, B.J. Volicer, L. 1992, Effect of antibiotic treatment on outcome of fevers in institutionalized Alzheimer's patients. *Journal of the American Medical Association, 263,* 3168-3172
Kübler-Ross, E. (1969). *On death and dying.* New York: Macmillan.
National Hospice Organization, Standards and Accreditation Committee. (1996). *Medical guidelines for determining prognosis in selected non-cancer diseases* (2nd. ed.).

Effects of Hospice Interventions on Nursing Home Residents with Later Stages of Dementia*

Christine R. Kovach

S pecial Care Units for people with dementia are increasing in number in nursing homes across the country (Leon, 1994). Although there are no uniform guidelines or standards for what makes a unit "special," the 1992 study of Special Care Units conducted by the U.S. Office of Technology Assessment (Maslow, 1994b) offers the following broad statements that can serve as guiding principles:

- Something can be done for persons with dementia.
- Many factors cause excess disability in persons with dementia.
- Individuals with dementia have residual strengths.
- The behavior of individuals with dementia represents understandable feelings and needs, even if individuals are unable to express their feelings or needs.
- Many aspects of the physical and social environment affect the functioning of individuals with dementia.
- Individuals with dementia and their families constitute an integral unit (Maslow, 1994).

*This study was funded by a grant from the Helen Bader Foundation.

A National Survey of Special Care Units in Nursing Homes (NSSCUINH) found that the features most often present in Special Care Units included modified physical environments (67%), physically separated units with controlled on/off access (78%), admission criteria limited to people with a diagnosis of dementia (82%), extra staffing (76%), special staff training (76%), and specialized programming (88%) (Leon, 1994). Most facilities do not, however, have all of these features, and, since there are not accepted definitions for what constitutes a feature such as special training or special programming, there may be great diversity in how these features have been operationalized.

Most Special Care Units have admission and discharge criteria. The units are usually designed for the person with mid-stage dementia who needs a quiet and controlled environment, interventions to manage behavioral symptomatology, and a program designed to maintain maximum functional independence (Kovach & Stearns, 1994). The person with end-stage dementia has needs for total, or close to total, assistance with all self-care needs: bathing, toileting, dressing, eating, and grooming. Impaired communication creates several other needs. First, because the person is often unable to articulate discomfort or other physical symptomatology, there is a need for increased physical assessment of the resident to prevent and treat physical problems. Also, staff must learn new communication strategies and must often slow down the communication process to accommodate the person with later-stage dementia. As physical and self-care needs increase during the later stages of a dementing illness, behavior problems tend to decrease and change. The person does not respond as severely to extraneous and multiple stimuli from the environment. Activity disturbances change from a decrease in wandering to an increase in perseverant behavior and increased null and somnolent behavior.

Since the person with end-stage dementia may not meet criteria for being admitted or remaining on a Special Care Unit (Riter & Fries, 1992), often such a resident will be found on a general long-term care unit. These units have competing, and at times conflicting, agendas: cure, palliation, and rehabilitation. With this mix of goals on a unit and the limited resources found in most nursing homes, the person who has needs for increased comfort care may be neglected in favor of residents who have cure and rehabilitation needs.

This chapter will describe a project that was undertaken to determine the efficacy of opening hospice households on traditional nursing home units for people in the later stages of dementia. The chapter is divided into two sections: "Development of the Households" and "Research Report."

DEVELOPMENT OF THE HOUSEHOLDS

Five hospice households in three long-term care facilities were designed for people specifically with later stages of dementia. These households were planned through an interdisciplinary team effort over a 5-month period. The hallmarks of hospice care—comfort, dignity, and quality of life—were the guiding force behind the development of interventions. The program was developed with the following key elements: admission criteria, specific hospice household interventions, environmental modifications, use of a hospice nurse as a case manager, and specialized staff education.

ADMISSION CRITERIA

Criteria for admission of a resident to the program through the study period were (1) diagnosed with irreversible dementia; (2) score on the Short Portable Mental Status Questionnaire (SPMSQ) indicated severe cognitive impairment (Pfeiffer, 1975); (3) identified by staff as usually unable to engage in group programming; (4) had at least two of the following symptoms: aphasia, apraxia, agnosia, and constructional difficulty; and (5) had advance directives that requested no cardiopulmonary resuscitation be initiated.

The line that divides mid stage and end stage is debated in the literature, and for practical purposes, the criteria used in this project were designed to capture those residents who were no longer functioning well or were having their needs met on the mid-stage special care unit. Since there is a fair amount of prognostic uncertainty regarding when death will occur in this group, there was much discussion about the ethics of requiring certain advance directives. The group did not want to place family members in a position of deciding between enhanced palliative care and feeding/hydrating a resident or treating an uncomplicated acute illness. By accepting only those residents who had an advance directive requesting no CPR, there was a belief that family members and staff would at least both be focusing primarily on comfort rather than on cure or rehabilitation efforts.

Since the study was completed, the criteria have been altered to include a Functional Behavior Profile (FBP) score below 40 (Baum, Edwards, & Morrow-Howell, 1993). The SPMSQ has been replaced by the Mini Mental Status Examination (MMSE) (Folstein, Folstein, & McHugh, 1975), and the four symptoms of agnosia, aphasia, apraxia, and constructional difficulty are considered to be adequately captured in the MMSE so are not assessed separately. The FBP measures strengths in three functional factors: problem solving, social interaction, and task performance. Staff use this tool to develop appropriate therapeutic activities, and the tool helps staff to objectively determine when mid-stage activities will no longer be successfully accomplished by the resident. Most residents in the hospice program score 0 to 3 on the MMSE.

HOSPICE HOUSEHOLD INTERVENTIONS

In order to have staff at the three facilities feel ownership of the project, interdisciplinary team meetings were held every other week to design interventions for the project. These meetings were led by two nurse researchers from a nearby university. The initial meetings were designed to be broad and philosophical so that staff would consider the person with later-stage dementia from a less task-oriented and more meaningful perspective. Staff were asked to talk in small groups about the daily life of people they care for with later-stage dementia, what the resident might be feeling, and what their own feelings are about the illnesses that lead to progressive and irreversible dementia. Examples of the descriptive reports given by these groups are shown in Table 15.1. These poignant exercises helped to develop group cohesiveness and a shared commitment to improve the lives of the residents.

The group became more concrete in its work and decided to focus on five main areas: comfort, quality of life, dignity, support for family, and support for staff. A booklet was developed that operationalized these five areas into a set of goals, actions, and quality indicators. The quality indicators for each area are presented in Table 15.2. This booklet became, in essence, the contract the staff made with the researchers regarding the enhanced care that would be provided.

COMFORT

Staff were educated in enhanced physical and behavioral assessment skills to recognize discomfort. When there was a change in behavior that might indicate discomfort (e.g., increased agitation without a known trigger), staff followed several steps in a protocol: nursing assessment for source of discomfort, behavioral intervention, medication with acetaminophen or psychotropic, and referral to medicine.

The nursing assessment involved screening for urinary tract infection, constipation, impaction, and other common sources of physical discomfort. If a source of discomfort was found that might have explained the change in behavior, appropriate interventions or consultations were initiated.

TABLE 15.1   Examples of a Staff Group Exercise

Group 1:	Confusion and unrest are present. There is some understanding that things are not right, and this makes residents uncomfortable. Residents seem very alone; there is a lack of mobility and confinement. There is a lot taken away from residents because of their poor mentation. We really don't know how they feel; there is a lot of guessing. We don't know how frightened or lonely they are. Perhaps there is pain and they can't tell us; perhaps they feel hopeless. Their life and world are very narrow. Things happen on a routine basis. It could be very frustrating when we don't understand what they want. Socializing is very limited. It's a boring, pretty blank existence with decreased options. Residents are very dependent and deteriorating slowly, both physically and cognitively.
Group 2:	Residents with end-stage dementia live in a world of uncertainty. They tend to be very fearful of people, activities, objects, and situations. They are totally dependent on others to meet all daily needs without being able to express desires or choices. In fact, they may not even be aware of what their needs are. Every aspect of their environment is potentially dangerous to them. Dealing with these frustrations may lead to acting-out behaviors. Families often have trouble coping with the situation and may project these frustrations on the staff.
Group 3:	Life for residents with end-stage dementia is filled with multiple emotions that they cannot explain. They can be frustrated, bewildered, happy, sad, helpless, weepy, bored, withdrawn, sleepy, and exhausted. Their family interactions can be strained. Families often feel helpless and guilty. Responses by residents to their surroundings may be exaggerated. They often respond well to smiles, hugs, touch, etc., however, caregivers need to be aware of overstimulation.

If a source for the agitated behavior could not be discerned, staff used behavioral interventions to attempt to calm the resident. Examples of behavioral interventions are distraction, decreasing the stress in the environment, one-on-one communication, and music therapy.

If behavioral interventions were unsuccessful, staff were encouraged to medicate the person with two regular-strength acetaminophen. The medical director at each facility wrote an order that acetaminophen could be given when necessary (i.e., prn). Staff were discouraged from giving prescribed prn chemical restraints unless all other options were unsuccessful. Staff also always had the option of seeking consultation from the resident physician or another member of the health care team.

Each resident in the program had an individualized comfort plan. Examples of interventions used include massage, flannel sheets, silk pillowcases, positioning, rummage boxes, and empathic communication. Because phys-

TABLE 15.2 Quality Indicators for the Hospice Program for Later Stage Dementia

Comfort Quality Indicators
1. All residents have an updated, individualized comfort care plan.
2. All residents have a primary CNA unless contraindicated.
3. Discomfort is documented and treated with appropriate interventions or referrals.

Prevention of Physical Iatrogenic Problems
1. All residents have a weekly assessment documented.
2. The care plan is implemented.

Sensory-Stimulating and Sensory-Calming Activities
1. All residents have an activity schedule.
2. All residents have a balance of sensory-stimulating and sensory-calming activities.
3. Extraneous environmental stimulation is decreased.

Human Dignity
1. All residents are addressed using a respectful name of their choice or of the family members' choice.
2. All residents are clean and odor free.
3. All residents are offered choices based on the person's functional level.
4. All residents are spoken to in a positive manner.
5. All residents have their privacy maintained during bathing, dressing, toileting, etc.
6. All residents have at least one sensory-stimulating activity per day involving sustained human interaction (above and beyond ADL cares).

Psychosocial/Educational Support for Families
1. Family members complete a survey once a year regarding satisfaction with resident care.
2. All residents who have a consent from their guardian have a biographical sketch framed in their room.
3. Family are updated with information regarding support group meetings, other activities and caregiver and dementia educational information through the family bulletin board.
4. Families have a biannual family night that focuses on friendship, fun, education, and support.

Psychosocial/Educational Support for Staff
1. CNAs are assigned to four or fewer residents in the households project.
2. CNAs work with a buddy for at least a portion of each day.
3. CNAs have classes before the start of the project and semiannually.
4. CNAs and nurses communicate a daily assessment and plan for each resident.
5. Staff have special external reward recognition four times a year.
6. Staff work at full staffing levels 95% of the time.

From "Hospice Concepts in the Care for End-Stage Dementia," by S. A. Wilson, C. P. Kovach, and S. A. Skarns, 1996, *Geriatric Nursing, 17,* pp. 6–10. Copyright 1996 by Mosby. Reprinted with permission.

ical iatrogenic problems become an increased concern as the person's condition deteriorates, plans for preventing problems such as decreased mobility, skin breakdown, constipation and impaction, sleep problems, and iatrogenic infection were reviewed and enhanced as needed.

QUALITY OF LIFE

Before the project began, the researchers toured one of the facilities and found that each resident who met admission criteria for this study was still in bed at 10:30 a.m. in nightclothes, and was displaying either null or somnolent behavior. When the nurse manager was asked why the low-functioning demented residents seemed to be the only group who were still in bed, she honestly replied, "Well, this is the group that can't complain, so we do them up last." Interventions surrounding quality of life therefore necessitated some massive changes in the daily routine. All residents were expected to be up in the hospice multipurpose room for breakfast. A daily schedule for each resident was developed that outlined activities for each half hour. This schedule was kept in the resident's room and in a binder at the nurse's station. The schedules were an essential tool for balancing sensory-stimulating and sensory-calming activities. The schedules also helped staff to see more clearly how much of the resident's day was truly therapeutic and focused on quality of life. Staff were educated in individual therapeutic activities designed for low-functioning people with dementia.

HUMAN DIGNITY, SUPPORT FOR FAMILY AND STAFF

The goals that staff established for maintaining human dignity were (1) all residents will be treated in a kind and caring manner and will be clean and odor-free; (2) residents' choices and preferences will be followed whenever possible; and (3) at least one formal sensory-stimulating activity per day will involve sustained human interaction. Even though it was somewhat offensive to think meaningful human interaction would need to be prescribed and quantified, because people with end-stage dementia have compromised and challenging communication needs, this is an often ignored human need. The current realities of long-term care necessitated that a formal communication model be incorporated into each resident's plan of care.

Family support took on various forms: providing satisfaction surveys, including family interventions on nursing assistant assignment cards;

holding support meetings; constructing biographical sketches of the resident with family members; providing an informational bulletin board for family members; and holding a biannual family night that focused on friendship and fun.

In order to plan a realistic program, staffing levels were not increased for this project. Because of concern about staff burnout, the project initially involved assigning a certified nursing assistant (CNA) to only two to four residents in the project. The remainder of the CNA's assignment came from residents with other needs. Once the project started, CNA's quickly began requesting that their entire assignment consist of hospice residents. CNA's chose their own assignment and kept this assignment for at least 4 months. If a resident was identified as psychologically straining to staff, care of this resident was rotated more frequently.

Staff received support through daily reports and monthly individual meetings with the case manager. The CNAs role was expanded to include activity therapies and CNAs received more assistance from nurses with tasks such as feeding and transferring residents. Probably the most important and tangible support came from a strong commitment to replacing staff when there was an absentee. Staff members reported that they were unable to provide quality care when the workload was excessive. Weekly planned employee appreciation activities occurred, including giving a small gift from the project directors to an employee each week whose name was drawn from a hat. Pizza parties and doughnuts provided at coffee break time also were expressions of appreciation for participation in the project.

ENVIRONMENTAL MODIFICATIONS

Rooms were made more homelike through decorations, afghans, pillows, plants, and family pictures. Lounges and a chapel were converted into multipurpose rooms for the project. These rooms were cheerfully decorated and were the hub for most daily activities. Meals, therapeutic activities, and religious services occurred in the multipurpose rooms. The rooms were well stocked with activity supplies for low-functioning people, had a preferences book that outlined each resident's likes and dislikes, and had an abundant supply of nonalcoholic wine, a favorite of residents during afternoon socials. The multipurpose rooms were used for a maximum of 16 residents, but 8 to 12 was a more manageable number. Extraneous environmental stimulation was controlled through strategies such as such as turning off the television, isolating housekeeping activities to certain times, and replacing pill crushers with noiseless pliers.

CASE MANAGER AND STAFF EDUCATION

Strong role modeling from the case manager was an essential component of this project. The case manager worked within the facility to refine and operationalize plans for opening the households. The case manager also assisted in implementing care plans and served as a role model, direct caregiver, coordinator of services, and advocate for residents, family, and staff.

Case managers received updated classes on the hospice program, care planning, assessment techniques, and case management. An all-day conference was held at the university for all staff involved in the project. Over 80 people attended. Classes focused on hospice concepts, dementia, treatment of behaviors, activity programming for low-functioning residents, and family and spiritual care. In addition, nurses attended a class that focused on improving recognition of commonly occurring physical conditions. Educational efforts focused on making staff aware of the importance of their work and helping staff to make a paradigm shift from task-oriented, rigid, institutional, and illness-oriented care to a more holistic, flexible, and life-affirming model of care. The day was an energizing and transforming experience for many staff members, who stated they felt a renewed commitment to their role in end-stage dementia care.

RESEARCH REPORT

One hundred eighteen residents at the three facilities met the sampling criteria explicated earlier in the chapter. Consent was obtained from 92 of the subjects' guardians. Seventeen subjects died during the 5-month planning phase of the project. Three other subjects were dropped because two family members refused to make necessary room changes and one person moved to another city. When the households opened, 35 subjects were in the treatment group and 37 were in the control group. Two months later, when posttesting was done, 5 subjects had died in both the treatment and control groups, leaving a sample size of 62 for posttesting. Table 15.3 describes the sample. Tests of differences between sample characteristics of the treatment and control groups support that random assignment was effective in yielding equivalent groups.

DESIGN

A pretest–posttest experimental design was utilized. Using a table of random numbers, subjects were assigned to the treatment or control group.

TABLE 15.3 Description of Sample

Variable	Treatment group	Control group	Test statistic	p
Age	x̄ = 88.06	x̄ = 87.78	t = .181	.857
Sex	Female = 30 Male = 5	Female = 28 Male = 9	x^2 = 1.56	.210
Length of stay	x̄ = 40 months	x̄ = 36 months	t = .419	.677
Marital status	Widowed = 26 Married = 7 Single = 1 Divorced =1	Widowed = 22 Married = 12 Single = 2 Divorced = 1	x^2 = 4.33	.228

From "Effects of Hospice Interventions on Behaviors, Discomfort, and Physical Complications of End-Stage Dementia Nursing Home Residents," by C. Kovach, S. Wilson, and P. Noonan, 1996, *American Journal of Alzheimer's Disease, 11* (4), 7–15. Copyright 1996 by Prime National Publishing Corporation. Reprinted with permission.

Two months before the households opened, measurements of discomfort, behaviors associated with dementia, and physical complications were obtained. Subjects in the treatment group received the enhanced hospice care, and subjects in the control group received the traditional care provided by the facility. Two months after the households were opened, measurements of study variables were again taken. Two months was chosen as the time frame for posttesting because of the high mortality rate of this population. Individual interviews with a convenience sample of 15 staff and were also conducted before and after the interventions were implemented to assess satisfaction and identification of changes. All measurements and interviews were done by two graduate nursing students who had experience in gerontology but were not directly involved in the project.

MEASUREMENT

Cognitive Impairment

The presence and degree of cognitive impairment were assessed using the SPMSQ. This 10-item instrument compares with results of a clinical psychiatric diagnosis of organic brain syndrome with 92% agreement when the SPMSQ indicated definite impairment and 88% when the SPMSQ indicated either no impairment or mild impairment (Reisberg et al.,

1987). Sclan, Reisberg, Franssen, Torossian, and Ferris (1990) found agreement between a rater and the BEHAVE-AD tool total score was .96. Patterson et al. (1990) found that for 20 of the 25 items, kappa scores were .619 to 1.00 and agreement was fair on the 5 remaining items.

Comfort

The Discomfort Scale for Dementia of the Alzheimer's Type (DS-DAT) is an objective scale for measuring discomfort in people with advanced dementia who have lost communication abilities. Discomfort was operationally defined as "the presence of behaviors considered to express a negative emotional and/or physical state that are capable of being observed by a trained rater unfamiliar with the usual behavior pattern of the patient" (Hurley, Volicer, Hanrahan, Houde, & Volicer, 1992). Ratings on the 9-item scale were made by assessing the magnitude of its defining characteristics on a 100mm horizonal line visual analogue scale (VAS) from absent (0) to extreme (100). The rater waited for 15 minutes after any event that might induce discomfort (e.g., a position change) and observed the subject for 5 minutes. The possible range of scores was from 0 to 900. The tool has a content validity index of 1.0 and an internal consistency reliability of .86 to .89 (Hurley et al., 1992).

Physical Complications

Physical problems commonly experienced in the end stages of a dementing illness were determined through consultation with three nurse administrators in long-term care and through a review of the literature. Based on this compilation, a data collection form was constructed that was used during a chart review. The major categories of problems in the tool were nutrition, elimination, sleep, mobility, and infection.

RESULTS

Because the groups were so similar at the pretesting period, there was no need for a covariate with pretest or posttest scores. The scores on all variables were normally distributed enough that a between group independent t-test was appropriate and used to analyze results. As seen in Table 15.4, at posttest, the treatment group had significantly less discomfort than did the control group. Table 15.5 shows the frequency of behavior problems and physical complications assessed. The most common behavior problems of this sample were social interaction difficulties, diurnal rhythm disturbances, activity disturbances, and aggression.

**TABLE 15.4 Differences Between Treatment
and Control Groups at Posttesting**

	Treatment group		Control group			
Condition/variable	M	SD	M	SD	t	p
Behaviors	4.52	5.2	6.58	6.0	1.44	.155
Discomfort	218.10	142.1	368.88	168.3	3.88	< .001*
Physical complications	1.68	1.74	1.66	1.3	.054	.957

*Statistically significant result.

From "Effects of Hospice Interventions on Behaviors, Discomfort, and Physical Complications of End-Stage Dementia Nursing Home Residents," by C. Kovach, S. Wilson, and P. Noonan, 1996, *American Journal of Alzheimer's Disease, 11* (4), 7–15. Copyright 1996 by Prime National Publishing Corporation. Reprinted with permission.

At posttesting, the treatment group showed improvements in all behavior problems except delusions and hallucinations. The control group showed a more moderate decrease in prevalence of some behavior problems, but increased frequency of hallucinations, delusions, and phobias. The differences between the treatment and control groups on the BEHAVE-AD tool were not large enough to be statistically significant. Due to the loss of subjects, a Type II error may account for this lack of statistical significance.

This sample had a high frequency of physical complications, and there was no statistically significant difference in the incidence of these complications between the treatment and control groups. At posttesting, the treatment group did, however, have only 4 iatrogenic infections, while the control group had 15 infections.

Interviews with staff members revealed what may be the most compelling findings from the study. Staff members expressed improved job satisfaction, increased empathy and caring, and recognition that there was an observable improvement in many residents.

Comments from nurse case managers included:

It was good to see the changes that developed. At first, I was a little leery, you know; how can you change someone that's been like a vegetable for years and years and years? But then we saw [residents] would try to help and move their arms when they were dressing and even . . . say good morning. Otherwise they wouldn't say anything. Just to see responses like that was really great.

TABLE 15.5   Frequency of Behaviors Associated with Dementia and Physical Complications for Treatment and Control Groups at Pre- and Posttesting

Variable	Pretesting		Posttesting	
	Treatment group (N = 35)	Control group (N = 37)	Treatment group (N = 30)	Control group (N = 32)
Behaviors				
Activity disturbances	18	21	12	16
Aggression	22	22	10	17
Diurnal rhythm disturbances	20	22	12	16
Affective disturbances	14	11	8	6
Phobias	14	13	8	16
Delusions	4	5	4	6
Hallucinations	2	2	2	6
Social interaction difficulties	29	24	16	23
Physical complications				
Nutrition	11	15	9	4
Elimination	17	20	9	13
Skin	15	16	14	11
Mobility	13	19	7	9
Infections	10	12	4	15

From "Effects of Hospice Interventions on Behaviors, Discomfort, and Physical Complications of End-Stage Dementia Nursing Home Residents," by C. Kovach, S. Wilson, and P. Noonan, 1996, *American Journal of Alzheimer's Disease, 11* (4), 7–15. Copyright 1996 by Prime National Publishing Corporation. Reprinted with permission.

It's changed how I look at those with dementia. They're not those poor unfortunates. There's lots we can do and they can laugh and have their quality of life and not just be stuck in a wheelchair looking out a window somewhere. Every once in a while there's just a little glimmer . . . you can hop inside and reach them. And when those little golden moments happen they are just beautiful. We have one lady where all the staff was just crying one day, because she kinda came to for just a little bit, but we were there for her when she was back. That's very rewarding. Very rewarding.

All this theory was in my head, but I didn't know it would work. And it does. For some. To see residents kind of go through awakenings . . . just blows you away. So I learned . . . we can make a difference.

I think it's made a grand difference. . . . We've seen very definite changes in some residents. One lady who was really nonverbal is speaking. Another is feeding herself when she hadn't before. One lady . . . just before she died was playing cards. . . . I never would have expected that she could do that. But that happened to be something she retained and she could do it. And so I think [the hospice project] has made a change . . . it's improved their quality of life and when residents are treated as people, the real people in them come out.

Comments from CNAs included:

This program makes me feel good, and the families love it. You have more time to talk to the residents. Before you were too busy with tasks. This makes me rich; I love it.

This project helped tremendously. I mean, I never thought there was a program like this. I always wondered what we could do with the residents, what we could do for them. When this came up I thought, Oh God, this is the best thing that has happened since I've been a nurse, and I've been doing this for 15 years and have never seen anything like it. It gives residents the opportunity to learn so much, you know, and to help.

Well, like with my Anne, she will . . . attempt to help me dress her, . . . put her arms in [the clothes], and if you tell her to stand, she will try. With the little stuffed animals—once I put one in her chair . . . her eyes [went] to it immediately. She touched it and she wanted contact with it. And we've achieved something there. There's recognition there. I can turn on the TV in the room, which I don't do too often—they're noise makers— and she will respond to the TV. She responds, I think, a little bit more. I know when it comes nap time—I know if she doesn't want to go down for a nap. She holds on to the side of her chair and she gets real stubborn. Because I do the same thing, the same routine, I don't even have to some- times tell her, okay, we are going to do this. She will move her body in that position. But if she doesn't want to get up, she won't. She'll be stiff. She'll get very difficult. [Interviewer asks if resident was like this before the project.] [Before the project,] it was just the same everything—you know, get up, get in the chair, and the days the priest would come up and do a blessing. Not much of a response. Her nurse manager made up little booklets with prayers. Sometimes when I feed her, . . . I'll read her one of the prayers and I'll get her full attention, and a couple times she's gone and she's folded her hands. It's things I have never seen with her. Maybe she would have done it all along—I don't know—but you know, we didn't have this type of program going. Maybe it's the benefit of the program. I don't know. But just to see the changes from before and now. It's like I said in the beginning, the littlest things, the smile, the recognition, and you can tell with the residents' eyes, because they do smile with their eyes. And Anne will hold my hand, and, you know, she looks to have her arm rubbed.

It's made a difference with all—even Gloria. We had residents who didn't do anything. They'd just sit there. When this lady spoke to me, I almost choked because I didn't know she would speak. So, yes, [the project] has made a big difference. [Before somebody [was always] rushing in and doing what they had to do and walking out and leaving the residents.[Now] I can go around to each individual and talk to him or her, and they will respond to me. So that's the difference. [Before] I would say hi every morning and tell residents what day it is and they would just sit there and say nothing. . . . This is what residents need. They don't need to be pushed aside. They need to enjoy their last days. And sometimes I look at them in that room and they smile, they seem happy. So, yes, [the project] has made a big change in residents here.

CONCLUSIONS

This chapter began with a presentation of the guidelines from the Office of Technology Assessment, which state that something can be done for people with dementia and that many factors can cause excess disability for those with dementia. This study supports the theory that these statements apply to nursing home residents with later-stage dementia. Research in this field continues to be hampered by the lack of adequate assessment tools. Even though the discomfort scale appears to capture the difference between treatment and control groups, some of the anecdotal observations of increased engagement in meaningful activities, increased wakefulness, communication, and positive affect were not fully captured in these assessments.

Because the interventions used in this study were multifaceted, it is not known which of the interventions used were helpful. Even though the delivery system, daily schedules, and specific interventions utilized involved large changes from previous care, it is not known how much of the difference in care received could be attributed to enhanced care provided by staff because of a Hawthorne effect rather than because of actual differences between the households and the traditional units.

Studies are needed that involve more sites, larger sample sizes, and more discreet interventions. This study did not demonstrate differences in physical complications between the treatment and control groups. In the midst of implementing multiple interventions for this study, the physical portion of the interventions planned were probably given the least amount of attention. Future research is needed that focuses specifically on prevention and early treatment of physical problems commonly seen in this group. A prevention and early treatment project may reduce utilization of high-cost medical and inpatient services while maintaining a high quality of care.

There is a need for innovation, research, and reflection regarding the care options that are available across the continuum of dementing illnesses. The medical model of delivering care with a focus on the treatment of illness is a limited and inadequate model for providing services to people with dementia. As the disease progresses and the individual enters the later phases of the illness, there is a consensus that palliation should be the major emphasis of care. Defining optimum palliative interventions, and ensuring that comfort care is not operationalized to mean "little or no care" are challenges for the future. It is said that a society may be defined by its treatment of vulnerable groups. Hospice concepts provide an opportunity for the care provided to people with end-stage dementia to be life-affirming, dignified, and holistic.

REFERENCES

Baum, C., Edwards, D. F., & Morrow-Howell, N. (1993). Identification and measurement of productive behaviors in senile dementia of the Alzheimer type. *Gerontologist, 33*, 403–408.

Folstein, M. F., Folstein, S. E., & McHugh, P. R. (1975). Mini-mental stage: A practical method for grading the cognitive state of patients for the clinician. *Journal of Psychiatric Research, 12*, 189–198.

Hurley, A. C., Volicer, B. J., Hanrahan, P. A., Houde, S., & Volicer, L. (1992). Assessment of discomfort in advanced Alzheimer patients. *Research in Nursing & Health, 15*, 369–377.

Kovach, C. R., & Stearns, S. A. (1994). DSCUs: A study of before and after residence. *Journal of Gerontological Nursing, 20*(12), 33–39.

Leon, J. (1994). The 1990/1991 national survey of special care units in nursing homes. *Alzheimer Disease and Associated Disorders, 1*(Suppl. 1), S72–S87.

Maslow, K. (1994a). Consumer education, research, regulatory and reimbursement issues in special care units. *Alzheimer Disease and Associated Disorders, 8*(Suppl. 1), S429–S433.

Maslow, K. (1994b). Current knowledge about special care units: Findings of a study by the U.S. Office of Technology Assessment. *Alzheimer Disease and Associated Disorders, 8*(Suppl. 1), S14–S40.

Patterson, M. B., Schnell, A. H., Martin, R. J., Mendez, M. F., Smyth, K. A., & Whitehouse, P. J. (1990). Assessment of behavioral and affective symptoms in Alzheimer's disease. *Journal of Geriatric Psychiatry and Neurology, 3*, 21–30.

Pfeiffer, E. (1975). A short portable mental status questionnaire for the assessment of organic brain deficits in elderly patients. *Journal of the American Geriatrics Society, 23,* 433–441.

Reisberg, B., Borenstein, J., Slaob, S. P., Ferris, S. H., Franssen, E., & Gergotas, A. (1987). Behavioral symptoms in Alzheimer's disease: Phenomenology and treatment. *Journal of Clinical Psychiatry, 48*(5), 9–15.

Riter, R. N., & Fries, B. E. (1992). Predictors of the placement of cognitively impaired residents on special care units. *Gerontologist, 32,* 184–190.

Sclan, S. G., Reisberg, B., Franssen, E., Torossian, C., & Ferris, S. H. (1990, December). *Remediable behavioral symptoms of Alzheimer's disease: A cognitive independent syndrome.* Paper presented at the annual meeting of the American College of Neuropsychopharmacology, San Juan, Puerto Rico.

Index

Index

Index